EMOTIONAL DEVELOPMENT ACROSS THE LIFESPAN

Emotional Development across the Lifespan

Linda A. Camras

THE GUILFORD PRESS
New York   London

Library of Congress Cataloging-in-Publication Data

Names: Camras, Linda A., author.
Title: Emotional development across the lifespan / Linda A. Camras.
Description: New York, NY : The Guilford Press, [2022] | Includes
    bibliographical references and index.
Identifiers: LCCN 2022008649 | ISBN 9781462549764 (paperback) |
    ISBN 9781462549771 (hardcover)
Subjects: LCSH: Emotions. | Emotions in children. | Child psychology. |
    Developmental psychobiology. | Social work with children. | BISAC:
    PSYCHOLOGY / Developmental / Child | SOCIAL SCIENCE / Social
    Work
Classification: LCC BF531 .C2877 2022 | DDC 155.4/124—dc23/eng/20220330
LC record available at https://lccn.loc.gov/2022008649

To my husband, Jerry, and my daughter, Justine,
both of whom inspired me—but in very different ways

Preface

After decades of neglect during the early and middle parts of the 20th century, the importance of emotion in daily life is being increasingly recognized both within and outside of academia. Since 2006, the Gallup organization has conducted yearly polls of emotional well-being within the United States and across the globe. Similarly, the UN-affiliated Organisation for Economic Co-operation and Development has included subjective well-being among the measures it has tracked since 2010. Reflecting (and perhaps inspiring) this increased interest, articles and books on emotion and emotional development are proliferating within academia. Currently there are three peer-reviewed journals devoted solely to emotion (*Emotion, Affective Science,* and *Emotion Review*). A PsycInfo search using the term *emotional development* yielded 553 entries for the 20 years between 1960 and 1980 but more than 5,000 entries for the last 20 years. Although this proliferation of scholarly material is a welcome contribution to our knowledge, it also can be overwhelming. Thus the present volume is intended to provide an introduction to the ever-expanding universe of research on emotion and emotional development across the lifespan.

As in any academic field, controversy abounds within the field of emotion, particularly with regard to the nature of emotion itself. Somewhat surprisingly, this controversy is rarely acknowledged within the developmental literature. In fact, some developmentalists and clinicians may be unaware that it exists. Yet understanding the fundamental nature of emotion is essential to our efforts both to understand its typical and atypical development and to design interventions that seek to foster children's emotional well-being. Thus this book begins with an overview of current emotion theories extant in the adult literature, as well as models of emotional development. Both here and throughout the book, I have made an attempt to present a balanced exposition of scholars' and researchers' different views. However, at the same time, current trends in the literature in favor of one position or another will inevitably be discernable to the reader (possibly reflecting in part my own personal leanings). Feel free to ignore these subtextual messages and take a deeper dive into the literature so as to decide for yourself. References cited throughout each chapter will be a convenient place to start.

The role of theory in psychological research (indeed in any scientific field) may itself be subject to debate. Within psychology, scholars largely adhere (at least in principle) to the well-known axiom attributed to Kurt Lewin, namely, that there is nothing so practical as a good theory. Yet much research on emotional development has paid only lip service to this principle. Rather than seeking to test hypotheses derived from a particular theory of emotional development, researchers may often identify a topic of interest (e.g., emotion recognition, emotion regulation) and attempt to identify the age at which it emerges, its different forms at different ages, and/or its ties to possible precipitating or contextual factors (e.g., family background, parent attitudes and behavior) or to socioemotional outcomes (e.g., emotional or behavioral adjustment). Hypotheses are typically tested, but they are not necessarily tied to an overarching theory. Still, the value of such research is unquestionable. In fact, it raises questions regarding the necessity of having a theory at all. As with many interesting questions, providing a definitive answer is not the purpose of this book. Instead, my goal is to introduce readers to the extensive literature on emotion and emotional development within the field of psychology. Commensurate with the limitations inherent in a short introductory text, coverage of each subject area is not comprehensive. Again, readers are encouraged to explore further on their own.

Regarding organizational structure, authors of any developmental text are confronted with the difficult choice of taking a topical or a chronological approach to their subject matter. Neither choice is ideal; topical approaches make it more difficult to keep in mind the inextricable links among different research areas (e.g., emotion expression, emotion socialization), whereas chronological approaches must impose artificial boundaries upon a continuous lifespan. Furthermore, with the current emphasis on longitudinal investigations, assignment of many studies to a single age group is problematic. Perhaps to finesse this issue, the present volume takes a hybrid approach. After an initial chapter devoted to theories, Chapters 2 through 6 cover a set of conventionally designated age periods, each with a range of topics typically included in general descriptions of emotional development. These include emotional expression and experience, temperament, attachment, emotion socialization, emotion regulation, culture and emotion, gender and emotion, neurobiological underpinnings, and emotion understanding. Chapter 7 covers some specific emotions in more depth, and Chapter 8 focuses on subject areas related to emotional adjustment and maladjustment. Chapter 9 concludes with some final comments and thoughts about future research.

I have attempted to institute a parallel structure within chapters such that roughly equal space is allotted to the same set of subjects covered at each age range. However, fully imposing such a structure would misrepresent the state of the science, as some topics have been investigated most thoroughly within a particular developmental period (e.g., attachment in infancy). Therefore, readers can expect to find something of an imbalance in the attention paid to certain subject areas across chapters. An additional goal of this book is to introduce readers to various methodologies used in developmental research. Thus readers will find many examples of studies for which the participants, measures, and procedures are described in some detail. At the same time, single studies—no matter how well conducted—can never provide sufficient evidence for the validity of a proposed principle, relationship, or conceptual model. Therefore, wherever possible, **meta-analyses** (i.e., statistical analyses that combine results from multiple studies) are presented in order to evaluate a body of research related to a particular question or issue. Admittedly, meta-analyses themselves may be subject to criticism (e.g., regarding the criteria used to identify and select studies included in the analysis). However, meta-analyses have emerged in recent decades as an important step forward in allowing us to determine what we can legitimately conclude based on the (often conflicting) findings of multiple studies on a single topic.

Although I have attempted to be comprehensive, I must extend my apologies to the many excellent scholars whose work may not be represented (or may appear oversimplified) in this introductory volume. In addition, readers may find that some areas of potential interest have been neglected. For example, the role of fathers in infants' and children's emotional development is not specifically addressed. Unfortunately, recruiting fathers as research participants remains difficult, even in this age of increasing gender equality. In addition, emerging research on special groups such as the LGBTQ community or particular ethnic groups will require more extensive and careful attention than could be provided in this short text.

As this is a book designed for a broad audience, I have made an effort to minimize expectations regarding readers' prior familiarity with all of the concepts and technical terminology used by developmental, clinical, or emotion researchers (e.g., **internalizing behaviors** and **externalizing behaviors**). Thus, when a possibly arcane concept or term is first introduced, I have included a brief explanation in the text and a corresponding entry in the Glossary. Terms in the Glossary are boldfaced in the text when they are first introduced. In addition, if a term in the Glossary is discussed more in depth after it is first mentioned in the text, it will appear in boldface again. Readers also may refer to the online APA *Dictionary of Psychology* (American Psychological Association, 2020).

To conclude on a personal note, writing this book provided me with a much appreciated opportunity to explore a wide range of subjects that extended beyond my own research area (i.e., development of emotional facial expressions). Although I covered many of these subjects in my university teaching, I found that I enjoyed considering them anew in light of more recent research. I hope that some of my enjoyment will come through in the pages of this book. Keeping in mind that emotional development is a continually evolving field, this text attempts to represent a moving target in a way that will be maximally useful—and hopefully interesting—to a wide range of readers.

Acknowledgments

I would like to express my appreciation to the many scholars who generously responded to my email queries about their work, including Karen Barrett, Lisa Feldman Barrett, Karen Budd, Susan Calkins, Joseph Campos, Pamela Cole, E. Mark Cummings, Jean Decety, Susanne Denham, Nancy Eisenberg, James Green, James Gross, Megan Gunnar, Amy Halberstadt, Paul Hastings, Tom Hollenstein, Dacher Keltner, Michael Lewis, Vanessa LoBue, Mara Mather, Martha McClintock, Dan Messinger, George Michel, Joe Mikels, Seth Pollak, Sharon Portman, James Russell, Stefanie Shields, and Sherri Widen. Of course, responsibility for any misrepresentation of their research or thinking remains with me. I would also like to thank Susan Campbell and Pamela Cole, who reviewed the prospectus for this book, and both Stuart I. Hammond and Ashley Maynard, who reviewed an early draft. All four offered constructive comments and suggestions that improved the manuscript. C. Deborah Laughton merits particular thanks for her support and invaluable editorial advice provided throughout this project. Last, I thank Jerry Seidenfeld, my husband and the first critical reader of this book.

Contents

1. Theories of Emotion and Emotional Development   1
    - Theories of Emotion 2
    - Theories of Emotional Development 11
    - Summary and Final Thoughts 26

2. Infancy: The First 2 Years   29
    - Emotional Expression and Experience 29
    - Temperament 35
    - Attachment 40
    - Socialization and Regulation 44
    - Culture and Emotion 45
    - Gender and Emotion 49
    - Neurobiological Underpinnings 51
    - Infant Discrimination, Categorization, and Recognition
      of Emotional Expressions 55
    - Summary and Final Thoughts 63

3. Childhood: 2–9 Years   65
    - Emotional Expression and Experience 65
    - Temperament 69
    - Attachment 71
    - Emotion Socialization 72
    - Emotion Regulation 78
    - Culture and Emotion 85
    - Gender and Emotion 88

- Neurobiological Underpinnings 90
- Emotion Recognition and Knowledge 95
- Summary and Final Thoughts 100

4. Adolescence: 10–17 Years   103
- How Old Are Adolescents? 103
- Emotional Experience 104
- Temperament 108
- Attachment 110
- Social Interactions 113
- Emotion Regulation 118
- Acculturation and Emotion 125
- Gender and Emotion 126
- Neurobiological Underpinnings 128
- Emotion Understanding 133
- Summary and Final Thoughts 136

5. Adulthood: 18–65 Years   139
- Emotional Experience 139
- Emotional Facial Expressions 141
- From Temperament to Personality 145
- Adult Attachment 147
- Socialization of Emotion-Related Parenting Behaviors 149
- Emotion Regulation 152
- Culture and Emotion 158
- Gender and Emotion 165
- Neurobiological Underpinnings 167
- Emotional Intelligence (EI) 173
- Summary and Final Thoughts 175

6. Later Adulthood: 65+ Years   178
- Emotional Experience and Expression 178
- Personality 184
- Attachment 187
- Emotion-Related Information Processing 191
- Emotion and Decision Making 192
- Emotion Regulation 196
- Culture and Emotion 199
- Gender and Emotion 202
- Neurobiological Underpinnings 203
- Emotion Understanding 209
- Summary and Final Thoughts 211

7. Some Specific Emotions   215
- Self-Conscious Emotions 216
- Empathy 221

- Positive Emotions 229
- Threats and Fear 233
- Anger 238
- Disgust 244
- Culture-Specific Emotions 247
- Summary and Final Thoughts 248

8. Adversity, Adaptation, Problems, and Interventions   251

- Adversity 251
- Environmental Sensitivity 252
- Childhood Maltreatment 255
- Psychopathology 260
- Anxiety 262
- Depression 267
- Disruptive, Aggressive, and Antisocial Behavior 272
- Culture and Psychopathology 279
- Intervention Programs 282
- Summary and Final Thoughts 287

9. Some Final Considerations   291

Glossary   297

References   317

Index   381

About the Author   392

CHAPTER 1

Theories of Emotion and Emotional Development

Younger scholars may be surprised to learn that the ontological status of emotion as an independent entity has not always been recognized within the scientific community and, in fact, has shifted greatly over the years. Scientists have debated—and, indeed, some scientists continue to debate—whether emotion is really a "thing"! This chapter presents a brief history of emotion theory to illustrate this point, followed by consideration of prominent contemporary theories of both emotion and emotional development. Although these differ from each other in important ways (at least in the eyes of their creators), there is considerable agreement regarding some of the broader aspects of emotion and emotional development. For example, most theorists agree that emotion involves a process that includes elicitation of a set of constituent components that encompass expressive, neurophysiological, and behavioral responses. However, adult-oriented theories tend to differ among themselves in terms of what components of the emotion process receive the most attention and how those components are characterized. Developmental theories differ chiefly in their portrayal of the origins and emergence of distinct emotions. These differences are reflected in the organization of this chapter, in which theories are grouped accordingly. Still, readers should not be surprised to find considerable overlap among many of these theories.

THEORIES OF EMOTION

Early Days

Although emotion has long been a subject addressed by philosophers, art-ists, writers, and scholars from many disciplines, the James–Lange theory (James, 1884, 1890/1950; Lange, 1885/1992) is widely considered to be the most influential early theory of emotion within the field of psychology. According to this theory, emotion is the perception of bodily changes (most importantly, changes in the **autonomic nervous system [ANS]***) that them-selves are a direct response to the experiences, thoughts, or memories that elicit the emotion. This theory is commonly exemplified by the statement: When I see a bear, I do not run because I am afraid; rather, I see the bear, I start to run, and then I know I am afraid.

Despite William James's personal prominence, the theory he advo-cated was soon subjected to a number of telling criticisms. In particular, the physiologist Walter Cannon (1927) suggested that ANS responses are too slow to account for the experience of emotion. In addition, Cannon pointed out that no emotion-specific patterns of ANS responding (i.e., dif-ferent patterns of response among the several ANS-controlled organs) had been identified to distinguish among the different emotions. Furthermore, an increase in ANS activity did not always result in the experience of emo-tion at all. In contrast, Cannon argued that emotions originate in neu-ral impulses that begin in the thalamus and are relayed to the cortex and various motor systems, resulting in both emotion feelings and emotional behaviors. As is discussed later in this chapter, the debate regarding the neurobiological underpinnings of emotion and their role as causal agents continues to this day.

During the early and middle 20th century, two other prominent fig-ures included treatments of emotion in their theories of human psychology and behavior. John Watson, the father of behaviorism, demonstrated that emotion could be elicited in human infants through classical conditioning in a famous (or infamous) experiment involving "Little Albert" (Watson & Rayner, 1920). In this experiment, 11-month-old Albert was conditioned to fear a previously neutral stimulus (a white rat) by pairing its presenta-tion with a loud, aversive noise. However, Watson's focus was on behavior rather than phenomenological experience (i.e., feelings), and thus he made no effort to develop a more comprehensive emotion theory.

---

* Terms in **bold** appear in the Glossary at the end of the book.

A second prominent figure, Sigmund Freud, embedded emotion within his larger theory of motivation and the unconscious origins of psychopathology. According to Freud, emotions may arise when our id-based impulses come into conflict with our ego or superego. For example, fear and guilt may arise when our id-based sexual attraction to a parent conflicts with our ego- or superego-based standards of appropriate behavior (Freud, 1930). Although Freud's larger theory has fallen into disfavor, the idea that emotions may be elicited when one's goals are obstructed appears in most contemporary models of emotion.

With the advent of psychology's cognitive revolution in the late 1960s, a major change in the ontological status of emotion occurred. The most popular theory of emotion at that time actually considered emotion to be an epiphenomenon of cognition. According to the **Schachter–Singer theory** (Schachter & Singer, 1962), emotion was merely a particular set of cognitions that one attributes to a generalized state of physiological arousal experienced in the context of emotion-related situational cues. As exemplified in their most famous (or, again, infamous) experiment, undergraduate research participants who experienced arousal due to an injection of norepinephrine rated themselves as significantly angrier when seated in the company of confederates expressing anger than when seated in the company of confederates expressing positive high spirits. Schachter and Singer's epiphenomenal view of emotion was enshrined in the majority of psychology textbooks for many years.

Nonetheless, despite the dominance of this perspective, in the middle and late 1960s, some researchers began to revive an earlier Darwinian view of emotion as presented in his 1872 volume, *The Expression of the Emotions in Man and Animals* (Darwin, 1872/1998). Darwin had argued that human emotions evolved from our nonhuman ancestors and are universally expressed primarily via configurations of facial movements (i.e., facial expressions) but also through vocalizations and other behaviors. Darwin's principal purpose was to provide further support for his proposal regarding man's evolutionary origins. Although earlier scholars had been familiar with Darwin's work (e.g., James, 1884; Dewey, 1894/1971; see Garrison, 2003), they had largely diverged from his evolutionary focus. However, in the late 1960s, his work inspired Silvan Tomkins (1962) to generate an emotion theory largely consistent with Darwin's views. In turn, Tomkins (as well as Darwin) inspired a set of systematic studies on emotion **recognition** using facial configurations similar to those that had been described by Darwin (e.g., Ekman, Sorenson, & Friesen, 1969; Izard, 1971; see Figure 1.1 for examples). This research culminated in a landmark investigation by Ekman and Friesen (1971) that reported significant recognition of these facial expressions in a number of literate and preliterate cultures.

These cross-cultural studies launched a new era of emotion theorizing and research that continues to this day. Literally thousands of studies have been conducted using the configurations of facial movements proposed by Ekman and by Izard to be prototypical emotional facial expressions. However, at the same time, new questions are being raised that challenge the status of these configurations as unique and universal expressions of emotion (e.g., Barrett, Adolphs, Marsella, Martinez, & Pollak, 2019; Fernández-Dols & Crivelli, 2013; Fernández-Dols & Russell, 2017). Accordingly, readers should note that this book uses the term **prototypic emotional facial expressions** to refer to these configurations only because they are commonly so designated in the literature; however, no commitment to their status as

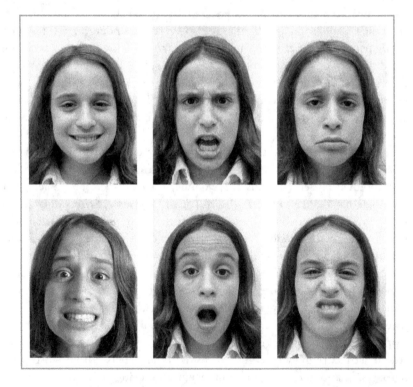

FIGURE 1.1. Prototypic emotional facial expressions. Top row from left: happiness, anger, sadness. Bottom row from left: fear, surprise, disgust.

uniquely emotional should be inferred. In addition to new views of facial expression, new theories, models, and perspectives on emotion itself are being proposed in the adult literature. In the following section, several prominent examples are briefly reviewed.

A Note on Theories

A scientific theory is commonly understood to consist of a set of broad organizing principles proposed to account for a larger set of observations. In addition, theories should be falsifiable (or at least refinable) via a process of testing hypotheses (i.e., specific predictions) that are based on the theory. Within the fields of emotion and emotional development, many scholars have been hesitant to formally confer upon their views the status of a theory. Instead, they may use the terms *model, perspective,* or *approach*. However, because many of these approaches, perspectives, and models have greatly contributed to our current understanding of emotion and have inspired both thinking and research, they are presented in this first chapter.

Current Adult-Oriented Theories of Emotion

Emotion theorists widely agree that the process of experiencing emotion involves a number of components, including elicitation by internal or external objects or events (e.g., memories, encounters with other persons), expressive behaviors (e.g., facial expressions, vocalizations), **instrumental actions** or action tendencies (e.g., fighting or fleeing), neurobiological reactions (e.g., ANS responses), and subjective experiences (i.e., feelings). To illustrate, a person might see a bear (i.e., an elicitor), gasp and widen his eyes (i.e., display expressive responses), run with a racing heart (i.e., produce instrumental and neurobiological reactions), while at the same time feeling afraid. However, any general consensus regarding the characteristic components of emotion quickly breaks down when questions about whether these components are unique, necessary, or sufficient constituents of the emotion are considered.

In their brief review of the scientific literature, Gross and Barrett (2011) identified 30 different explicit theories or general perspectives on emotion going back to William James (1884). To compare these perspectives, the authors organized them into four general categories: **basic emotion theories, appraisal theories, psychological construction theories,** and **social construction theories.** These categories provide a useful framework for discussing the current landscape. However, as will be shown, theories from different categories often share some key features, although they differ in their relative emphasis on these features or in the detail with which they are described (e.g., the role of **appraisal** in the generation of emotion). Because extensive review of all 30 theories is beyond the scope of this volume, the following sections focus on some prominent exemplars.

Basic (or Discrete) Emotion Theories

Following their groundbreaking studies of expression recognition across cultures, Ekman and Izard each offered a theory of emotion intended to both account for their findings and embed them within a more general theorical framework. Following Darwin and also consistent with then-current views of neurobiology, they proposed that humans have evolved a set of brain-based **affect programs** (Ekman, 1971; Izard, 1977) that are distinct for different basic emotions. When these programs are activated, they are presumed to automatically generate a distinct emotion-specific set of physiological responses, expressive behaviors, and subjective experiences. Both theorists proposed a relatively restricted set of basic emotions based on their evaluation of the evidence for cross-cultural universality in the recognition of their corresponding facial expressions. However, interestingly, the number of basic emotions identified by each differed slightly and has changed over the years (see Ekman, 1971; Ekman & Cordaro, 2011; Izard, 1977, 1991). Still, both theorists consistently included happiness, surprise, anger, fear, sadness, and disgust in their set of basic emotions (herein referred to as the **Big Six**). In addition, both theorists agree that basic emotions are products of evolution that have important short-term motivational functions and long-term survival value. According to both theorists, these motivational functions can be enacted via a variety of instrumental behaviors depending on the situational context and personal characteristics of the person experiencing the emotion. However, only Izard explicitly considered emotional development in his theory (see further details below).

Ekman's and Izard's affect program theories were met with fierce resistance by sociologists and anthropologists who objected on principle to accounts that emphasized any innate determinants of human behavior (e.g., Birdwhistell, 1970; Mead, 1975). With particular respect to facial expressions, anthropologists highlighted the cultural variability they had observed in expressive behavior (e.g., cultures whose members smiled and acted happy at funerals). In response to this challenge, basic emotion theorists readily

acknowledged that the automatic (involuntary) expressive responses generated by an affect program may sometimes be overridden by a voluntary control system that could suppress or mask the response in the service of cultural norms (i.e., **display rules**; Ekman, 1971; Ekman & Friesen, 1969). Still,
current cultural psychologists have continued to argue that basic emotion
theories fail to adequately capture the role of culture in emotion generation
(Mesquita, De Leersnyder, & Boiger, 2016).

Appraisal Theories

In yet another experiment that probably could not be conducted today,
Richard Lazarus and colleagues (Speisman, Lazarus, Mordkoff, & Davison,
1964) showed undergraduate research participants a documentary movie
depicting young adolescent boys from a non-Western culture undergoing
a coming-of-age circumcision ceremony. In one condition, the accompanying narrative emphasized the boys' pain and suffering, whereas in a second
condition, the narrative emphasized the happiness and pride experienced
by the boys at the conclusion of the ceremony. Lazarus found that viewers'
emotional responses differed across the two conditions; not surprisingly,
those who heard the pain-and-suffering narrative reported significantly
more stress than those who heard the happiness-and-pride narrative.

Lazarus's experiment set the stage for modern appraisal theories of
emotion (e.g., Lazarus, 1991; Roseman, 2013; Scherer, 1984; Scherer &
Moors, 2019; Smith & Ellsworth, 1985—but see Magda Arnold, 1960, for
an even earlier version). Appraisal theories share the assumption that emotional responses depend on one's interpretation (i.e., appraisal) of the emotion elicitor rather than the elicitor itself. For example, an appraisal theorist
would emphasize that a bear will only elicit fear if one appraises it as dangerous. In point of fact, most contemporary theories of emotion have come to
acknowledge the importance of appraisal in the elicitation of emotion. However, self-identified appraisal theories have the particular goal of carefully
delineating the nature of the appraisal process and the appraisal features
that are related to each emotion.

In considering the landscape of appraisal theories, Agnes Moors (2014)
identified two general categories: those that start with a set of emotions
and those that start with a set of appraisal components. Lazarus's cognitive-
motivational–relational theory (Lazarus, 1991) falls into the first category.
Beginning with a set of familiar emotions, Lazarus sought to identify
each one's corresponding appraisal pattern characterized in terms of six

components and a relational theme. The appraisal components were (1) perception of the eliciting event as goal relevant, (2) perception of the event as goal congruent or incongruent, (3) type of ego involvement (i.e., perception of its relevance to one's self-concept), (4) credit or blame (i.e., assignment of responsibility to oneself, another, or circumstance), (5) coping potential (i.e., perception of one's ability to manage the event), and (6) future expectancy as to whether the situation will become better or worse depending on how one acts. To illustrate, the emotion of anger is characterized by the appraisal of an event as goal relevant, goal incongruent, potentially threatening one's ego identity, caused by another rather than the self, remediable by removing the goal impediment, and likely to improve if that takes place. To provide a hypothetical example, if a child has her favorite toy grabbed away by a peer, the child might interpret (i.e., appraise) that event as both relevant and incongruent with her goal of playing with the toy and as threatening her self-concept as the toy's rightful possessor. If the child also believes that remediation is possible, she would become angry and attempt to regain possession.

Relational themes are brief statements representing the abstraction of a prototypical event for that emotion. For example, the relational theme for anger is "a demeaning offense against me or mine" (Lazarus, 1991, p. 122) that is deliberate or at least inconsiderate. The theme for sadness is "an irrevocable loss." One important feature of Lazarus's theory is the requirement that the object or event is deemed significant (i.e., goal relevant) by the experiencer. Thus not every irrevocable loss will elicit sadness, but only a loss that is also appraised as significant.

Appraisal theories falling into Moors's (2014) second category have shifted their focus away from explaining a preset list of emotions and instead attempt to understand appraisal as it more generally operates to mediate between objective reality and human experience. Sometimes the appraisal process may generate a state corresponding to one of those identified as a basic emotion, but this is not necessarily the case. Sometimes it may generate a more diffuse affective response (e.g., pleasant or unpleasant feelings) or something that may not be considered emotional at all (e.g., feeling powerful).

Currently, the most active researcher to adopt this latter perspective is Klaus Scherer. Like Lazarus, Scherer (2001) proposes that humans continually scan and appraise their environment. For Scherer, this process involves implicitly going through a list of appraisal checks to determine how they apply to the object or event being encountered. This list includes a check for novelty–expectedness, goal relevance, **valence** (pleasantness–unpleasantness), agency, intentionality, control, power, and fairness (Scherer

& Moors, 2019). Scherer proposes that specific appraisals will influence specific physiological and expressive responses and specific action tendencies. These may coalesce such that the emerging state will be considered an emotion (basic or otherwise). However, this will not necessarily be the case; emotions are only one subset of states that can result from the appraisal process.

Psychological Construction Theories

In some sense, all current theories of emotion can be considered to be constructivist theories. That is, as indicated earlier, all consider emotion to have various components that come together in an emotion episode (e.g., expressive responses, neurobiological underpinnings, **instrumental actions** or action tendencies). However, those theories that are identified as constructivist (see Gross & Barrett, 2011) are characterized by their radical abandonment of the idea that emotion responses are controlled by an innately provided emotion-specific affect program or neural network. Instead, constructivist theories (e.g., Russell, 2003) propose that emotions emerge from domain-general processes that sometimes produce a set of co-occurring responses that may be categorized as an emotion (basic or otherwise).

Historically, one of the most popular psychological construction approaches was the Schachter–Singer theory noted above—that is, that emotions were constructed by overlaying an emotion label (i.e., emotion name) on a physiological state of arousal in a cognitive act of interpretation. More recently, James Russell and Lisa Barrett (Russell & Barrett, 1999) developed a similar approach that added *valence* as a second factor. **Valence** is a dimension of feeling running from high positivity to high negativity (i.e., pleasantness to unpleasantness). Their model of **core affect** proposes that both arousal and valence may vary in intensity and that humans thus experience differing combinations of these two experiential dimensions. Some of these affective experiences may be labeled as emotional depending upon the circumstances under which they take place. For example, a state of high negative arousal that occurs before receiving an inoculation may be interpreted as fear or merely anticipation, depending on whether the procedure is undergone voluntarily or involuntarily. Readers should note that Russell and Barrett use the term *core affect* in a very specific way that differs from how others often use the word *affect*. In this book, the term *core affect* is used when referring to feeling states as conceptualized by these authors, that is, in terms of the dimensions of both arousal and valence. Otherwise, the term **affect** (alone) will be used in conformity to various authors' own usage. Most often, the term is used to refer to a wide range of positive and negative feeling states that may include but also go beyond what are considered classic discrete emotions (e.g., strong, inspired, and determined; Watson, Clark, & Tellegen, 1988).

BARRETT'S THEORY OF CONSTRUCTED EMOTION

In separate work, Lisa Barrett has developed what she currently calls the **theory of constructed emotion** (Barrett, 2017a, 2017b). This theory goes beyond pure psychological constructivism in that it embeds emotion within a larger model of brain functioning. More specifically, Barrett adopts a predictive processing model that views the brain as responding to the world in a way that maximizes growth, survival, and reproduction through a process of **allostasis**, that is, the body's "regulating of the internal milieu by anticipating physiological needs and preparing to meet them before they arise" (Barrett 2017b, p. 6; see also Hutchinson & Barrett, 2019; Köster, Kayhan, Langeloh, & Hoehl, 2020). In the service of allostasis, the brain generates embodied models of the events it encounters (i.e., neural representations and bodily states that include core affect) and compares them with past experiences (similarly represented). In a Bayesian fashion, the previous models are updated, are instantiated in the organism's current mental and behavioral activity, and at the same time serve to predict future experiences (that will themselves lead to further updating). For example, you may start your day of hiking expecting a relaxing encounter with the beauties of nature. Instead, you encounter a grizzly bear. This causes you to update your currently functioning model of the world and produce a set of neurobiological reactions consistent with a flight response. Because you are experiencing these neurobiological reactions in a context involving perceived danger, you may assign the emotion label of "fear" to your experience.

According to Barrett, "emotion" consists of those mind–body experiences that come to be conceptualized as emotion through a process of socialization that emphasizes the linguistic labeling of children's experiences over the course of development (see the next section for further details of her proposal regarding development). That is, emotions are actually abstract concepts that we develop in order to provide an organizational structure for our experiences that allows us to predict and respond (i.e., understand and behave) in an adaptive manner. Similar to other abstract concepts (e.g., justice, honor, and patriotism), specific events that exemplify emotion concepts may share little in the way of concrete features. For example, elicitors of anger may involve insults or physical attacks, and anger responses may involve counterattacks or simmering plots of revenge.

Social Construction Theories

Social construction theories may be considered a type of constructivist approach that places culture in the forefront. However, not all culturally oriented researchers adhere to a strictly constructivist point of view. For example, some scholars retain the concept of innate basic emotion programs and focus on how culture may dictate the specific objects and events that activate them or the display rules that govern their expression (e.g., Matsumoto & Hwang, 2012). Some appraisal theorists may reject the idea of innate programs but still posit that links between particular appraisals and particular emotions are consistent across different cultures (Scherer & Fontaine, 2019). True social constructivists, however, hold a more radical point of view. For example, Mesquita et al. (2016) assert that relationships between appraisals and emotions are themselves socially constructed and may differ across cultures. For example, anger in Western cultures might typically involve blaming others (as exemplified by Lazarus's relational theme for anger, as described above). However, in Japan, anger might more often involve self-blame (e.g., when one forgets to show proper respect to an elder). Most recently, Mesquita and her colleagues have adopted a population-based approach that seeks to empirically identify sets of appraisals and action tendencies that are associated with different emotions in different cultures (Boiger et al., 2018). At the same time, appraisal–action relationships may differ among individuals within a culture and also between cultures. This approach is particularly compatible with Barrett's view of emotion construction as rooted in an individual's particular set of experiences.

THEORIES OF EMOTIONAL DEVELOPMENT

To some extent, adult-oriented emotion scholars and those focusing on emotional development have proceeded on relatively separate tracks. Compared with adult-oriented scholars, debates about the nature of emotion have concerned developmentalists to a lesser extent, especially in recent years. At the same time, questions of development have been neglected within many (but not all) adult-oriented theories. In addition, fewer competing theories of emotional development have been proposed in comparison with adult-oriented theories. Therefore, a more comprehensive review of both early and contemporary developmental theories, models, approaches, and perspectives can be presented. As is shown in this section, these sometimes differ from each other in emphasis and sometimes in substance.

Early Days

As previously noted, both Freud and Watson touched upon emotion in their work, although emotion was not the primary focus of either theory. Similarly, Piaget only briefly considered affect as it related to his cognitive-developmental theory. Still, some implications for development and behavior could be discerned in all three cases. For example, Piaget viewed affect as an energizing force underlying the development and operation of one's cognitive structures (Inhelder & Piaget, 1958). Both Freud's and Watson's theories implied that individual differences in emotion responding will emerge due to an individual's experiential history (i.e., conditioning experiences according to Watson, family influences according to Freud). Development was virtually ignored within William James's physiological feedback proposal and also the proposals of his critics. However, the relationship between physiology and emotion was considered by one of the earliest explicitly developmental theorists of emotion, Katherine Bridges.

In the early 1930s, Bridges (1930, 1932) conducted extensive observations of expressive and behavioral responses of infants and preschool children. Bridges was one of the first to argue that the same observable physiological response (e.g., increased respiration) can occur with different emotions and that different visceral changes can occur in different episodes of the same emotion. Regarding development, Bridges proposed a process of differentiation and integration through which emotional responses gradually become more distinct over time. As described by Bridges, newborn infants express (and presumably experience) only diffuse excitement, but this quickly differentiates such that expressions of distress and enjoyment are also observed. By 24 months, Bridges identified 11 different emotions in infants (e.g., affection, anger, disgust, fear, jealousy) and noted that additional emotions emerge during childhood and adolescence. Bridges also emphasized that even the early-emerging emotions change in form as development proceeds such that they involve the integration of increasingly complex and organized behaviors (e.g., instrumental behaviors as well as expressive responses). To illustrate, she described anger in a 3-month-old as involving screaming and diffuse vigorous leg thrusts, whereas an 18-month-old showed more targeted behavior, that is, hitting and pulling the anger-eliciting impediment (Bridges, 1932). Bridges also noted that at least some emotion-related behaviors will vary across individuals because of "constitutional and environmental differences" (Bridges, 1930, p. 499). As will be seen, many of these ideas also appear in contemporary theories of emotional development.

Current Developmental Theories

Perhaps because fewer exist, contemporary theories of emotional development are not typically assigned to more general categories. In fact, all developmental theories share one important (albeit obvious) feature: They all agree that emotion changes with age. Still, an important distinction can be made between theories that propose the existence of at least some basic discrete emotions at birth and those proposing that infants initially experience only broad distinctions in affective or behavioral states (e.g., positive vs. negative affect) that serve as precursors of true emotions. Because most developmental theories can be placed into one of two categories based on this distinction, it will be used to frame much of the discussion of developmental emotion theories presented herein. At the same time, one important theory eschews taking a stand on the question of whether basic emotions or precursors to true emotions exist in early development. Inspired by Dewey's (1894/1971) earlier functional approach, Campos and Barrett's (1985) theory focuses on the interpersonal functions of emotions rather than the intrapersonal mechanisms (i.e., internal constituents) of emotion. Beyond these considerations, all extant developmental theories acknowledge that both cognitive and social factors are drivers of emotional development. However, as is discussed later in the chapter, they may also differ greatly in their depiction of the cognitive and/or social factors that are key to development and their relative emphasis on one or the other.

Basic (or Discrete) Emotions as Foundations of Development

CARROLL IZARD'S DIFFERENTIAL EMOTIONS THEORY (DET)

As noted above, Carroll Izard provided an elaborate treatment of basic emotions as foundations of development. Izard (Izard & Malatesta, 1987) proposed that "preadapted genetic programs" (p. 507) for distinct emotions emerge during infancy and early childhood via a biologically determined process of maturation. As also noted earlier, Izard asserted that these programs involve distinct emotion-specific neurobiological networks and generate a coordinated set of responses that include emotion-specific facial and vocal expressions and subjective experiences (i.e., feelings). According to Izard (2009), feelings are elemental qualia (i.e., subjective experiences) that "arise from the integration of concurrent activity in brain structures and circuits that may involve the brain stem, amygdala, insula, anterior cingulate, and orbito-frontal cortices" (p. 5). Feelings may not always reach conscious awareness, but they always retain their motivational force.

With respect to the emergence of emotions, Izard originally asserted that an emotion can be assumed to have emerged when its corresponding facial expression can be observed (Izard & Malatesta, 1987). Thus a newborn infant who smiles while sleeping would be considered to be experiencing happiness. However, in later years, he acknowledged that the invariant links between facial expressions and other emotion components may not exist in **neonates** (Izard, 1997). Irrespective of this, Izard recognized that emotions undergo profound changes during the course of development in terms of what elicits them and how they are expressed. These changes rest in part on changes that occur in infants' and children's cognitive abilities and skills. Still, for Izard, cognitive status is not a requirement for experiencing emotion, as it is in some developmental theories (described later in the chapter). Rather, it is the presumed activation of an emotion system that exists independent of cognition and may sometimes be activated by perceptual input (rather than cognitive appraisal) early in life (Izard, 2011). For example, according to **differential emotions theory (DET)**, fear in infants might be directly evoked by a sudden loud noise rather than by an appraisal that the noise is dangerous.

Regarding further development, Izard proposed that basic emotions become components of **emotion schemas**, that is, mental structures involving interactions among emotion feelings and higher order cognition that may include images, thoughts, strategies, and goals (Izard, 1977, 2007, 2011). These links are presumably formed based on associations experienced by the person. For example, one of an infant's earliest emotion schemas might involve the association between feelings of joy and viewing mother's face (Izard, 2007). Later in development, language plays an important role in establishing links between emotion feelings and behaviors, events, objects, intentions, and goals. For example, a fear-of-dogs schema might be formed if a child is frequently told that dogs can cause them harm. Although emotion schemas are largely adaptive, maladaptive schemas may arise when the person is exposed to adverse environments, and these may lead to behavior problems or psychopathology (Izard, Youngstrom, Fine, Mostow, & Trentacosta, 2006). For example, children who are exposed to household violence may themselves become prone to anger and aggression. Personality characteristics are also viewed as involving emotion schemas that arise in the context of an individual's own personal experiences (Abe, 2015; Izard, 2007; Izard, Libero, Putnam, & Haynes, 1993). For example, some children may have a greater propensity to react happily during social interactions, and this propensity would contribute to their developing extraverted personalities.

Conceptualizing emotional development as involving emotion–cognition interactions provided Izard with the means to account for other important phenomena. For example, some emotions that do not appear until later in infancy (e.g., shame) are linked to the development of their associated cognitive components (Izard, 2007, 2011). In addition, Izard's view of emotion–cognition relationships can account for the plethora of nonbasic emotions that emerge even later, some of which may be recognized across many cultures (e.g., love) and some of which may be culture specific (e.g., *schadenfreude, amae*). According to Izard, nonbasic emotions are emotion schemas that link specific basic emotions to particular classes of events as they are conceptualized within a particular culture or by a particular individual (Izard, 2011). Note that by emphasizing the crucial importance of emotion schemas (i.e., cognition–emotion interactions), Izard includes a constructivist element in his theory.

MANFRED HOLODYNSKI'S SOCIOCULTURAL INTERNALIZATION MODEL

Although his model emphasizes the role of sociocultural factors in emotional development, Holodynski and his collaborators align themselves with traditional basic emotion views (e.g., Izard's DET) by asserting that neonates start with a set of biologically given emotions (Holodynski & Friedlmeier, 2006; Holodynski & Seeger, 2019). However, Holodynski differs from Izard by proposing that the infant facial expressions corresponding to these emotions are shaped by caregivers rather than emerging on their own via a process of biological maturation. Holodynski acknowledges this disagreement and also notes that considerable controversy exists regarding the timeline for and mechanisms underlying emergence of the emotions themselves (Holodynski & Seeger, 2019). Still, drawing upon the literature (albeit somewhat selectively), he proposes that distress, disgust, interest, pleasure, and fright are present in neonates, as indicated by their facial and nonfacial reactions in situational contexts presumed to evoke these emotions. Following Michael Lewis (see discussion later in the chapter), Holodynski asserts that **self-conscious emotions** (e.g., embarrassment, shame, guilt, pride) emerge during the first years. However, in addition, he emphasizes the existence of culturally specific forms of emotion that develop in the course of cultural socialization (e.g., *tahotsy*, an indigenous form of fear observed among the Bara people of Madagascar that is related to being punished for wrong behavior; Holodynski & Seeger, 2019).

Holodynski proposes three broad phases in the development of emotion. In the first phase (*acquisition of sign-mediated emotions*), infant emotions are initially enacted in the form of rather diffuse expressions and overt behaviors. For example, young infants simply cry when they are either angry, sad, or afraid. However, infants' expressive behavior is gradually shaped into distinct culturally appropriate forms during the course of social interactions with caregivers (and others). Using contextual cues, caregivers may infer which specific emotion is being experienced, and their emotion-appropriate response to the infant may include a demonstration of the emotion-appropriate facial expression. For example, mothers may show a sad facial expression when picking up a crying infant whom they believe is experiencing sadness rather than fear or anger. During this first phase, infants' overt expressive behavior (in combination with contextual cues) serves as a signal to others, communicating the needs and desires of the infant. This is similar to Vygotsky's depiction of verbal language arising in children as a means of social communication rather than an instrument of thought (as was proposed by Piaget).

In the second phase (*emergence of self-regulation*; starting around 3 years of age), children begin to use emotional expression to guide their own behavior as well as to communicate to others. That is, the feelings associated with the child's emotional expression provide the child with information about his or her own goals and may be used to guide his or her own behavior. For example, an infant who is frustrated by an impediment (e.g., the cellophane wrapper tightly enveloping her new toy) might simply cry, whereas a 3-year-old child would show an anger expression and attempt to pull off the wrapper. Holodynski considers this emotional self-guidance phenomenon to be equivalent to Lev Vygotsky's (Vygotsky, Rieber, & Carton, 1934/1987) depiction of **egocentric language** (i.e., self-talk) that is often used by children (and sometimes by adults) to focus their attention and guide their behavior while engaging in a difficult task.

Finally, in the third phase (*internalization of expression signs in self-regulation*; starting around 6 years of age), Holodynski proposes that expressive signals are internalized and that their associated feelings may now guide behavior without being overtly manifested; that is, the subjective feelings associated with the expressions are still experienced, but no overt expressive behavior need be shown. This is equivalent to Vygotsky's proposal that children's language becomes internalized in the form of inner speech at around the same age.

As acknowledged by Holodynski, one important aspect of emotional development is learning to recognize others' emotions. Emotion recognition contributes to one's ability to communicate effectively with others, for example, to understand and sometimes predict their behavior. In addition, emotion recognition is involved in emotion socialization—that is, children learn how to appraise and respond to objects and events in the environment by observing others' emotional reactions. According to Holodynski, infants have no innate understanding of the expressive behaviors that correspond to emotion feelings. Instead, they must learn to recognize these expressive signals (in their culturally appropriate forms), and this learning takes place primarily in the context of social interaction with other persons. Holodynski identifies four processes that are involved in emotion socialization: (1) context selection, in which adults determine the type of experiences to which infants and children are exposed; (2) affect mirroring/modeling, in which adults respond to infants' relatively diffuse signals (e.g., crying) by showing (in somewhat exaggerated form) the appropriate emotion-specific expression; (3) **social referencing**, in which the infant or child looks to another person for information about how to interpret an emotionally ambiguous situation; and (4) acting as if the emotion has already occurred, in which adults interpret the child's ambiguous behavior as reflecting a particular emotion and reinforce that emotion by labeling it, praising it, and/or responding in an emotion-appropriate manner. Exemplifying this fourth process, a parent might see her child momentarily hesitate when approaching an unfamiliar dog and then spontaneously tell the child that she is right to be afraid. According to Holodynski, an important feature of many socializing interactions (particularly during infancy) is coregulation, in which the caregiver helps the infant or child regulate his emotions by responding to the **appeal function** of his emotional expression, for example, by comforting a sad child or teaching an angry child how to effectively cope with the source of frustration.

Theories Proposing Affective and/or Cognitive Pre-Emotion Precursors

L. ALAN SROUFE'S ORGANIZATIONAL PERSPECTIVE

Although he is perhaps more widely known for his attachment research (see Chapter 2), Sroufe (1996) also articulated a model of emotional development focusing particularly on infancy and toddlerhood. After considering how emotion is conceptualized by other researchers, Sroufe (1996) provides a tentative definition of emotion as "a subjective reaction to a salient event, characterized by physiological, experiential, and overt behavioral change" and as a "complex reaction . . . which includes cognitive, affective, physiological and other behavioral components" (p. 15). Sroufe uses the term *affect* to refer to "both the feeling component of emotion and the facial and postural expressive components of emotion" (pp. 15–16).

Sroufe designates his approach as *organizational* so as to emphasize that behaviors become hierarchically organized in more complex ways as development proceeds. Reflecting the influence of cognitive-developmental theories, he is particularly concerned with identifying links between emotional development and cognitive development and how both emotions and cognitions play a role in accomplishing the normative tasks of socioemotional development that are salient at different ages (e.g., developing attachments, mastery, autonomy, and a sense of self; Sroufe, 1979). Regarding development, Sroufe maintains that affect is present from birth, as indicated by infants' expressive reactions (e.g., crying). However, as previously indicated, Sroufe also requires a particular degree of cognitive development before he is willing to assign the term *emotion* to infants' affective reactions. This emphasis on the interrelatedness of cognitive and emotional development is reflected in Sroufe's description of the process through which emotions emerge.

Infant emotional development proceeds through a series of three presumably universal phases. In the first developmental phase (*pre-emotion reactions*), neonates respond reflexively with smiling or distress to dynamic quantitative features of stimuli (e.g., distress in response to a sudden high-intensity stimulus such as a loud noise; smiling in response to stimuli having low but variable intensity, such as gentle rocking). However, because their cognitive abilities are minimal, neonates are unable to ascribe meaning to a stimulus, which Sroufe considers a necessary qualification for the presence of an emotion. In the second phase (*precursor emotions*), post-neonatal infants up to approximately 6 months of age can experience pleasure, wariness, and frustration. These result from simple cognitive processes relating a stimulus to past experience. Thus pleasure results from stimulus recognition (e.g., seeing mother's face), wariness from recognition failure (e.g., encountering a stranger), and frustration from one's inability to execute a familiar (i.e., recognized) behavioral routine (e.g., inability to grasp a familiar toy that has now been placed out of reach). In the third phase (*basic emotions*), Sroufe considers mature emotions to be present in that infants are capable of making more cognitively sophisticated ascriptions of meaning to the encountered stimulus (e.g., an appraisal of danger for fear). This phase begins at around 18 months.

Importantly, Sroufe does not rely exclusively on expressive signaling to identify a particular emotional response in the infant. Rather than relying on the presence of specific emotion-related behaviors (e.g., prototypic facial expressions), Sroufe asserts that the presence of an emotion must be inferred by interpreting the meaning of the individual's behavior within the context in which it occurs. For example, in the second phase, he distinguishes wariness and frustration according to the nature of the stimulus and notes that the infant's expressive response in both cases may be the same, that is, crying. Similarly, in the third phase, anger may be inferred based on an infant's negative reaction to an obstacle, whereas fear may be inferred based on her reaction to a presumed threat.

One key feature of Sroufe's model is his emphasis on the role of tension in eliciting emotion (Sroufe, 1982, 1996). Tension may involve physiological arousal produced by physical stimulation (in young infants) and/or cognitive arousal produced by the need to respond to an encountered object or event (at older ages). The emotion that is engendered depends on the dynamics of arousal in young infants and how the older infant or child appraises the emotion-eliciting event. Also important is the older infant's or child's ability to manage the experience of tension (and sometimes modulate it). Thus the development of **emotion regulation** is an important aspect of emotional development.

MICHAEL LEWIS'S THEORY OF EMOTION AND CONSCIOUSNESS

Like Sroufe, Michael Lewis (2014, 2016a) does not believe that all of the defining features of an emotion are present in young infants. According to Lewis (2014), emotion involves a precipitating event, the bodily changes associated with that event, and, importantly, the conscious experience of the bodily changes. As described further below, the developmental emergence of conscious experience is evidenced by infants' demonstration of **objective self-awareness** (i.e., awareness of the self as a potential object of others' attention). This level of self-awareness is not seen until the middle of the second year of life (Lewis & Ramsay, 2004).

Before the advent of objective self-awareness, Lewis observes emotion-relevant behaviors in younger infants that he originally referred to as primary emotions. Although he continues to use this label, more recently Lewis has emphasized that these are contextually embedded *innate action patterns* rather than emotions per se (Lewis, 2014, 2016a). These action patterns may consist of facial and body movements, vocalizations, and physiological processes. Their function is to enable infants to begin to engage with their environment in an adaptive manner. For example, when given a drop of sour-tasting liquid, even newborn infants produce a facial expression that adults interpret as indicating disgust and that might serve to expel the unwanted fluid. When presented with a human face, 2- to 3-month-old infants will gaze and smile at the person and thus attract his or her attention. Infants will even smile at nonhuman objects (e.g., stuffed animals) that are depicted with a face. These action patterns are innate automatic responses, but they prepare the way for the subsequent development of true emotions.

Lewis proposes a developmental sequence for the emergence of emotion-related action patterns. Following the thinking of some prominent early scholars (e.g., Schneirla, 1959), Lewis (2014, 2016a) proposes that infants initially have two basic action patterns: approach and withdrawal. However, by 2–3 months, these differentiate into patterns related to more specific emotions. That is, the general approach pattern differentiates into joy-, anger-, and interest-related patterns, and the withdrawal pattern differentiates into disgust and sadness. A fear-related pattern also emerges that represents a combination of approach and avoidance. One interesting feature of this developmental scheme is that it is not based on valence (i.e., positivity vs. negativity). For example, two action patterns related to negative emotions are derived from the initial withdrawal pattern (disgust and sadness), but one negative pattern (anger) derives from the approach pattern and one negative pattern (fear) derives from both initial action tendencies. Anger is considered an approach emotion because it may be associated with attack. According to Lewis (2014, 2016a), fear may be related to interest and also an impulse to flee.

To investigate infant action patterns related to anger and sadness, Lewis and his colleagues have used a creative *contingency-learning procedure*. In the first step of this procedure, infants learn to produce a desirable result (i.e., the appearance of an attractive picture) by waving their arms. After the infant learns the contingency between arm waving and the appearance of the picture, the procedure may be modified in a number of ways, for example, by removing the picture altogether or by removing the contingency so that the picture still appears but is no longer controlled by the infant's arm waving. Across a number of studies, Lewis and his colleagues (e.g., Lewis, Alessandri, & Sullivan, 1990; Lewis, Ramsay, & Sullivan, 2006; Lewis, Sullivan, Ramsay, & Alessandri, 1992) have found that vigorous arm waving is typically (though not always) accompanied by a facial configuration proposed as an unique expression of anger according to Izard's DET (see Izard, Dougherty, & Hembree, 1983); lower levels of arm waving are associated with a facial configuration proposed to express sadness. According to Lewis, these facial-plus-arm action patterns may be considered early instantiations of these two emotions. However, although this may be the case within the context of Lewis's contingency studies, it should also be noted that the presumptive anger facial expression itself occurs in many other negative emotional contexts (see Camras, 2019, for a review). Thus, as will be emphasized later, inferences regarding the presence of a discrete emotion may require more than just observing a particular facial expression.

Although initial action patterns are presumed to be innate, Lewis (2014, 2016a) also emphasizes that infants may differ in their propensity to produce these responses. At first, these individual differences derive from differences in **temperament** (i.e., behavioral and emotional dispositions that are biologically based yet modifiable over the course of development; see Chapter 2). However, infants' action patterns soon come to be shaped by their social and nonsocial environments (e.g., caregivers' reactions to the infants' smiles). Environmental influences—particularly social influences—continue to shape emotion responses throughout development. For example, children learn what they should consider disgusting, and their set of learned disgust elicitors typically goes well beyond the sour or bitter tastes and smells that initially evoke disgust expressions.

As noted above, Lewis believes that consciousness (including objective self-awareness) emerges sometime in the middle of the second year. The emergence of consciousness is considered to be a biologically determined maturational event and marks a critical transition in the development of emotion. According to Lewis (2014, 2016a), at this point infants can be said to have true emotional experiences (i.e., to be aware of their own emotions). In addition, a new set of **self-conscious emotions** emerge (i.e., emotions that require self-awareness). The development of these new emotions is described more fully in Chapter 8. However, in brief, the first self-conscious emotions include embarrassment, **empathy**, and jealousy. Sometime between 2 and 3 years of age, additional self-conscious emotions develop as children become aware of social **standards, rules, and goals (SRGs)** to which they may or may not successfully conform (Lewis, 2016b). Lewis refers to these as *self-conscious evaluative emotions*, and they include pride, shame, and guilt. Lewis believes that a child's particular social environment plays a crucial role in his or her development of SRGs related to self-conscious evaluative emotions. For example, depending on how they are raised, some 3-year-old children will experience shame or guilt when they get their clothing dirty, whereas other children will not.

LISA BARRETT'S THEORY OF CONSTRUCTED EMOTION

As noted earlier, Lisa Barrett views emotions as abstract concepts rather than innate biologically based mental modules or emotion programs. She and her colleagues (e.g., Hoemann, Xu, & Barrett, 2019) propose that children construct their emotion concepts using the same processes that are used to construct other abstract categories. These processes include: (1) constructive-thinking mechanisms (e.g., seeking explanations, perceiving analogies, experimenting via mental imagery), (2) Bayesian inductive learning (e.g., updating one's initial interpretations and expectations based on new input), and, most importantly, (3) linguistic labeling (e.g., using others' emotion-related language to anchor a set of experiences that may differ in their physical features and immediate situation-specific goals). In recent years, constructive-thinking mechanisms and Bayesian learning have received increasing attention by investigators of infants' and children's (non-emotion-related) concept development (e.g., Gopnick & Wellman, 2012; Xu & Kushnir, 2013). In addition, studies of language and concept development have suggested that infants can form a novel category for objects that differ greatly in appearance (e.g., dinosaurs) if they hear each exemplar labeled with the same word (Fulkerson & Waxman, 2007).

Barrett and her colleagues consider studies of the latter type to be particularly relevant to the learning of emotion categories; that is, they propose that children develop emotion concepts on the basis of how they hear other persons talk about the world. More specifically, children observe (or participate in) various events that are given the same verbal emotion labels by those around them (e.g., *angry, yucky,* or *scary*), and these labeled instances of experience become exemplars for their model (or concept) of each emotion. Of importance, common emotion labeling provides the basis for the child's considering the various exemplars to be members of an abstract emotion category (e.g., anger), despite the fact that the exemplars of each category may share virtually no behavioral features. Using constructive-thinking mechanisms (e.g., making analogies), children may come to perceive a common, higher order goal-based function for at least some exemplars of an emotion (e.g., removing an obstacle for anger). To provide a hypothetical example, a toddler might drop a cookie in the dirt and find that his mother takes it away and calls it "yucky." Mother similarly interferes when the child reaches for a piece of candy found on the playground but does not object when the child picks up a discarded toy. In this way, the child gradually learns an ever-expanding set of "yuck" elicitors and may draw some general inferences based on these experiences (e.g., dropped food items are yucky but other things may not be). Thus, when the child next drops a lollipop in the dirt, she herself may call it "yucky," look to her mother for confirmation, and then throw the lollipop away.

As acknowledged by Hoemann et al. (2019), little empirical research has yet been conducted to evaluate these proposals regarding emotional development. However, their thought-provoking nature and parallels in the cognitive and language literature suggest them as fruitful targets for future investigation.

A DYNAMICAL SYSTEMS PERSPECTIVE

Another type of constructivist approach to emotional development is the **dynamical systems (DS) perspective**. This perspective was first developed in the fields of physics, chemistry, and biology to explain the emergence and functioning of complex systems of various sorts (Haken, 1983; Kelso, 1995). Applications within the area of biological motion attracted the attention of Esther Thelen and Alan Fogel, who themselves applied DS principles to both motor development and some aspects of emotional development (e.g., Fogel et al., 1992; Thelen & Smith, 2006). Subsequently, other developmentalists have applied the concepts and principles of DS to emotional development in somewhat different ways (e.g., Hollenstein & Lanteigne, 2018; M. D. Lewis, 2005; Lewis & Granic, 2000).

As applied to human behavior, the DS perspective rejects the notion that complex behavioral patterns (including emotions) are dictated by affect programs in the brain (i.e., basic or discrete emotion programs). Instead, emotions are the result of the self-organization of behavioral components partly via synergistic links among the components themselves and partly in response to the demands of the particular environmental circumstances in which the behavior is produced. To illustrate, smiling may be intrinsically linked to happy feelings—but this synergistic relationship can be overwhelmed by contextual circumstances. If a child smiles to disguise his fear while being confronted by a bully, happy feelings are unlikely to follow. One key feature of a dynamical system is that qualitative shifts from one pattern of responses to another pattern (termed *phase shifts*) will occur when some *control variable* reaches a particular threshold. Drawing a clear example from the realm of the physical sciences, a phase shift occurs when water turns to ice as the temperature drops below 32 degrees Fahrenheit. As applied to human emotion, one might consider a phase shift to occur when some powerful emotion elicitor (i.e., a trigger) evokes a sudden overwhelming emotional response (e.g., being overcome by grief when learning about a loved one's death). Another key feature of the DS perspective is the principle of **heterochronic development** (Fogel & Thelen, 1987; Thelen & Smith, 2006). This means that elements of a system may emerge at different times and only later become coordinated with others into a (relatively) stable pattern (i.e., an "attractor"). As applied to emotional development, this might explain the dissociations between emotional facial expressions and other components of the emotion process in the early development of young infants and children (as described in Chapters 2 and 3).

Elsewhere, I have provided a more detailed proposal that casts emotional development into a DS framework (Camras, 2011). This proposal also incorporates a number of ideas that have been advanced within some of the other theoretical perspectives reviewed above. To briefly summarize, the proposal asserts that components of the emotion process emerge heterochronically (i.e., at different times) during the course of development but eventually become loosely organized into emotion systems (i.e., conceptualized as DS attractors). Consistent with Russell and Barrett's (1999) construct of core affect, infants' emotion-related responses initially are distinguished primarily in terms of arousal and valence (positive or negative). However, as development proceeds, the set of responses available to serve as components of the emotion process grows larger. Using anger as an example, children's appraisal abilities, facial expressions, and motor behaviors develop independently but may eventually become linked in an anger episode, as children recruit their motor capabilities (e.g., hitting) in the service of an appraisal-related goal associated with that particular emotion (e.g., retrieving a toy when it is taken by another child without permission).

Like each of the other theoretical approaches described above, the DS perspective has challenges. However, some advantages can also be highlighted. In particular, the DS perspective acknowledges multiple influences on the development of emotion systems, some of which have not been considered within most other theories (e.g., synergistic relations among components). In addition, it potentially provides an alternative explanation for partial coherences among emotion components observed both early and later in development (i.e., the principle of self-organization). However, empirical research that applies a DS perspective to normative age-related changes in emotion is lacking. In particular, determining whether normative developmental changes can be properly characterized as qualitative phase shifts remains an open question.

CAMPOS AND BARRETT'S FUNCTIONALIST/RELATIONAL PERSPECTIVE

One of the first (and most influential) alternatives to Izard's DET was the **functionalist/relational perspective** proposed by Joseph Campos and his colleague Karen Barrett (Barrett & Campos, 1987; Campos, Barrett, Lamb, Goldsmith, & Stenberg, 1983). While acknowledging the evolutionary roots of emotion, Barrett and Campos (1987) pointed out that human behavior is highly flexible, certainly more so than the behavior of many species whose rigid response patterns seemingly provided the model for proponents of basic emotion theories. Campos and Barrett further emphasized that emotional responding occurs in the context of the emoter's interactions with the environment, often—but not always—with other persons. Therefore, emotion is defined as a relational process, that is, a "bidirectional process of establishing, maintaining, and/or disrupting significant relationships between an organism and the (external or internal) environment" (Barrett & Campos, 1987, p. 558). This definition of emotion is still widely used in the developmental literature, and this relational and functionalist view is identified as the theoretical framework in which many recent empirical studies are situated.

As embodied in the definition provided above, Barrett and Campos propose that emotional behavior is directed toward achieving a relational goal. Basic emotions are redefined in these terms rather than in terms of a rigid emotion program within the brain. For example, fear is a process related to avoiding harm, whereas anger is a process related to removing an obstacle to one's goal (Campos & Barrett, 1985). Although emotions may often be associated with particular responses (e.g., characteristic actions, facial expressions, physiological patterning), these are not mandatory but are instead subservient to the context-dependent selection of responses designed to achieve the individual's emotion goals.

With respect to development, Barrett and Campos concur with appraisal theorists in emphasizing that emotional responses are dependent on how the individual interprets the events and objects they encounter in the environment in relation to their own goals. In some cases, that relationship may be obvious even to an infant, but in many instances, there is ambiguity in the environmental event. Campos's well-known experiments with the "visual cliff" illustrate this point (e.g., Sorce, Emde, Campos, & Klinnert, 1985). When placed at the edge of a virtual cliff that appears to have a very deep drop-off, 1-year-old infants typically will avoid going beyond the edge, presumably interpreting it as potentially harmful. However, when confronted with a moderate drop-off, the infant's response will depend upon the emotional signals provided by the mother, typically crossing when the mother expresses happiness but not when she expresses fear. Thus infants' appraisals are guided by emotional information provided by social partners.

Regarding development, Barrett and Campos (1987) highlighted the role of changing goals and increasing skills and abilities that support the achievement and maintenance of goals. These include: (1) understanding how conditions in the environment relate to one's goals (e.g., that being called a "sissy" damages one's newly acquired goal of maintaining his or her reputation), (2) advances in motor development enabling the activities required to achieve one's goals (e.g., fighting), (3) advances in cognitive and language development that serve a similar function (e.g. to produce counter-insults), and (4) the development of strategies to regulate (i.e., reorganize) one's initial response (e.g., disguise one's distress at being insulted).

Campos's approach does not directly address the feeling component of emotion nor the question of whether emotions need always reach conscious awareness. In contrast, he argues that excessive (perhaps even obsessive) concern with these issues has diverted scholars from focusing on the more important relational nature of emotion and its functional role in guiding persons' interactions with social and nonsocial objects and events.

SUMMARY AND FINAL THOUGHTS

Emotion theorizing has come a long way from its sad neglect in the middle of the last century. For one thing, no current theory considers emotion to be an epiphenomenon having no causal effect on other psychological processes or behaviors. Furthermore, there is considerable agreement regarding some of the broader aspects of emotion and emotional development. For example, most adult-oriented emotion theorists agree that emotion involves a process that includes elicitation of a set of response components that encompass expressive, neurophysiological, and behavioral responses. Adult-oriented theorists also agree that emotion is typically elicited through some process of appraisal. However, beyond these points of general agreement are many disputative devils lurking in the details.

Consistent with contemporary views of neurobiology, most current adult-oriented theorists (save the basic emotion theorists) have abandoned the notion of dedicated emotion programs located in specific areas of the brain or even emotion-specific neural networks (i.e., neural networks whose distributed components are exclusively dedicated to particular emotions). However, abandoning this type of approach has its disadvantages. Basic emotion theories provided a straightforward mechanism-based definition of emotion (i.e., the emotion programs and the responses that they generated). Abandoning this conceptualization now opens the question of how emotion should be defined and measured.

One solution has been to seek a functional rather than a mechanistic definition. In that way, elicitor-response processes that serve goals having especially important adaptive functions would be designated as emotions. Those elicitor-response processes identified similarly in many cultures might be considered universal or basic emotions. At the same time, processes that may have adaptive significance in some particular cultures but not others might be recognized as culture-specific emotions. In fact, most appraisal, psychological construction, and social constructivist theorists appear implicitly willing to sign onto this type of functionally oriented conceptualization of emotion. Still, this conceptualization raises its own question, that is, what should be the criteria for determining which elicitation-response processes should be considered to have sufficient adaptive significance (either within or across cultures) so as to be legitimately categorized as emotions? This question has rarely been explicitly considered. However, implicit consensus has apparently been reached to use people's everyday language as the basis for identifying emotions within a particular cultural environment or across cultural environments. That is, emotions are whatever people say they are. This solution is most explicitly adopted by constructivists such as Lisa Barrett but also seems to be tacitly accepted in other theories. Of course, one problem with this solution is that people (including psychologists) do not always agree even within a particular culture. Is surprise an emotion or a cognitive evaluation? What about gratitude, jealousy, or even interest? Still, to their credit, investigators have boldly moved beyond these ambiguities to produce an important body of knowledge regarding emotion as we struggle to understand it. Representing that knowledge is the purpose of this book.

Regarding development, contemporary theorists agree that not all emotions are present at birth. Even those adhering to basic emotion theory (such as Izard) or some of its premises (e.g., Holodynski) propose that several of the emotion-defining neural programs do not become operational until later in development (e.g., those involved in the self-conscious emotions). Disagreements among other theorists revolve around both their definitions of emotion and their depiction of the pre-emotional states that precede it. Several developmental theorists (e.g., Sroufe, L. Barrett) require some level of cognitive development to take place before they are willing to ascribe emotion to infants. Still, they differ in the type of cognition that is required (i.e., "meaningful" appraisal of the elicitor for Sroufe; concept development for Barrett). Michael Lewis requires the development of objective self-awareness and consciousness. Campos requires evidence that infants are acting to achieve emotion-related functional goals. The DS perspective would require the emergence of attractors, that is, context-dependent configurations involving several of the responses considered characteristic of an emotion.

Developmentalists may also differ regarding the nature of the pre-emotional states that eventually evolve into mature emotions. Similar to Bridges's earlier differentiation and integration model, several current theorists propose a smaller number of initial states that differentiate to produce a larger set of emotions. These include Sroufe's precursor emotions, Lewis's approach and withdrawal action patterns, and Barrett's core affect. However, despite these theoretical disagreements, much research on emotional development has proceeded without requiring an investigator to explicitly commit to one or another theoretical position.

Beyond their disagreements, scholars generally do agree that emotional development does not take place in a vacuum but is embedded within social interactions and relationships with persons and objects in one's environment. As such, emotional development is inextricably entwined with developments in other conceptual domains that are typically considered (by convention) to be independent research areas, such as the areas of temperament and attachment. For example, some key temperamental constructs are emotional in nature (e.g., fearfulness). Likewise, some key distinctions among different types of attachment relations are characterized by differences in the individual's emotional interactions with attachment figures. Understanding how emotion functions within these domains is necessary in order to comprehend the full scope of emotional life and development. In addition (and reflecting the bidirectional integrated nature of development), individual differences (and sometimes cultural differences) in temperament and attachment importantly influence emotional development itself, for example, the development of emotion regulation. Thus, in order to provide a broader picture of the role of emotion in persons' overall development and functioning, research on temperament and attachment (as well as other emotion-related domains such as personality) are included in this volume. In addition, reflecting psychologists' increasing interest in the neurobiological underpinnings of human behavior, emotion-related functioning of the brain, autonomic nervous system, and **hypothalamic–pituitary–adrenal (HPA) system** are also covered.

In conclusion, students of emotional development today find themselves in a similar position as do students of cognitive development—that is, no dominant theory exists to provide a unified framework encompassing different investigators' research agendas. Whether this state of affairs should be considered anarchistic or liberating might depend on one's own emotional inclinations. Still, working under the DS assertion that order can eventually emerge out of chaos, this book carries forth under the assumption that the many different paths of research pursued by different emotion psychologists can each make a worthwhile contribution to our thinking about emotion and emotional development.

CHAPTER 2

Infancy

The First 2 Years

Although few people would still argue that a person's future is entirely determined during his or her first years of life, infancy does lay down an important foundation for later emotional development. But how best to characterize that development? Infants' expressive behavior provides the primary window into their emotional lives. Individual differences in infants' tendencies to express (and presumably experience) positive and/or negative affect or emotion result from many sources, including differences in infant temperament, as well as in their attachment relationships to and social interactions with their caregivers. In turn, these social interactions are influenced by caregivers' cultural backgrounds and the gender of the infant. Infant emotional behavior is also rooted in neurobiological processes that include the functioning of the brain, autonomic nervous system (ANS), and hormonal networks. Lastly, emotional development also includes developing the ability to perceive and understand other persons' emotions. All of these areas of development are explored in this chapter.

EMOTIONAL EXPRESSION AND EXPERIENCE

How do we determine when an affective or emotional response has been elicited in an infant and what type of response has been evoked? This is a thorny question because infants cannot verbally report their feelings. Neither is there agreement regarding any nonverbal gold standard to measure infant emotion (e.g., a unique pattern of ANS responses or brain activity). As noted in the previous chapter, differential emotions theory (DET) attempted to solve this problem by asserting an invariant relationship between facial expressions and discrete emotions in infancy. Thus researchers (and parents) could identify discrete basic emotions by examining infants' facial behavior. How has this hypothesis held up over time?

Do Infants Show Discrete Emotional Facial Expressions?

To aid researchers (and parents) in their efforts to identify infant emotions, Izard and his colleagues described a set of facial configurations, each presumed to correspond to a specific basic emotion. These expressions resembled—but were not entirely identical to—the prototypic emotional expressions described for adults by Ekman and his colleagues (e.g., Ekman & Friesen, 1975; see also the "Investigator's Guide" in Ekman, Friesen, & Hager, 2002). Coding systems for these infant expressions were developed (i.e., Maximally Discriminative Facial Movement Coding System [MAX; Izard, 1995] and the System for Identifying Affect Expressions by Holistic Judgments [AFFEX; Izard, Dougherty, & Hembree, 1983]), and these coding systems are still used by some researchers today.

Izard considered the validity of these expressions to be demonstrated via the observation of "predictable relations between particular incentive events and specific expressions" (Izard et al., 1995, p. 998). For example, Izard and his colleagues (Izard, Hembree, Dougherty, & Spizzirri, 1983; Izard, Hembree, & Huebner, 1987) found that 2- to 18-month-old infants showed the MAX/AFFEX-specified expressions for pain/physical distress and anger in response to routine (but painful) medical inoculations. However, mismatches between some MAX-specified expressions and appropriate incentive events subsequently were observed by other researchers.

For example, in a cross-cultural study involving 11-month-old infants from China, Japan, and the United States, Camras et al. (2007) showed that similar facial expressions were produced in response to both arm restraint (an anger elicitor) and a disembodied growling toy gorilla head (a fear elicitor). In particular, MAX/AFFEX-specified anger expressions were most often produced in both situations, and MAX/AFFEX-specified fear expressions were almost never seen. Of importance, the researchers provided evidence that the two situations did indeed elicit anger and fear by obtaining emotion ratings from untrained undergraduate observers who watched videotapes of the infants' nonfacial actions (produced by electronically obscuring the infants' faces; Camras et al., 1997). In addition, objective coding of the infants' nonfacial actions showed that they produced different (and emotionally appropriate) behavioral responses to the two elicitors: behavioral stilling (i.e., "freezing") in response to the growling gorilla and struggling in response to arm restraint.

Based on the body of data produced in this and other studies, my colleagues and I concluded that up to at least 11 months of age, infants do not produce the MAX/AFFEX-specified expressions for negative emotions as would be predicted by basic emotion theories, including DET (see Camras, 2019; Camras & Shutter, 2010, for more detailed reviews). As is discussed in subsequent chapters, whether prototypic facial expressions become uniquely tied to specific negative emotions later in development remains an open question.

Do Infants Show Expressions of Core Affect?

Although infants' facial behavior may not be consistent with the predictions of DET, neither is it random. Studies of infants' smiling and crying suggest consistency with a core affect perspective. That is, smiling and crying appear to reflect positive and negative affect, respectively, and these expressions may be produced at different levels of intensity (Green & Gustafson, 2016; Messinger, Mattson, Mahoor, & Cohn, 2012). Beyond these theoretically important generalizations, an extensive body of research has produced a more nuanced picture of the development of these expressive behaviors.

Crying

As every mother knows, infant crying is present at birth. Crying is accompanied by a set of infant facial configurations that can include the MAX/AFFEX-specified expressions for distress/pain, anger, and sadness (Camras, 1992; Oster, 2005). In fact, these expressions all tend to occur during any bout of crying (Camras, 1992). Recent advances in 4-D ultrasound technology have even allowed researchers to identify these infant **cry faces** in fetuses (e.g., Dondi et al., 2014). Fetal cry faces appear to occur at random in the womb rather than in response to a discernible perturbing stimulus. In line with a dynamical systems (DS) perspective, they have been interpreted as exemplifying the heterochronic emergence of an emotion component (i.e., facial expression) that is not yet linked to other components of the emotion system (Mitsven, Messinger, Moffitt, & Ahn, 2020).

During the first few months of life, infants occasionally will produce brief cry faces during rapid eye movement (REM) sleep, but crying generally occurs in circumstances that may be plausibly interpreted as causing physical discomfort (i.e., hunger, pain, cold, wet diapers; Sroufe, 1996; Wolff, 1987). Because it evokes such a strong perception of distress in listeners, unexplained crying is typically attributed to internal discomfort (Sroufe, 1996). That is, parents, physicians, and researchers generally concur that crying represents distress rather than being a meaningless expressive exercise, such as babbling (Mitsven et al., 2020). Variations in the morphology of infant cry faces do occur, including (but not restricted to) the DET-specified configurations discussed above. Several alternative interpretations of these expressive variations have been offered. For example, Oster (2005) has proposed that some configurations (termed *pouts*) may reflect infants' efforts to self-regulate their own crying. Camras (1992) noted that some variations correspond to the intensity of the vocal cry and thus may represent the intensity of distress. In addition, different facial configurations may be produced as the infant takes a breath in the midst of a bout of crying.

In post-neonatal infants, any attempt to generate a comprehensive list of cry elicitors would inevitably fail. In part, this is because crying can be elicited by an almost infinite number of undesired objects or events, in addition to physical pain or discomfort. Furthermore, not all infants respond the same way to any specific potential elicitor. Building upon the work of others (e.g., Kagan, 1974; Wolff, 1969) as well as his own research, Sroufe (1977, 1996) instead proposed a more general principle, that is, that distress (including crying) results when tension is generated in infants due to their inability to assimilate a stimulus in the Piagetian sense (i.e., to recognize or act upon the stimulus in a familiar or expected way; Piaget, 1952). Importantly, Sroufe also noted that the tension produced by failed assimilation efforts may vary depending on the infant's temperament or on contextual factors, for example, familiarity of the environment, presence of the mother, fatigue, or illness (Sroufe, Waters, & Matas, 1974). For example, when a person wearing a mask approaches an infant, the infant may or may not cry, depending on whether the mask wearer is his mother or a stranger. In all cases, tension must reach a relatively high level to evoke crying. Lower levels of tension may evoke a lower level of negative response that is manifested in sobering, brow frowning, and gaze aversion (Sroufe, 1977).

Several investigators have noted that the different facial configurations that may accompany crying are associated with different forms of body activity. For example, Camras, Sullivan, and Michel (1993) found that adults rate the body movements of an infant displaying the MAX/AFFEX-specified expressions of pain/physical distress or anger as being highly active, jerky, and rigid, whereas MAX-specified sadness expressions are accompanied by more depressed body activity. Michael Lewis and his colleagues (e.g., Lewis et al., 1990, 1992, 2006) have observed a similar association between MAX-specified anger expressions and vigorous arm waving in their studies of infants' contingency learning. These findings are consistent with Lewis's current view that approach and withdrawal patterns of expression and action are the first forms of emotion-related behaviors (see Chapter 1). Whether the patterns reflect discrete basic emotions or different levels of core affect depends largely on one's theoretical perspective and definition of emotion.

Smiling

Smiling (defined as contraction of the *zygomaticus* muscle) can be observed even in neonates. Many neonatal smiles occur during REM sleep in the absence of any external stimulation. These have been called **endogenous smiles** and are considered to reflect spontaneous activity in subcortical areas of the central nervous system (Emde & Koenig, 1969; Wolff, 1963). In addition, neonatal smiles can sometimes be elicited in response to gentle external stimulation (e.g., stroking the cheek), but only when infants are in a sleep state. These are considered the first form of **exogenous** (i.e., externally elicited) **smiling**. Lastly, although unconfirmed by extensive empirical research, some neonatal smiles may be produced when infants burp or pass gas.

Because neonatal smiles do not generally occur in response to plausible elicitors of positive affect, they are not generally considered to be expressions of emotion (Emde & Koenig, 1969; Sroufe, 1996; Wolff, 1987). Although a strong version of DET would assert that the feeling component of joy must accompany a smile, Izard, in the face of skepticism by other scholars, eventually acknowledged that the circuitry linking smiles to other emotion components (particularly feelings) may not yet be developed in neonates (e.g., Izard & Abe, 2004).

Starting at 6–8 weeks of age, infants begin to produce **social smiles** in response to human faces and voices (Wolff, 1963). Many mothers can distinctly remember their babies' first social smiles in response to their faces. Because smiles are now linked to presumably rewarding stimuli, there is general agreement that social smiles are expressions of positive emotion. However, smiles are also elicited by nonsocial objects and events (Zelazo & Komer, 1971). In particular, infants often smile when mastering and practicing a new developmental task (e.g., walking; Mayes & Zigler, 1992). Over time, smiling decreases as the stimulus becomes more familiar or the behavior becomes more routine. Harking back to Piaget (1952), researchers appear to concur that this decline in smiling reflects a decline in the effort needed to assimilate the object or event. Sroufe (1996) incorporated this idea into his tension model, arguing that both social smiles and mastery smiles are produced by a tension profile that involves a moderate increase followed by a decrease or relaxation.

Recently, some researchers have become interested in different forms that smiling may take. All smiles involve contraction of the zygomatic muscle, but they may also involve (or not involve) mouth opening and/or contraction of the muscle surrounding the eye (i.e., *orbicularis oculi*). In the adult literature, *orbicularis oculi* contraction has been hypothesized to distinguish genuine smiles (called **Duchenne smiles**) that express true emotion from nongenuine smiles that may be produced as deliberate social signals or for purposes of deception (Ekman, Davidson, & Friesen, 1990). However, careful observation of infants' facial behavior has led Dan Messinger and his colleagues (e.g., Messinger et al., 2012) to propose that *orbicularis oculi* contraction instead serves as an intensifier that can signal a greater degree of either positive affect (if co-occurring with a smile) or negative affect (if occurring in the context of a cry face). Open-mouth smiles have been called *play smiles* because they resemble a similar expression produced by chimpanzees during play. Open-mouth smiles can occur alone or in combination with *orbicularis oculi* contraction. Between 1 and 6 months, all four possible types of smile (i.e., open mouth, closed mouth, Duchenne plus open mouth, and Duchenne plus closed mouth) are produced more often when infants gaze at their mothers during face-to-face interaction than when they gaze elsewhere, suggesting that they all reflect positive affect (Messinger, Fogel, & Dickson, 2001). By about 1 year of age, Duchenne-plus-open-mouth smiles become the most common form seen during tickling and active physical play (Dickson, Walker, & Fogel, 1997; Fogel, Hsu, Shapiro, Nelson-Goens, & Secrist, 2006).

At around 9 months of age, infants begin to intentionally use their smiles as deliberate social signals. For example, they will sometimes smile while looking at a toy and then continue to smile as they turn to look at their caregiver. This has been termed **anticipatory smiling** and has been interpreted as an early form of affect sharing. Other forms of intentional communication (e.g., pointing) also begin to emerge at around 9 months of age (Venezia, Messinger, Thorp, & Mundy, 2004). Although intentional crying has not received the same research attention, examples are readily observed and sometimes have even been captured in popular YouTube videos (e.g., *www.youtube.com/watch?v=Yz-iwwhJueo*).

TEMPERAMENT

What Is Temperament?

Temperament is conceptualized as a set of personality-related behavioral and emotional dispositions (Shiner et al., 2012; American Psychological Association, 2020). These characteristics may differ across individual infants. To illustrate, mothers who join infant play groups will readily observe that some babies tend to be fearful, whereas others are more outgoing. Although temperamental dispositions are believed to be biologically based, they also are modifiable during the course of development.

Although theories may differ somewhat in the set of characteristics considered to be constituents of temperament, virtually all models include some aspect of emotion responding. In fact, some researchers conceptualize temperament purely in emotion terms. Focusing on infancy, this section reviews the models of several prominent researchers and highlights the place of emotion in each.

Goldsmith and Campos's Model

Inspired by the groundbreaking research on discrete basic emotions that arose toward the end of the last century, Goldsmith and Campos introduced a model that defined temperament as "individual differences in the probability of experiencing and expressing the primary emotions and arousal" (Goldsmith et al., 1987, p. 510; see also Goldsmith & Campos, 1982, 1986). Based on this perspective and focusing on the behavioral manifestations of temperament, Goldsmith and his colleagues have developed a set of age-appropriate laboratory procedures (Laboratory Temperament Assessment Battery [Lab-TAB]) in which infants or young children are confronted with potential emotion elicitors and their responses are objectively coded. In the infant version (Goldsmith & Rothbart, 1996), fear, anger, sadness, joy, and interest (as well as activity level) are assessed via procedures such as the approach of a stranger, restraint in a car seat, and a peek-a-boo game. Facial, vocal, and body activity are coded so as to generate scores for each emotion. Of note, scoring is weighted so as to assign equal importance to each behavioral modality.

Recent infant research using Lab-TAB and related emotion-eliciting procedures has generated a number of interesting findings. As a representative example, Planalp and Goldsmith (2020) applied latent profile analysis to the behaviors of monozygotic and dizygotic twins who participated in the Lab-TAB at 6 and 12 months of age. The researchers identified four temperament types that they labeled as (1) typical (characterized by average levels of emotion and activity), (2) withdrawn/inhibited (characterized by high levels of fear and sadness), (3) low negative affect (characterized by low levels of anger), and (4) positive/active or low reactive (at 6 months and 12 months respectively; characterized by average levels of negative emotion at both ages but also higher levels of positive affect and activity at 6 months). Further analyses showed significant stability across age for the first three temperament types but not the fourth. In addition, comparisons between twins suggested a significant genetic influence on membership in the second (i.e., withdrawn/inhibited) category. Lastly, potential relations to parenting were examined, although relatively few significant findings emerged. However, among these were the findings that fathers of inhibited/withdrawn infants reported higher levels of parenting stress than other fathers, whereas mothers of inhibited/withdrawn infants reported higher levels of their own negative affect. Of course, the causal direction of these relationships could not be determined in this study, although reciprocal influence might seem likely (i.e., infants and parents each having an effect on the other).

Mary Rothbart's Model

A second influential approach to temperament has been developed by Mary Rothbart and her colleagues (see Rothbart, 2011). Within this perspective, temperament is defined as "constitutionally based individual differences in reactivity and regulation in the domains of affect, activity, and attention" (Rothbart, Sheese, Rueda, & Posner, 2011, p. 207). Thus emotion is embedded within this model but does not provide its overarching structure. Rothbart has identified three broad temperament factors that are manifested in infancy and provide the roots for the later development of temperament in childhood: **surgency, negative reactivity**, and **orienting/regulation**. Within infancy, surgency (defined as positive emotion, rapid approach to potential rewards, and high activity level; Rothbart, 2011) is manifested in behaviors such as actively smiling, laughing, and vocalizing during play or routine caregiving activities. Negative reactivity includes showing sadness when separated from the caregiver, anger/frustration when confined, fear (i.e., startle or distress) to novel stimuli, and a slow rate of recovery from these negative emotions. Orienting/regulation includes showing pleasure in quiet play, cuddliness, soothability, and ability to attend to a single stimulus for an extended length of time. Parent questionnaires are used to provide ratings on behaviors considered to reflect these temperamental variables (e.g., frequency of crying or fussing when left in a crib). Because the broad temperamental factors may be manifested via different behaviors at different ages, a number of age-appropriate questionnaires have been created (e.g., Infant Behavior Questionnaire [IBQ]; Gartstein & Rothbart, 2003).

One important feature of the Rothbart model is its portrayal of the development of self-regulation. From a neurobiological perspective, Rothbart proposes that an important part of this development involves a transition in attentional control from an orienting neural network during early infancy to a (more voluntary) executive attention network during later infancy and early childhood (Posner & Rothbart, 2007; Rothbart et al., 2011). Thus, at older ages, the orienting/regulation factor in temperament questionnaires is replaced by an **effortful control (EC)** factor that includes variables reflecting "the ability to voluntarily regulate behavior and attention as seen in the inhibition of a dominant response and activation of a subdominant response" and "to detect and correct errors" (Posner & Rothbart, 2007, p. 11).

Research using Rothbart's infant temperament questionnaire has shown that higher scores on the Orienting factor are related to lower scores on Negative Affect and higher scores on Surgency/Positive Affect (Rothbart et al. 2011; Gartstein & Rothbart, 2003). Somewhat surprisingly, high scores on Orientation in infancy are not related to high scores on EC at 3-4 years of age. One possible explanation for this disconnection is that different neural systems underlie orienting and executive (i.e., controlled) attention and that the development of executive attention in particular can be influenced by environmental variables. For example, Rothbart has proposed that sensitive parenting, including stimulation via exposure to novel objects during play, can facilitate the development of executive attention (Rothbart et al., 2011). In support of this proposal, Bernier, Carlson, and Whipple (2010) found that greater maternal sensitivity and autonomy support at 15 months of age was indeed related to children's greater executive functioning at 18-20 months. Illustrating the detrimental effect of insensitive parenting, Thomas et al. (2017) found that infants rated high on temperamental negativity coped poorly with the mildly stressful Lab-TAB procedures—but only if their mothers were rated low on sensitivity.

Kagan and Behavioral Inhibition (BI)

Rather than presenting a general model of temperament, Jerome Kagan and his colleagues have focused on the development of a temperamental disposition related to fearfulness that they term **behavioral inhibition (BI**; Kagan, 1997). Their research program has primarily utilized laboratory observations and psychophysiological measures rather than parent reports. For example, Kagan and Snidman (1991) observed 4-month-old infants' motor activity and crying responses during several laboratory procedures that involved the introduction of somewhat intense novel stimuli (e.g., mobiles with varying numbers of colorful objects, audiotaped voices speaking at various levels of loudness). These same infants were again observed at 9 months and 14 months during procedures that also involved potentially fear-producing novel stimuli (e.g., an unfamiliar experimenter speaking in an angry voice at 9 months or introducing the baby to a noisy toy robot at 14 months). Data analyses showed that infants who displayed both high levels of motor activity and frequent crying at 4 months (i.e., 23% of the group) showed more fear-related behaviors (i.e., fretting, crying, refusal to approach the stimulus) later in infancy than those who displayed little motor activity and little crying (18% of the group). Those 4-month-old infants who showed either high motor activity or high levels of crying (but not both) later displayed intermediate levels of fear.

In a subsequent study involving a larger number of infants, Kagan, Snidman, Arcus, and Reznick (1994) further examined stability of the high and low categories of fear-related reactivity. Infants were again categorized at 4 months of age as showing high, intermediate, or low levels of reactivity. At 14 and 21 months, they were categorized as highly fearful, moderately fearful, or minimally fearful based on their crying and/or avoidance of novel persons and objects presented in the lab. Approximately a third of the highly reactive 4-month-olds were categorized as highly fearful at the older ages, whereas only 3% were minimally fearful. Approximately a third of the low-reactive 4-month-olds were categorized as minimally fearful at later ages, whereas only 4% were highly fearful. Similar results were found in separate longitudinal studies (see Fox, Snidman, Haas, Degnan, & Kagan, 2015, for analyses that combined three separate investigations). Thus about two-thirds of the 4-month-olds in each of the extreme inhibition categories (i.e., high or low) became more moderate in their fear-related reactivity over time, although few moved to the other extreme.

Why Isn't Temperament More Stable?

In everyday parlance, temperament is commonly considered to represent a person's inherent nature. Yet researchers ascribing to all three models described above have found temperament to be only moderately stable across development. That means that the relative ranking of individuals in their temperament scores can change considerably over time. Why is this the case? One possibility is faulty measurement. Perhaps greater stability would be found if researchers measured different (presumably more appropriate) behaviors or used more valid or reliable measurement techniques. Indeed, the limitations of each measurement strategy described above have been acknowledged even by those who use them. For example, parent report measures may be biased by some parents' idiosyncratic definition of "fussing," or a laboratory visit may capture an atypical sample of an infant's behavior—after all, even babies can just be having a bad day. Thus multimethod measurement strategies have often been recommended. However, even the results of studies using such multimethods (e.g., parent report together with laboratory observations) can raise questions, as agreement across methods is itself modest.

A second possibility lies in an apparent paradox within the conceptualization of temperament itself—or rather a contradiction between the everyday view of temperament and psychologists' understanding. Temperament is thought to have genetic foundations (Rothbart & Bates, 2006) and has been shown to have a heritable component in studies of twins (e.g., Scott et al., 2016). However, psychologists also have identified a variety of environmental factors that can influence its development. For example, in a short-term longitudinal study, Calkins (2002) found that difficult 18-month-old infants who received positive parental guidance (e.g., affection and support) showed lower levels of anger/frustration at 24 months than those infants who received less positive guidance. Sheese, Voelker, Rothbart, and Posner (2007) found that parenting quality appeared to influence the development of 18- to 21-month-old infants who carried a dopamine allele linked to attention-deficit/hyperactivity disorder (ADHD). For those infants, high-quality parenting was associated with lower levels of sensation seeking (including impulsivity) in comparison with infants receiving low-quality parenting, that is, less supportive, more hostile, and overly intrusive parenting in which parents exert excessive control rather than allowing the child an age-appropriate degree of autonomy.

Both overly intrusive and overprotective parenting have been linked to the maintenance of BI across infancy and early childhood. Both of these different forms of parenting may discourage children from developing coping strategies that allow them to effectively deal with unfamiliar situations (Pérez-Edgar, 2019). Somewhat ironically, nonparental caregivers may be less likely than parents to engage in these problematic forms of caregiving. To illustrate, Fox, Henderson, Rubin, Calkins, and Schmidt (2001) found that highly reactive 4-month-old infants who received nonparental care (e.g., day care) were less likely to be classified later as inhibited in comparison with highly reactive infants who were exclusively cared for by their parents in the home. Behaviorally inhibited children in day care also may be repeatedly exposed to a wider range of initially unfamiliar situations and thus become more familiarized with and less fearful of them.

From a neurobiological perspective, Kagan has proposed that BI derives from an inherently overreactive amygdala (Kagan, Reznick, & Snidman, 1988). However, some research suggests that environmental experiences may sometimes be able to alter development of the underlying neurobiological substrates of temperament. For example, results of one recent study (Montirosso et al., 2016) suggested that stress experienced in a neonatal intensive care unit may result in increased methylation of an infant's serotonin transporter gene, interfering with normal gene expression and influencing the development of several temperamental variables (e.g., duration of orienting, positive approach).

Cultural values may also affect temperament development through their influence on infants' experiences. For example, Krassner et al. (2017) documented a number of differences in infants' temperament across the United States, Chile, South Korea, and Poland that they suggest are linked to variations in caregiving behaviors reflecting differing cultural values. Thus the future of temperament research may lie in investigations that seek to further document environmental factors leading to temperamental stability or change.

ATTACHMENT

Emotional expression and behavior take place mostly in the context of social interactions and relationships rather than during laboratory experiments. In infancy, the first and (arguably) the most important emotional relationships are parent–child attachments. In contrast to some earlier views, these initial attachments do not completely determine the future of one's emotional relationships. Still, they provide an important foundation for later development.

John Bowlby's Theory

Although his views have been reinterpreted and modified over the years, John Bowlby's theory continues to dominate attachment scholarship. Drawing from the fields of ethology, cognitive development, systems theory, and psychoanalysis, Bowlby (1969) proposed that human infants have evolved a predisposition to seek physical proximity to an attachment figure when experiencing physical or emotional distress. Infants and young children use their attachment figure as a **secure base** for both coping with distress and exploring the world. Perhaps somewhat counterintuitively, Bowlby himself initially emphasized physical security (i.e., protection from danger, provision of necessities for survival) more than the emotional benefits of maintaining proximity to an attachment figure. Yet underlying his description of attachment as a proximity-seeking system was recognition that the proximity set point was maintained by emotional processes (i.e., distress at separation under threatening circumstances, relief when contact is reestablished, exchanges of positive emotion when in close proximity). Real-life examples of these emotional processes can be readily observed in shopping malls or amusement parks where young children who have wandered away from their families will typically show distress that can only be alleviated when reunion with their parents takes place. From the perspective of Bowlby's theory, the child's distress at separation motivates both herself and her caregiver to reestablish contact so that the child's needs can be met. The positive emotion experienced during day-to-day caregiver–infant exchanges also provides reward for both caregiver and infant.

One important premise of Bowlby's (1969) theory is that infants will form their primary attachment to the person who is their primary caregiver. Despite laudable advances in gender equality with respect to parenting, infants' primary caregivers still are typically their mothers. This gender imbalance is reflected in attachment studies, although some effort has been made (with limited success) to recruit fathers as research participants. Therefore, most investigations of attachment (and indeed other areas of emotion-related development) have involved mothers. Alas, this gender imbalance is reflected in the research reviewed below (but see Bakermans-Kranenburg, Lotz, Alyousefi-van Dijk, & van IJzendoorn, 2019, and Dagan & Sagi-Schwartz, 2018, for discussions of fathers' role).

Although the emotionally rewarding scenario described above portrays an ideal attachment relationship, Bowlby recognized that such ideal conditions often are not met. In fact, the original impetus for his work came from observations (by Bowlby and others) of circumstances in which quite the opposite was true—that is, circumstances in which the mother–child relationship was disrupted for extended periods of time (e.g., by hospitalization or imprisonment of the mother; Bowlby, 1969). Bowlby (1969, 1973) described a progression of responses to extended separations that are primarily emotional in nature: protest (characterized by active distress), despair (characterized by apathy and withdrawal), and finally detachment (characterized by seeming uninterest in the mother when she returns after a lengthy separation). However, much of the subsequent work on nonoptimal attachments has focused on individual differences in the quality of attachments that may be formed in the context of an intact family.

Are Some Attachments Better Than Others?

Systematic research on individual differences in the attachment of family-raised infants was pioneered by Mary Ainsworth, who developed a theory-based laboratory paradigm for studying attachment (Ainsworth, Blehar, Waters, & Wall, 1978). The **Strange Situation procedure** involves seven episodes in which the infant is introduced to a number of stressors theoretically expected to activate the attachment system: the unfamiliar environment of a laboratory, meeting an unfamiliar person (the researcher), being left in the unfamiliar room with the researcher, and being left alone in the unfamiliar room. Based on their responses in this situation, infants are classified into one of four categories, each with particular emotion-related features. **Secure** infants typically show distress at separation but are readily comforted when reunited with their mothers (or other major caregivers). **Avoidant** infants are typically not distressed when separated from their mothers and tend to avoid or ignore the mothers upon their return. **Resistant/ambivalent** infants show distress at separation but are not readily comforted upon reunion. **Disorganized** infants display behaviors interpreted as suggesting some degree of fear when their mothers return after separation—avoiding the mothers' gaze even while approaching them, freezing briefly in the midst of their approach. Infants in the avoidant, resistant/ambivalent, and disorganized categories are considered insecurely attached (rather than nonattached). This interpretation reflects an important principle of Bowlby's (1969) evolution-based theory, that is, that infants will become attached to a primary caregiver given any opportunity to do so—irrespective of the quality of care they receive. From an evolutionary point of view, then, poor care is better than no care at all. Thus only infants for whom no primary caregiver can be identified (e.g., some institutionally raised infants) can be considered nonattached.

Ainsworth attributed the source of attachment insecurity to nonoptimal care by the infant's attachment figure(s). In a seminal study (Ainsworth et al., 1978), she conducted home observations of 23 mother–infant pairs during the infants' first year of life. Based on these observations, Ainsworth identified (and scored the mothers on) several features of their caregiving behaviors: **sensitivity** (i.e., noticing, correctly interpreting, and responding appropriately to the baby's signals regarding his or her wants and needs), **acceptingness** (i.e., maintaining positive feelings about the infant while also realistically recognizing the challenges of parenting), **cooperativeness** (i.e., supporting the baby's autonomy by not exerting excessive and unnecessary control over his or her behaviors), and **accessibility** (i.e., being consistently "tuned in" to the infant so that she can perceive the baby's signals). Babies who were later classified as secure in the Strange Situation procedure had mothers who scored higher on these parenting variables than the mothers of insecure infants. Mothers of avoidant and resistant/ambivalent babies differed only in that the latter were more accepting than the former. As the disorganized category was not developed until after this initial study (Main & Solomon, 1986), no disorganized infants were identified. Maternal sensitivity was highlighted as a particularly important feature of caregiving, and the association between sensitivity and attachment security was later confirmed by meta-analysis in a systematic review (de Wolff & van IJzendoorn, 1997). Of additional importance, a further meta-analytic study (Booth, Macdonald, & Youssef, 2018) found that maternal sensitivity is itself significantly influenced by maternal anxiety and depression, as well as social and economic stressors.

From a theoretical perspective, infant attachment status sets the stage for later social-emotional development by establishing an initial **internal working model (IWM)** of attachment. The IWM is an (initially implicit) mental representation of one's attachment relations and establishes expectations about future social and emotional relations that may become self-fulfilling prophecies through their influence on one's own behavior (Bowlby, 1969; Sherman, Rice, & Cassidy, 2015). Importantly, IWMs may be modified during the course of development in response to later experiences. Thus contemporary researchers view early attachment as providing the foundation for later social and emotional adjustment rather than being its sole determinant (Thompson, 2016). In a study exemplifying this view, Belsky and Fearon (2002) reported that infants' attachment status at 15 months and their mothers' sensitivity measured at 24 months were both related to their children's social competence and school readiness at 3 years of age. Of particular note, children categorized as secure at 15 months whose mothers later scored high in sensitivity showed more competence than children categorized as secure at 15 months whose mothers later scored lower in sensitivity. In a recent set of meta-analyses, Cooke, Kochendorfer, Stuart-Parrigon, Koehn, and Kerns (2019) found that securely attached children subsequently show more positive and less negative affect than less secure (or insecure) infants and are better able to regulate their emotions.

SOCIALIZATION AND REGULATION

Although attachment is not typically assessed until the end of the infant's first year, the socialization processes leading to security or insecurity operate from early on. Therefore, differences in the interactions of infants with sensitive versus insensitive caregivers can be observed well before the age at which they are studied in the Strange Situation procedure. Of particular importance, sensitive mothers appear to be more effective in helping infants regulate their distress (i.e., calming down), and this ability may provide a foundation for the further development of emotion regulation.

Because home observations of natural caregiver–infant interactions are both labor intensive and difficult to standardize, a number of researchers have instead studied laboratory interactions intended to distill significant features of such interactions with a focus on infants' responses to their caregivers' behaviors. The **still-face paradigm** (Tronick, Adamson, Wise, & Brazelton, 1978) is a widely used procedure in which infants under 1 year of age (typically 4 to 6 months old) and their caregivers (almost always their mothers) are seated face-to-face and caregivers are instructed to play with their infants as they might normally do for several minutes. This is followed by a short episode in which the caregiver is instructed to maintain a neutral expression and not respond to the infant. Lastly, the caregiver returns to her normal style of interaction. Meta-analysis has confirmed the existence of a robust *still-face effect* characterized by infants' decreased smiling and increased negative affect and gaze aversion during the still-face episode (Mesman, van IJzendoorn, & Bakermans-Kranenburg, 2009). During the final reunion episode, reparation of the interaction occurs, with positive affect increasing and negative affect decreasing, although not typically restored to baseline levels. Further meta-analyses (Mesman et al., 2009) found that greater maternal sensitivity is associated with more positive infant behavior during the still-face procedure. Higher positive affect and lower negative affect during the procedure are associated with secure attachment later assessed at 12 months of age.

The still-face paradigm is thought to capture several important processes related to infant emotion communication and development. According to Tronick's **mutual regulation model** (Tronick & Beeghly, 2011), parent–infant interaction involves the reciprocal communication of affect, intentions, and relational goals. As in adult–adult interactions, misunderstandings (i.e., affective mismatches) are common and to be expected. In well-adjusted pairs, however, they are readily repaired by means of both parties' behavior. For example, if a mother's vigorous play (or her still face) causes her infant to be overly aroused or distressed and to turn away (an early attention-based form of self-regulation; Kopp, 1989), then a sensitive mother normally will modify her activity to reestablish a more mutually reward-ing interaction. Learning to successfully repair interactional mismatches is considered the key to optimal development. Thus a moderate level of coor-dination and synchrony is considered more desirable than exceedingly high levels because it creates opportunities for reparation. Indeed, such moder-ate levels have been found to predict optimal-level attachment development (Granat, Gadassi, Gilboa-Schechtman, & Feldman, 2017; Jaffe, Beebe, Feld-stein, Crown, & Jasnow, 2001).

Although the above description applies to most infants and their major caregivers, a particular interest of some researchers is identifying atypical patterns of interaction that may characterize infants at risk for poorer devel-opment due to the caregiver's emotional problems, abusive/neglectful behav-ior, or stressful living conditions. One purpose of this research is to identify points of possible intervention by pediatric professionals, as well as patterns of behavior that might be observed by such professionals and thus indicate that the caregiver–infant pair might benefit from intervention. Much of this research has focused on mothers with depression and their infants, perhaps because these pairs might be expected to be more negative or less expressive overall than pairs without depression. Indeed, some researchers have found such differences (e.g., Field et al., 2007). However, results have been inconsis-tent across studies. In fact, no significant difference between mothers with and without depression and their infants was obtained in Mesman et al.'s (2009) meta-analysis of still-face studies. Thus some—but not all—mothers with depression and their infants may respond atypically during face-to-face interactions, and identifying their particular characteristics would be use-ful. Similarly, findings in individual investigations of other at-risk mothers (e.g., those with postpartum anxiety disorders; Reck, Tietz, Müller, Seibold, & Tronick, 2018) would benefit from replication studies so as to be better understood.

CULTURE AND EMOTION

Are Infants WEIRD Worldwide?

As in many areas of psychology, research on infant emotional development has largely been restricted to studies of babies from **WEIRD** (i.e., **Western, educated, industrialized, rich, democratic**) populations (Henrich, Heine, & Norenzayan, 2010). This is somewhat surprising given that the influential basic emotion theories at the turn of the century rested on the assumption that emotional experience, expression, and recognition are universal across cultures. Furthermore, infants were considered to be ideal subjects for studying basic emotional processes because they were assumed to be minimally influenced by cultural norms that might obscure the underlying commonalities. Thus those studies that have included infants from non-Western cultures are of particular interest. These studies suggest that the influence of cultural values can already be seen in several aspects of infant emotional development.

Infant Emotional Expression

To date, most research comparing infant emotional expressions across cultures has focused primarily on quantitative similarities and differences (i.e., similarities and differences in the amount of expressive behavior produced) rather than qualitative similarities and differences (i.e., in the morphology of expressive responses associated with particular emotions). Emerging from this research is a thought-provoking picture in which cultural differences in infant behavior are seen to derive from cultural differences in parents' beliefs, values, and behaviors related to emotion in infancy and beyond (Keller, 2017).

Both recent research and earlier studies have suggested that European American mothers value an active, expressive baby, whereas mothers from non-Western cultures value a calm, quiet baby. For example, Keller and her colleagues (Keller & Otto, 2009; Otto & Keller, 2015) found differences consistent with this view when they interviewed both German and Nso Cameroonian mothers of 1-year-old infants about their attitudes toward babies. The Cameroonian mothers valued an even-tempered infant who did not cry easily, whereas German mothers valued an expressive baby, especially one who expresses positive emotion. Additional research showed that parents from each culture behave in ways that encourage the type of infant they value (Lavelli, Carra, Rossi, & Keller, 2019). For example, corresponding to differences in their valuing of positive emotional expression, German mothers smile more toward their infants than do Nso Cameroonian mothers (Wörmann, Holodynski, Kartner, & Keller, 2012, 2014). Although social smiling emerges at the same age for infants in both cultures, German infants produce more social smiles than do Cameroonian babies.

Asian mothers also have been described as both valuing and encouraging emotional expression less than mothers from Western societies (Chao & Tseng, 2002; Chen, 2000; Wu, 1996). Correspondingly, studies have shown that Chinese infants are typically less expressive than European American infants. For example, Camras et al. (1998) found that 11-month-old European American infants produced intense (i.e., Duchenne) smiles more often than did Chinese babies from Beijing during play with an experimenter from their own culture. They also cried more quickly in response to non-painful arm restraint. Japanese infants fell between the other two groups on measures of both smiling and crying. Importantly, these findings demonstrated that differences may occur between different Asian groups, as well as between Asian and Western infants.

Perhaps because of the labor-intensive nature of facial behavior coding, only one study thus far has systematically examined cultural differences in the morphology of infant facial expressions focusing particularly on expressive responses to negative elicitors. As described above, in their study of infants' responses to anger and fear elicitors, Camras et al. (2007) showed that similar facial expressions were produced in response to both arm restraint (the anger elicitor) and a disembodied growling toy gorilla head (the fear elicitor) by 11-month-old Chinese, Japanese, and European American infants. Separate comparisons across the two procedures for each group of babies showed that key findings for the DET-specified anger and fear expressions held for all three cultures. That is, in each cultural group, the MAX-specified anger expression was produced more often than the MAX-specified fear expression in response to both arm restraint and growling gorilla.

Attachment

One of the most controversial aspects of attachment theory and research is its presumed generalizability across cultures and even across U.S. families with caregiving arrangements that differ from those initially studied by Ainsworth (e.g., dual-worker families that rely on nonparental care; Clarke-Stewart, Goossens, & Allhusen, 2001). Some researchers have voiced concerns that cultural differences in infants' typical experiences (e.g., with separations from their mothers) may produce differences in their behaviors that will affect their attachment classification (e.g., producing nonchalance regarding separations or extreme distress that makes comforting difficult; van IJzendoorn & Sagi, 2001; Keller, 2013; Otto & Keller, 2014; Rothbaum, Weisz, Pott, Miyake, & Morelli, 2000). These differences may result in a disproportionate number of infants from such backgrounds being classified as insecurely attached. Still, recent research appears to show that the proportion of babies categorized as secure in most non-Western samples is comparable to the proportion found in European and American samples (around 65%; Kondo-Ikemura, Behrens, Umemura, & Nakano, 2018; Mesman, van

IJzendoorn, & Sagi-Schwartz, 2016). However, the distribution of insecure infants across the several insecure categories may differ.

With respect to parenting, caregiver sensitivity (considered the key feature of desirable parenting by Ainsworth) also may be manifested differently across cultures. For example, as earlier noted, maternal smiling is more frequent in Germany than in Cameroon. However, as pointed out by Mesman and her colleagues (Mesman & Emmen, 2013; Mesman et al., 2018), several recently developed measures of caregiver sensitivity may be problematic because they include the scoring of maternal positive affect (e.g., smiling). In point of fact, emotional expressivity was not considered an indicator of sensitivity as originally conceived and measured by Ainsworth. That is, a sensitive mother might be attentive and responsive to her infant without necessarily producing many smiles. Therefore, Mesman has recommended that attachment researchers exclude emotional expressivity from their sensitivity measures or evaluate it separately from the more central indices of sensitivity (i.e., prompt and appropriate responding to infants' signals).

Cultural differences in expressivity might also affect mother–infant behavior in the still-face paradigm, making it inappropriate for use in many non-Western societies. In fact, Tronick himself suggested that this might be the case for Gusii mothers in Kenya who actively discourage infant smiling and engage in less face-to-face interaction with their infants (Tronick & Beeghly, 2011). These mother–infant pairs might be less expressive during the initial and final episodes of the still-face procedure, tempting researchers to inappropriately judge their relationship to be problematic and meriting intervention. Overall, the message is that care must be taken when developing clinical applications based on research conducted solely with European or American families and then attempting to use them with non-Western families (including immigrants to the United States).

One important limitation of the research on attachment across cultures is the lack of studies investigating associations between infant attachment status and later social-emotional adjustment. A key premise of Bowlby's (1988) theory is that secure attachment provides the foundation for the development of healthy social and emotional relations with other people. Investigating this premise across cultures presents a thought-provoking challenge in that cultures may differ in how they conceptualize a healthy social or emotional relationship. For example, in cultures that value loyalty to the family more than emotional bonding, infant attachment may not be a good predictor of later relationship satisfaction. Without further research to address this question, conclusions about the generalizability of attachment theory across cultures must be viewed with caution.

GENDER AND EMOTION
How Important Are Gender Differences?

Americans' views regarding gender differences in emotion have shifted radically in recent decades in part because of changes in Western cultural values. At the same time, this shift has been empirically corroborated by research showing only minimal gender differences in infants' emotions along with potential social determinants of such differences.

What Differences Have Been Found in Infants?

Meta-analyses have been conducted that examine gender differences in infants' and children's temperament (Else-Quest, Hyde, Goldsmith, & Van Hulle, 2006), emotional expressivity (Chaplin & Aldao, 2013), and emotion processing (McClure, 2000). These meta-analyses interpreted the **effect size** for each significant gender difference in terms of conventionally accepted criteria (i.e., whether an effect size reached the lower level cutoff point for a small, medium, or large effect; Cohen, 1988, 1992; Hedges & Olkin, 1985). Several statistically significant gender differences were found for infants. For example, in their investigation of temperament, Else-Quest et al. (2006) found that infant boys (up to 12 months of age) were rated as more difficult and emotionally intense but less fearful than girls. Boys also were rated higher for high-intensity pleasure and activity, whereas girls were rated higher for less intense positive approach. However, only the gender difference in high-intensity pleasure met the criterion corresponding to a small effect size. Effect sizes for all other differences were trivial (i.e., less than "small"). In the meta-analysis of emotional expression, Chaplin and Aldao (2013) reported that infant girls (up to 17 months of age) showed significantly more sadness, fear, and anxiety (analyzed together as a group) than did boys; however, again, the effect size was less than small.

For her meta-analysis of expression processing by infants, children, and adolescents, McClure (2000) analyzed facial expression studies that included age-appropriate outcome measures (e.g., preference, **discrimination** or social referencing for infants, and recognition or labeling for children and adolescents). For infants, a significant gender difference was found indicating better emotion processing by female babies (up to 18 months of age). However, again, the effect size was unimpressive. Along with other findings in both the developmental and adult literature, these results have led one prominent scholar to propose the **gender similarity hypothesis** (Hyde, 2014) to replace psychology's earlier emphasis on presumed gender differences.

Where Do Gender Differences Come From?

Those gender differences that do exist may reflect differences in how parents interact with their infant sons and daughters. This possibility was illustrated almost 50 years ago when Condry and Condry (1976) presented viewers with the videotape of a 9-month-old infant responding to the presentation of several toys, including a teddy bear, a doll, and a jack-in-the-box. Half of the viewers were told that the infant was a boy, and half were told that the infant was a girl. Viewers rated the baby on a number of characteristics, including pleasure, anger, and fear. Results revealed a significant gender-labeling effect consistent with stereotypical views of gender differences. That is, when labeled as a boy, the infant was judged to be more active, more angry, and less fearful in response to the jack-in-the-box than when the infant was labeled as a girl. In discussing their findings, Condry and Condry suggested that differential gender labeling might well produce differential caregiver behavior. That is, caregivers might respond to girls who cry (e.g., when startled by a jack-in-the-box) with more comfort and cuddling than boys because the girls are perceived as being afraid while the boys are perceived as being angry. Condry and Condry's study was widely interpreted as demonstrating a predominance of social influences (i.e., society-generated stereotypical beliefs) on the shaping of gender role behaviors, including the development of gender differences in emotion.

Subsequent research has produced a more nuanced picture. In a review of 17 gender-labeling studies, Stern and Karraker (1989) found that differences in ratings were not always found (i.e., were found in only 12 studies) and were consistent with gender stereotypes in only seven of those studies. Seven studies directly examined adults' behavioral responses to gender-labeled infants. A gender-labeling effect was found in only three of these studies and for only 18% of the comparisons that were made overall. However, those effects that were found conformed to predictions made based on gender stereotyping. Thus, as had been originally suggested by Condry and Condry (1976), gender labeling may influence caregiver responses only in some ambiguous situations, for example, situations in which an infant's or child's crying might plausibly reflect either anger or fear. Still, this may be sufficient to significantly influence later gender role development.

In addition to gender-labeling studies, some investigations of parents' interactions with their own infant sons and daughters have found potentially relevant variations in parent behavior. For example, in a home observation study of mothers and their 3-month-old infants, Lewis (1972) found that mothers responded more to daughters' than to sons' affect behaviors (i.e., both smiling and crying/fretting). In a laboratory study involving mothers and their 6-month-old infants, Malatesta and Haviland (1982) reported nonsignificant trends for mothers to respond contingently to sons' smiles more than daughters' smiles and to imitate sons' expressions more than daughters' overall. In contrast, when the infants were 22 months of age, mothers were found to smile more at daughters and to be more expressive with daughters overall (Malatesta, Culver, Tesman, & Shepard, 1989). These findings suggest that mothers' socialization of greater emotional expressivity in girls relative to boys (via modeling and **contingent responding**) may increase during the first 2 years.

Infants' own behaviors also may play a role in their emotion socialization. For example, Brody, Hall, and Stokes (2016) have suggested that infant girls' tendency to stay closer to and attend more to their mothers than do boys (see Bornstein et al., 2008; Buss, Brooker, & Leuty, 2008; Goldberg & Lewis, 1969) may contribute to their developing slightly greater sensitivity to others' emotional expressions. Still, given the sparsity of relevant data, more research is needed before conclusions can be drawn with confidence regarding gender-related emotion socialization in infancy.

NEUROBIOLOGICAL UNDERPINNINGS

During the last several decades, there has been an increasing emphasis on understanding the neurobiological bases of human behavior and development. Emotion is no exception. At the same time, research has been constrained by limitations in our technology for studying brain activity and physiological functioning (especially in infants and children), as well as by interpretative difficulties. Depictions of behavior and neurobiology take place on essentially different levels of analysis, and when associations are found, inferences regarding causal relations require caution. Still, plausible inferences (or at least hypotheses) can often be made based on associations found between behavior and neurobiological activity. These may set the stage for future research leading to a better understanding of brain–behavior relations and possible translational applications.

Brain Functioning

How Do We Study the Brain?

Currently several technologies are available to study brain functioning. **Magnetic resonance imaging (MRI)** produces images of the anatomical structure of the brain, whereas **functional MRI (fMRI)** produces images that represent small changes in blood flow associated with neural activity in various brain areas. However, both techniques require research participants to stay immobile in a scanner and thus can only be used with infants or very young children who are sedated or sleeping. **Electroencephalography (EEG)** is a low-stress procedure feasible for infants, children, and adults. EEG involves measuring electrical activity across the scalp in the form of brain waves (i.e., voltage fluctuations measured via electrical sensors) that vary in frequency and amplitude. Spikes of activity that occur in response to the presentation of stimuli (i.e., **event-related potentials [ERPs]**) can be measured on different areas of the scalp, and comparisons between adults, children, and infants can be made. **Near-infrared spectroscopy (NIRS)** is another low-stress procedure that involves measuring blood flow in the cerebral cortex. A relatively new procedure, NIRS is used less often than the others to study emotion and emotional development.

Brain Functioning and Emotion in Infancy

Models of brain functioning in relation to emotion have historically emphasized the amygdala (a subcortical structure), the prefrontal cortex (PFC), and the bidirectional interconnections between them. Although early studies focused on associations between amygdala activity and fear responses (in adults), currently the amygdala is viewed more broadly as responding to ambiguity or uncertainty (including but not exclusively associated with emotional stimuli) and as facilitating learning (including affective learning) more generally (Adolphs, 2008; Madarasz et al., 2016).

Whereas the amygdala is well developed at birth, MRI studies of sleeping infants have shown that cortical and other subcortical areas of the brain undergo substantial expansion in size during the first year and a lesser degree of growth during the second year (Gilmore et al., 2012; Hodel, 2018). However, functional activity of brain regions is more difficult to assess because fMRI studies cannot be conducted when babies are awake. Extrapolating from animal research, as well as research comparing children, adolescents, and adults, one plausible recent model (Gee et al., 2013; Tottenham & Gabard-Durnam, 2017) posits that functional connections between the amygdala and PFC develop during infancy and are largely "positive," that is, with influence running from the amygdala to the cortex. As development proceeds, "negative" connections (i.e., with influence running from the PFC to the amygdala) gradually increase during childhood and become dominant as children approach adolescence. The functional implications of these connections and their development is concisely captured in the title of Tottenham and Gabard-Durnam's (2017) article "The Developing Amygdala: A Student of the World and a Teacher of the Cortex." This means that during infancy, amygdala activation facilitates learning about the circumstances that produced it (with such learning presumably stored in the cortex). Later on, amygdala activation will itself be influenced by what has been learned. The proposed model is consistent with constructivist views of emotional development that emphasize the learning of relationships among emotion components (see Chapter 1). It is also consistent with popular theories that view the development of emotion regulation as involving increasing cortical control over subcortical emotion regions (including the amygdala). However, as is discussed later, making a sharp distinction between emotion and its regulation is somewhat problematic from both theoretical and methodological points of view.

Although fMRI studies of awake infants are infeasible, EEG can readily be used. However, EEG is limited in terms of its spatial resolution and cannot directly identify activity of particular subcortical structures. Still, inferences regarding cortically mediated processes with emotion relevance can sometimes be made. For example, some researchers (e.g., Harmon-Jones, Gable, & Peterson, 2010; Marshall & Fox, 2008) have found greater left hemisphere activity associated with approach-related emotions (e.g., happiness, anger) and greater right hemispheric activation associated with avoidance- or withdrawal-related emotions (e.g., sadness, fear). Other research has shown that 7-month-old infants generate a larger Nc component (a type of ERP) in response to presentation of prototypic facial expressions of fear compared with other emotional expressions. A larger Nc response is generally interpreted as indicating heightened attention, leading some to infer that infants are biased to attend to facial cues indicating threat (Morales & Fox, 2019). However, illustrating the potentially ambiguous implications of brain activity data, it is not clear whether infants perceive the fear expressions as reflecting threat or attend to them because of their novelty, given that fear expressions are rarely seen by infants in real life.

Autonomic Nervous System (ANS)

In addition to being connected to the cortex, the amygdala is also anatomically and functionally connected to the ANS via the vagus nerve and its connections to the heart (Smith, Thayer, Khalsa, & Lane, 2017). Because it is quite feasible to obtain heart rate and other autonomic measures from infants, much research on the neurobiology of their emotional responses has involved such measures (see Hastings & Kahle, 2019, for review). Although the two branches of the ANS bear a complex functional relationship to each other, the **sympathetic nervous system (SNS)** is generally described as preparing and sustaining bodily action (e.g., fight or flight), whereas the **parasympathetic nervous system (PNS)** sustains a state of lower arousal that allows the body to "rest and digest." At rest, the PNS exerts control over the SNS to maintain a relatively low but variable heart rate. When action might be required (e.g., during stressful circumstances), the PNS releases the vagal "brake," allowing for increased sympathetic activity. Sympathetic arousal can include a number of responses that facilitate action, including increases in heart and respiration rates, conversion of glycogen to glucose, and pupil dilation.

One commonly used measure of autonomic functioning is **respiratory sinus arrhythmia (RSA)**. RSA is a measure of heart rate variability in synchrony with respiration (i.e., increases in heart rate during inspiration and decreases during exhalation). Higher RSA generally (although not always) reflects greater parasympathetic control (see Beauchaine, 2001, for a more detailed discussion). According to Stephen Porges's **polyvagal theory** (Porges, 2007; Porges & Furman, 2011), higher parasympathetic control (i.e., higher RSA) is associated with relaxed engagement with social partners, whereas decreased parasympathetic control (i.e., lower RSA) facilitates orientation and active coping. Developmental researchers have often measured RSA in contexts in which higher RSA can be interpreted as a measure of emotion regulation (or alternatively conceptualized as an appropriate level of emotion-related arousal). For example, in a recent meta-analytic investigation including multiple studies, Jones-Mason, Alkon, Coccia, and Bush (2018) reported that RSA typically decreases during the mildly stressful disengagement episode of the still-face procedure (when mothers cease to interact with their infants) but increases again during the reunion episode.

Hypothalamic–Pituitary–Adrenal (HPA) System

A second physiological system involved in stress responding is the **hypothalamic–pituitary–adrenal (HPA)** system (Gunnar & Quevedo, 2007). Activation of this system results in the release of cortisol, which circulates through the body and facilitates attention, arousal, and energy—adaptive responses for coping with a stressor. Under optimal circumstances, some of this cortisol eventually circulates back to the hypothalamus and reduces excessive further production through a negative feedback loop. A normative diurnal rhythm of cortisol secretion has been identified that involves a sharp increase shortly after awakening (i.e., the **cortisol awakening response**

[CAR]) followed by a gradual decrease over the course of the day and then a gradual increase during the second half of the night. However, in response to some stressors, cortisol levels may temporarily increase at any time.

The HPA system is active in infants at birth, although the normal diurnal cortisol rhythm takes several years to become established (Gunnar & Donzella, 2002). Newborns react with both observable distress and elevated cortisol to physically induced stress (e.g., inoculations). However, the two responses typically become dissociated by 12 months of age, with infants showing observable distress but not elevated cortisol to physical stressors. Cortisol reactivity to social stressors also declines. In still-face studies, cortisol elevation is seen only if the procedure is extended so as to expose the infant to two episodes of maternal nonresponsiveness. Even so, cortisol reactivity decreases between 4 and 8 months of age (Provenzi, Giusti, & Montirosso, 2016). Elevated cortisol to unfamiliar people or events (e.g., stranger approach, clowns) is only seen under special circumstances. That is, infants with insecure attachments and/or higher levels of temperamental negative reactivity may show increased cortisol levels when threatened or frustrated. To illustrate, Nachmias, Gunnar, Mangelsdorf, Parritz, and Buss (1996) found that behaviorally inhibited infants with insecure attachments showed higher levels of cortisol than behaviorally inhibited but securely attached infants when they were confronted with a boisterous clown and a noisy robot in the presence of their mothers. In another example, Ahnert, Gunnar, Lamb, and Barthel (2004) found that insecurely attached 15-month-old infants produced higher levels of cortisol than did securely attached infants when adapting to day care accompanied by their mothers. These latter studies illustrate the phenomenon of **social buffering** (i.e., reduction in stress when in the presence of an attachment figure; Gunnar, 2017).

INFANT DISCRIMINATION, CATEGORIZATION, AND RECOGNITION OF EMOTIONAL EXPRESSIONS

Most contemporary scholars agree that emotion understanding is learned rather than innate, that such learning begins in infancy, and that infants can recognize valence-related differences in emotional expressions (i.e., positive vs. negative facial expressions) before the end of their first year. However, characterizing the preliminary steps leading to this achievement has proved difficult, in part because researchers have not always used key terminology in the same way.

Some Important Distinctions

Distinguishing between discrimination, categorization, recognition, and knowledge is critical to the accurate portrayal of infants' understanding of others' emotional expressions. These terms are often conflated or used interchangeably in the literature. Herein, the term **discrimination** refers to perceiving that different patterns of sensory input are indeed different from each other (e.g., a smile looks different from a frown). **Categorization** refers to the grouping together of expression exemplars that represent the same emotion but differ in their details (e.g., smiles with or without mouth opening, smiles posed by different models). Similar to the distinction made in Castro, Cheng, Halberstadt, and Grühn's (2016) EUReKA model, the term **recognition** denotes perceiving differences in meaning associated with different expressions. At a simple level, recognition denotes understanding that a particular expression is related to some other nonexpressive feature(s) of the emotion (e.g., characteristic elicitors, action tendencies, appraisals, or goals). **Emotion knowledge** is treated in the next chapter and refers to a more sophisticated comprehension of the mental states and experiential origins of the expressers' emotions (e.g., cultural background or history of **abuse**). The term **emotion understanding** is used as an umbrella label to include both recognition and/or knowledge.

Some Important Challenges

Infants' discrimination, categorization, and recognition of emotional expressions has been extensively investigated. However, methodological differences among studies make it difficult to reach generalizable conclusions. Typically, only a subset of emotions is studied, and that subset differs across investigations. Therefore, findings cannot be generalized so as to apply to all emotions. Other methodological differences abound. For example, some investigators employ a habituation procedure (in which discrimination is indicated by habituation to an initial stimulus followed by recovery of attention to a novel stimulus). Others use a preference procedure (in which the duration of infants' visual attention to simultaneously or sequentially presented stimuli are compared). Although each has its limitations, habituation procedures are generally considered more diagnostic in that infants may be able to discriminate between expressions yet have no preference for one or the other. However, when infants do show a preference, it can be assumed that they see a difference. Still, the basis for that preference may be unclear. In fact, in some cases, greater attention to an expression (e.g., an unfamiliar fear expression) may reflect uncertainty or wariness rather than a positive affective response.

Unfortunately, no meta-analyses have yet been reported that integrate this literature for the purpose of determining the ages at which discrimination, categorization, and recognition emerge for some or all emotions. Nonetheless, some excellent narrative reviews are available (e.g., Bayet & Nelson, 2019; Grossman, 2010; Quinn et al., 2011; Ruba & Pollak, 2020; Ruba & Repacholi, 2020). Although these reviews provide more extensive treatments of the topic than space permits herein, many empirical studies have yielded conflicting results, making it challenging to reach definitive conclusions.

Early Discrimination by Neonates (0–4 Weeks)

Perhaps because participant cooperation can be difficult to achieve when participants have only recently been born, few studies have investigated neonates' responses to emotional expressions. Beyond any lack of motivation to participate, newborn infants' limited visual acuity likely imposes severe restrictions on their capacity to perceive facial expressions. However, if care is taken when positioning the stimuli, discrimination might still be possible. In one often-cited study, Field, Woodson, Greenberg, and Cohen (1982) reported neonatal discrimination among (as well as imitation of) happy, sad, and surprised facial expressions posed by a live model. In contrast, Farroni, Menon, Rigato, and Johnson (2007) failed to find evidence for neonatal discrimination between fear and neutral expressions in a study that used a different set of emotions (i.e., happiness, fear, and neutral), still photographs rather than a live model, and a habituation procedure. At the same time, Farroni et al. (2007) did find a preference in neonates for happy over fearful expressions. Rigato, Menon, Johnson, and Farroni (2011) found a preference for happy over neutral expressions—but only when the photographic stimuli showed models with direct (as opposed to averted) gaze.

Field et al. (1982) interpreted their earlier findings as consistent with a theoretical model that posits an innate mechanism supporting both expression discrimination and imitation (see Meltzoff & Marshall, 2018). In contrast, Farroni et al. (2007) and Rigato et al. (2011) interpreted their findings in terms of Johnson's two-process model that posits a mechanism for learning to discriminate and prefer happy faces based on neonates' experiences during their first few days (Johnson, Senju, & Tomalski, 2015). In either case, these studies suggest the possibility that neonates discriminate between (and prefer) happy over some negative and neutral facial expressions.

Unfortunately, as is discussed below, studies of somewhat older infants cast doubt on the robustness of these findings or suggest a more complicated developmental story. In addition, some researchers have raised important questions about the existence of neonatal imitation (e.g., Oostenbroek et al., 2016; but see Meltzoff et al., 2018, for a defense of his position).

Considering psychology's historical emphasis on facial rather than vocal emotional expression, one might be surprised to learn that infants respond to the voice as early as or perhaps even earlier than to the face. However, given that the auditory system is more fully developed than the visual system at birth, such surprise might be unwarranted. To illustrate, Mastropieri and Turkewitz (1999) presented 3½-week-old neonates with scripted verbal statements spoken with happy, sad, angry, or neutral intonation by speakers of the infants' mothers' native language or by speakers of a different language. Infants responded with greater eye widening to happy speech—but only when it was produced in their mothers' native language. These findings suggest that by the end of the neonatal period, some degree of discrimination between vocal intonations for different emotions may have developed but may be restricted to intonations embedded within a familiar language. More generally, this suggests the possibility of very early discrimination and preference learning by newborns based on their auditory experiences.

Post-Neonatal Discrimination and Categorization

Studies of post-neonatal infants up to about 1 year of age have been remarkably inconsistent. For example, some studies find that infants discriminate between happy facial expressions and facial expressions of negative or neutral emotions by 6 months of age (e.g., Barrera & Maurer, 1981; LaBarbera, Izard, Vietze, & Parisi, 1976; Serrano, Iglesias, & Loeches, 1995). However, similar results have not been reported in all investigations (e.g., Schwartz, Izard, & Ansul, 1985). Still, infants' visual acuity has improved substantially by 6 months, making it seem highly unlikely that they are incapable of seeing differences between facial configurations that constitute expressions for different emotions (Grossman, 2010).

Because exemplars of any emotional facial expression can differ in their details (e.g., depending on the intensity of facial movements or the expressers' facial morphology), perhaps a more interesting question is, When do infants recognize that these different exemplars are members of the same expression category? To address this question, some researchers have creatively modified the habituation paradigm. For example, in one modified version, infants are habituated to multiple exemplars of an expression (e.g., a smile) produced by different models and/or at different intensities. Category formation for this emotional expression is demonstrated if infants fail to recover their attention in the test trials when a new and different exemplar of the initial expression is shown (e.g., a different smile) but do recover their attention when a new expression is shown (e.g., a frown). Again, findings for such studies have not been consistent. However, overall, they suggest that infants can form a general category for happy expressions (as distinct from various negative expressions) by 7 months of age (Caron, Caron, & MacLean, 1988; Caron, Caron, & Myers, 1982; Walker-Andrews, Krogh-Jespersen, Mayhew, & Coffield, 2011) although—again—this has not been found in all studies (e.g., Lee, Cheal, & Rutherford, 2015; Cong et al., 2019).

Few investigations have examined category formation when the habituation stimuli and the test stimuli are expressions of different negative emotions. However, two studies have reported significant results: Serrano, Iglesias, and Loeches (1992) for 4- to 6-month-olds' categorization of anger, fear, and surprise, and Ruba, Johnson, Harris, and Wilbourn (2017) for 10- and 18-month-olds' categorization of disgust and anger. The latter study is particularly interesting because anger and disgust are considered similar in terms of core affect (i.e., their levels of valence and arousal) and their expressions share some morphological features (i.e., lowered brows). The ability of these older infants to place disgust and anger facial expressions in separate perceptual categories suggests the possibility that they may also recognize other differences between the two negative emotions.

Recognizing Emotions

As indicated earlier, recognizing an emotional expression involves understanding something about the meaning of the expression, in particular, its link with at least one other component of the emotion process (e.g., elicitors, appraisals, feelings, action tendencies). In preverbal infants, such understanding must be manifested in a way that does not clearly allow an alternative explanation of the infant's behavior (e.g., simply liking the way the expression looks rather than understanding something about its emotion meaning).

A number of investigations of infants younger than 9 months have indeed examined their behavioral responses to emotional expressions. For example, Fernald (1993) found that 5-month-old infants smiled more to maternal vocalizations intended to express positive approval and responded more negatively to vocalizations intended to express scolding. However, given the harsher acoustic properties of mothers' scolding messages relative to their approval messages, it is not clear that infants' differential responding reflected anything beyond disliking the harsher sounds. Still, such perceptual preferences might provide an important basis for later learning. With respect to facial expressions, differential facial responses by infants have also been examined in some studies (e.g., Haviland & Lelwica, 1987; Serrano et al., 1995; Soussignan et al., 2018). For example, Serrano et al. (1995) found that 4- to 9-month-old infants smiled more to joy expressions than expressions of anger. However, as with the Fernald (1993) study, the differential behavior produced by the infants in these studies cannot be interpreted as clearly indicating anything beyond a positive (i.e., liking) response to the expressive configurations.

At the present time, the most convincing evidence for some level of expression recognition has been obtained in the context of **social referencing** studies. Social referencing refers to the process wherein a person encounters an emotionally or affectively ambiguous event and seeks information from another person to help determine how she should interpret and respond to the event. For example, an infant may be confronted with a stranger, may be unsure about whether to be afraid, and may look to his mother to find out what to do. Thus social referencing requires the ability to engage in **referential communication** (i.e., communication between two persons about a third object or event).

Development of Social Referencing

Social referencing can be observed in infants by around 9 months of age, the same age at which other forms of referential communication (such as pointing) begin to be seen. To illustrate, Boccia and Campos (1989) found that 8½-month-old infants responded more positively to a stranger if their mothers greeted the stranger in a cheery rather than in a stern manner and also responded more positively to a toy if their mothers vocalized toward the toy in a positive manner. Social referencing in response to facial expressions alone (i.e., without accompanying vocalizations) has been demonstrated in somewhat older infants. For example, as described in Chapter 1, Sorce and colleagues (1985) found that 12-month-old infants would typically cross a visual cliff in response to their mothers' smile but avoid crossing if their mothers showed a fear expression. Of importance, infants' behavioral responses to emotional expressions are referentially specific; that is, when mothers direct their negative expression to only one of two toys, infants will avoid the targeted toy but readily approach the other toy (Hertenstein & Campos, 2004; Mumme & Fernald, 2003).

Taken together, the social referencing studies convincingly demonstrate that by the end of their first year infants have a valence-based understanding that positive expressions signal the expresser's positive evaluation of something in the environment such that an appropriate response is approach, whereas negative expressions signal the opposite. However, whether infants make meaning-based distinctions among different negative emotions or among positive emotions is unclear from their behavior in studies that only measure approach and/or avoidance behavior. To illustrate, in the previously described study by Sorce et al. (1985), the investigators also found quantitative differences in the proportion of infants who crossed the visual cliff in response to different negative emotions. That is, the percentage of infants who crossed was 33%, 11%, and 0% in response to sadness, anger, and fear, respectively. These results might reflect the infants' ability to make qualitative distinctions among different negative emotions (e.g., associate them with different emotion-related appraisals such as loss vs. goal blockage vs. danger). However, a more parsimonious interpretation is that infants were responding to perceived differences in the intensity of negative affect indicated by the different facial expressions (see Martin, Maza, McGrath, & Phelps, 2014, for similar findings with older infants).

Recognizing Differences among Different Negative Emotions

More recently, several investigators have sought clearer evidence indicating when qualitative distinctions among negative emotional expressions can be made. Together, these studies suggest that differential recognition of negative expressions begins to emerge during the second year, but such knowledge is still quite fragile. To illustrate, Reschke, Walle, Flom, and Guenther (2017) presented 12-month-old infants with brief videos showing interpersonal interactions associated with happiness, anger, and sadness (i.e., receiving a toy, fighting over a toy, or breaking a toy, respectively). Subsequent to viewing each interaction, the infant saw either a happy, angry, or sad facial expression. Consistent with the researcher's prediction of a novelty preference, infants' looking time was shortest for the happy expression following the happiness-related (i.e., receiving) scenario and for the sad and angry expressions following the fighting scenario. However, infants did not respond differently to the three expressions when they followed the broken toy scenario. These results suggest that 12-month-old infants associate both sad and anger expressions with some types of negative events (e.g., fighting) but may not differentiate between them.

Using a somewhat similar procedure with older infants, Ruba, Meltzoff, and Repacholi (2019) conducted three related studies in which they presented 14- and 18-month-old babies with brief videos of a presumed anger-eliciting event (i.e., an unmet goal), a disgust-eliciting event (i.e., a new food), or a fear-eliciting event (i.e., a strange toy). Each was followed by another brief video in which the protagonist displayed a facial and vocal expression of either anger, disgust, or fear. As in Ruba et al.'s (2017) study, an important feature of this investigation was the inclusion of negative emotions that are similar in terms of core affect (i.e., valence and arousal) in order to preclude differential looking at the expressive displays based solely on their valence and arousal level. Results showed that infants associated the disgust expression with the new food in two out of two studies and the angry expression with the unmet goal in one of two studies, but they did not match the fear expression to the fear event in any of the studies.

In a subsequent investigation, Ruba, Meltzoff, and Repacholi (2020) presented 10-month-old infants with the same anger and disgust events used in their previous studies and found some minimal indications of emerging knowledge even at this younger age. Infants associated anger expressions with one of two types of anger-related events (i.e., having a toy taken away, but not inability to reach a desired object). However, they did not associate a disgust expression with the presumed disgust elicitor (i.e., a new food). Furthermore, they did not associate a happy expression with the presumed happiness-eliciting event (i.e., being given an attractive toy). Together these studies suggest that differential recognition of negative expressions may begin to emerge toward the end of the first year, but such knowledge is still quite fragile even during the infant's second year of life. However, research that involves a wider variety of emotion elicitors and dependent measures other than relative looking time might further clarify infants' understanding of emotional expressions.

Adopting a more naturalistic approach based on the functionalist perspective, Walle, Reschke, Camras, and Campos (2017) coded the spontaneous behavior of 16-, 19-, and 24-month-old infants who viewed an experimenter opening a box and expressing either happiness, sadness, fear, anger, or disgust (both facially and vocally) in response to contents that could not be seen by the infant. Their complex findings revealed emotion-appropriate differences across emotion conditions for a number of behaviors (e.g., greater avoidance of the experimenter in the anger condition by the 24-month-old infants). Still, some predictions were not confirmed, and other behavioral differences were somewhat difficult to interpret. Furthermore, as acknowledged by the investigators, the spontaneous behavior of infants in a relatively unconstrained situation is determined by multiple factors, and thus failure to find behavioral distinctions among emotions does not necessarily demonstrate infants' failure to comprehend their differences. In summary, the several studies reviewed herein are not conclusive but represent an important direction for future research on infants' differential understanding of distinct emotions.

SUMMARY AND FINAL THOUGHTS

Infants' expressive behavior provides the primary window into their emotional lives. Crying and the facial expressions that accompany it appear to map reliably onto negative affect, while smiling appears to map reliably onto positive affect (at least for post-neonatal infants). However, there appears to be no one-to-one mapping between specific facial expressions and specific negative emotions, at least during the first year and probably beyond. Still, all is not lost with regard to emotion communication between infants and adults. Adults seem able to make reasonable inferences about infants' affective or emotional states by interpreting their facial, vocal, and body activity together with contextual cues (e.g., a wet diaper, a painful inoculation).

Regarding temperament, substantial individual differences in behavioral dispositions can be seen early in infancy. Several influential theoretical models for characterizing these differences have been proposed that highlight emotion-related behaviors. All of these models agree that temperament rests upon a biological basis but is malleable in response to environmental influences. Understanding how, when, and why temperament may evolve over the course of development is an important challenge for future research.

Attachment theory continues to dominate thinking about early emotional relationships between infants and their caregivers. Early attachments can be secure or insecure depending importantly on infants' experience with sensitive caregiving. Secure attachments set the stage for later development of other healthy social and emotional relationships. Still, an insecure attachment does not necessarily consign the infant to later relational difficulties; infants' IWM of attachment can be modified over the course of development in response to more favorable experiences.

Infant–caregiver social interactions provide a context in which early forms of emotion regulation take place. When infants become overstimulated, overly aroused, or distressed, caregivers may alter their behavior so as to enable the infant to become calm. Infants can also make a contribution, for example, by looking away from the source of their overarousal.

Parents from Western and non-Western cultures may differ greatly in how much they value and encourage emotional expressivity in their infants. Cultural differences in attachment have also been found, although their interpretation has been the subject of debate. To better understand these differences, future research that examines relations between infant attachment and later adjustment in non-Western cultures will be important.

Gender labeling may influence caregivers' interpretation of infants' behavior, especially in situations in which multiple interpretations are possible. Parents may also interact differently with their infant sons and daughters, leading to small gender differences in infants' emotion-related behaviors and sensitivity to others' emotional expressions.

Recent decades have seen an increasing emphasis on the neurobiological underpinnings of human behavior, including emotion and emotional development. Models of brain functioning have been proposed that emphasize changes in the reciprocal relationship between amygdala and cortical functioning between infancy and childhood. Regarding the ANS, RSA has emerged as a measure interpreted to indicate emotion regulation. The HPA system is considered a stress-response system, and its relationship to affect- or emotion-related stress has been studied in infants.

Some early scholars interpreted basic emotion theories to imply that emotion recognition is an innate capacity. However, this position has been mostly abandoned in recent years. A clear picture of development during the first year has been elusive in part because consistent distinctions between expression discrimination, categorization, and recognition have not always been made. In addition to the terminological confusion, results across studies have also been inconsistent. Still, there is general agreement that by the end of the first year, infants show convincing evidence of understanding affective valence (i.e., positive vs. negative affect) as demonstrated in social referencing studies. Understanding of discrete basic emotions appears to be developing during the second year; however, infants' ability to recognize associations between facial configurations presumed to express basic emotions and their emotion-appropriate elicitors and associated behaviors is both limited and fragile. Further research in this area will be important.

CHAPTER 3

Childhood

2–9 Years

M ost scholars agree that a wide range of discrete emotions can be identified in children by early childhood. Although some normative trends in emotional development can be identified, individual differences among children are striking. Variability is seen in children's emotional expressivity, emotional experience, emotion regulation, and emotion understanding, as well as the neurobiological concomitants of these processes. Individual differences in emotion depend upon many factors, including children's temperament, attachment relations, socialization experiences, gender, and culture. Each of these is explored in this chapter.

EMOTIONAL EXPRESSION AND EXPERIENCE

As noted in previous chapters, investigating emotional development is complicated by the absence of a gold standard to determine the presence of an emotion and identify which type of emotion is present. As also noted, in infancy, expressive behavior is generally used for this purpose, although there is debate about when infants begin to experience and express discrete basic emotions as opposed to more general affective or pre-emotional states. When considering children, the role that facial expressions play in signaling their emotions continues to be debated.

How Pervasive Are Prototypic Emotional Facial Expressions?

Although infants' facial expressions do not appear to bear a one-to-one relationship with discrete basic emotions, perhaps such a relationship emerges during early childhood. Alas, evidence to support this proposal has been mixed at best (see Camras, 2019; Camras, Fatani, Fraumeni, & Shuster, 2016, for more detailed reviews). Exemplifying this state of affairs, a study by Gaspar and Esteves (2012) examined preschoolers' facial expressions during naturally occurring episodes of enjoyment, surprise, fear, and anger identified by the researchers on the basis of nonfacial contextual cues. On the positive side, smiling was the facial configuration most often produced during presumably enjoyable play interactions. However, the prototypic facial configurations of surprise, fear, and anger rarely were seen. Similarly, in a study of children's conversations with their mothers, Castro, Camras, Halberstadt, and Shuster (2018) found that 7- to 9-year-old children produced smiles most often in self-reported episodes of happiness. However, prototypic expressions for anger, fear, and sadness rarely occurred during self-reported episodes of these emotions.

From the perspective of traditional basic emotion theories, one limitation of both studies is that they took place in social situations during which expression **display rules** (i.e., norms regarding socially appropriate displays of emotion) might have been operating. For example, the children in Castro et al.'s (2018) study may have masked their negative emotions while being videotaped with their mothers. However, the plausibility of this argument is undercut by the fact that naïve observers who viewed the videotapes were able to identify children's self-reported emotions with significant accuracy. This indicated that the children were indeed effectively communicating their emotions but were doing so by nonfacial means (e.g., verbalizations, vocal tone, body movements). Still, it is possible that children were exerting control over their facial displays but failing to manage other communication channels.

Another limitation of both Gaspar and Esteves's (2012) and Castro et al.'s (2018) studies might be that only low levels of emotion intensity were evoked in the situations they observed. Perhaps observable prototypic expressions are produced only in high-intensity emotion situations. To explore this possibility, Wenzler, Levine, van Dick, Oertel-Knöchel, and Aviezer (2016) asked observers to view children's facial expressions taken from YouTube videos in which they experienced highly positive or negative events (i.e., receiving a surprise trip to Disneyland or being told that their parents ate all their Halloween candy). Observers were unable to distinguish between children's facial expressions produced in these two very different situations. In another investigation involving intense emotion, Shuster, Camras, Grabell, and Perlman (2020) coded YouTube videos of 4- to 7-year-old children engaged in a fear-producing Internet prank (i.e., "Scary Maze"; see also Camras, Castro, Halberstadt, & Shuster, 2017). Results showed that full prototypic fear expressions were produced by fewer than half of the children (i.e., 46.7%), although 82% of the children did produce at least one component (i.e., a fear-related brow or mouth movement).

Taken together, these findings indicate that prototypic facial expressions are seen considerably less often than researchers initially predicted based on basic emotions theories. Consequently, they cannot serve on their own as an adequate measure of children's emotions. This is especially true when the researcher's goal is to distinguish among different negative emotions. Nevertheless, these prototypic facial configurations should not simply be dismissed as useless or irrelevant. Indeed, sometimes they do occur in their corresponding emotion situations (e.g., almost 47% of the time for Scary Maze). Furthermore, recognition of these expressions constitutes an important element of many tests of emotion understanding that are significantly associated with other measures of children's social and emotional adjustment (see Chapter 8). Consequently, it would seem fruitful to seek a better understanding of the circumstances under which prototypic emotional facial expressions are produced and the mechanisms that underlie expression production. In the meantime, the use of multimodal emotion scoring systems that incorporate both facial and nonfacial emotion cues would seem prudent, and this approach indeed has been adopted by many developmental researchers.

Is It Good to Be Emotionally Expressive?

Independent of controversies about prototypic facial configurations are questions regarding the quantitative dimension of emotional expression, for example, the consequences of being more or less emotionally expressive. On the one hand, emotion expression provides information to others (and sometimes to oneself) regarding one's situational appraisals, goals, and possible future behaviors. In the context of social interactions, the exchange of such information can allow co-interactants to negotiate a mutually satisfying co-regulation of their exchange. On the other hand, emotional expression can sometimes cause damage. This may occur when it violates social norms, interferes with desired or desirable social relationships, is directed toward a target who is unwilling or unable to engage in mutual co-regulation, or reflects an unwillingness or inability to cooperate on the part of the expresser. To illustrate, if a child shows fear when invited by peers to ride a roller coaster, her social acceptance might be jeopardized. Similarly, if a child fails to smile in response to another's social initiative, she may eventually cease to receive many social invitations. Part of emotional development involves learning how to deploy (and sometime reorganize or regulate) one's emotional expressions so as to more effectively deal with life's challenges.

Studies of children's expressivity in the school environment illustrate its complex relationship to social outcomes. For example, Hernández et al. (2016) measured kindergarten children's positive and negative expressivity at school using a multimodal coding system that included facial expressions, physical movements (e.g., jumping up and down), vocalizations and vocal tone (e.g., whining), and verbal content (e.g., "That made me feel bad"). Findings showed that positive expressivity measured both inside and outside of the classroom (e.g., at recess or lunch) predicted greater peer acceptance. The relationship between positive expressivity and positive social outcomes (e.g., likability ratings, prosocial actions, cooperation) has been found in a number of other studies (e.g., Lindsey, 2017; Sallquist, DiDonato, Hanish, Martin, & Fabes, 2012; see Denham, 2019, for further examples). Negative expressivity both inside and outside the classroom was unrelated to peer acceptance. However, the relationship between negative expressivity and social outcomes may depend on the specific negative emotion being expressed. For example, in a later study, Hernández et al. (2017) found that anger expressivity in kindergarten was related to lower peer acceptance as well as greater teacher–student conflict. However, it would seem unlikely that sadness expressivity would have the same effects. That is, lumping together all forms of negative (or positive) affect may sometimes mask important differences in the functions of specific emotions.

Overall emotional expressivity may decline as children grow older; however, this has not been well studied. In support of his internalization hypothesis (see Chapter 1), Holodynski (2004) found that the intensity of children's expressive reactions to receiving a disappointing present declined between the ages of 6 and 8 years when the present was opened in private rather than in front of the gift giver. From a theoretical perspective, examining such private expressions is necessary to distinguish declines in spontaneous expressivity from declines that may be due to the operation of newly acquired display rules. Still, further investigations that include a range of ages, expressions, and expressive contexts would be necessary before generalizations can be made regarding normative age-related changes in expressivity.

TEMPERAMENT

As noted in Chapter 2, all current theories of temperament include emotion-related components. Within Rothbart's reactivity and regulation model of child temperament, these are: positive reactivity, sadness, fearful distress/fear, and frustration/irritability/anger (Putnam, Gartstein, & Rothbart, 2006; Rothbart & Bates, 2006). Individual differences in the manifestation of these emotions are attributed to both differences in reactivity (i.e., one's tendency to experience the emotion) and differences in children's ability to regulate their reactive tendencies. To illustrate, some children are more frustrated (i.e., reactive) than others when their team loses a ball game. Other children may also be frustrated but better able to control (i.e., regulate) their frustration. As conceptualized within the domain of temperament research, regulation may influence the emotional experience itself and/or the behavioral expression of emotion. These may be difficult to distinguish.

Numerous studies have investigated interactions between children's reactive and regulatory dispositions. For example, as part of a larger project, Kochanska, Murray, and Harlan (2000) examined the relationship between effortful control (EC) and anger reactivity in 33-month-old children. Children who demonstrated greater EC (e.g., ability to control their attention and behavior) also showed less reactive anger during a car seat-restraint episode taken from the Lab-TAB procedure. Eisenberg et al. (2001) found that both emotional reactivity and EC were related to the development of children's problem behaviors as measured using the **Child Behavior Checklist (CBCL**; Achenbach, 1991; see Chapter 8 for further description of this widely used measure). In particular, high anger reactivity and low regulation were associated with **externalizing behaviors** (i.e., rule breaking and aggression), whereas high sadness reactivity and low regulation were associated with **internalizing behaviors** (i.e., withdrawn, depression, anxious depression, and somatic complaints). The influence of temperament on emotion-related behavioral regulation is further considered in the section on emotion regulation later in this chapter.

One innovative line of research on children's temperament is recent work on fear by Kristin Buss. Buss (2011) contends that measures of fearfulness that do not consider its context fail to capture key individual differences among children that may predict later social and emotional adjustment. Instead, she argues for the importance of identifying children who show dysregulated fear, which she defines as high levels of fear in contexts that do not evoke fear in most children. Consistent with this proposal, Buss and her colleagues (e.g., Buss, 2011; Buss, Davis, Ram, & Coccia, 2018) have found that 2-year-old children who responded most fearfully in both low-threat and high-threat situations (e.g., a puppet show or being confronted by a giant toy spider) later showed more anxious behavior and social inhibition in preschool and kindergarten than did children who showed fear only in high-threat situations.

How Can Parenting Influence Temperament?

A number of studies have focused on how parenting may influence children's emotion-related temperamental behavior, particularly behavioral inhibition (BI). As noted in Chapter 2, both overly intrusive and overprotective parenting appear to contribute to the maintenance of BI (Pérez-Edgar, 2019; Rubin, Burgess, & Hastings, 2002). Overprotective parents of inhibited children tend to limit their exposure to potentially distressing contexts or may prematurely intervene when their child shows minimal signs of distress. For example, an overprotective parent might avoid bringing her or his fearful child to the home of a friend who owns an enthusiastically friendly Great Dane. Thus the child has no opportunities to desensitize (i.e., adapt) or learn to cope with such situations. In contrast, overly intrusive parents may force their inhibited child to confront a potentially distressing situation without providing effective emotional support. For example, such a parent might force his or her child to pet the Great Dane without first physically restraining it. In such cases, the inhibited child may be overwhelmed and consequently unable to cope or adapt. Illustrating these points, Rubin et al. (2002) found continuity in children's BI between 2 and 4 years of age if their mothers demonstrated high levels of intrusive control. Continuity was not observed for children with less intrusive mothers. Johnson et al. (2016) found that greater parent overprotection and less child positive emotion together predicted continuity of BI between 3 and 6 years. In contrast, appropriately sensitive and supportive parenting may help behaviorally inhibited children. To illustrate, Eisenberg, Spinrad, Taylor, and Liew (2019) found that mothers' self-reports of their supportive responses to children's negative emotions (e.g., comforting, encouraging problem solving) were positively related (albeit marginally) to lower levels of shyness/inhibition.

As suggested above, effective parenting may serve to teach children how to deal with stressful situations by regulating (i.e., modifying or reorganizing) their temperamentally influenced emotion responses. Nevertheless, early temperament can be a significant predictor of later socioemotional adjustment. For example, in one widely cited longitudinal investigation, Caspi and Silva (1995) found that undercontrolled 3-year-old children (i.e., children who showed more anger/frustration and less attentional control) were more likely to later report less satisfactory social and emotional relationships and more antisocial behavior during adolescence and adulthood.

ATTACHMENT

During infancy, children develop attachment relationships that include an **internal working model (IWM)**, that is, a representation of their experiences that influences expectations regarding future social and emotional relationships. Thus some children may expect an emotionally welcoming world outside the family, whereas others may expect rejection and strife. However, as previously noted, IWMs are modifiable in response to later experiences. For example, a child's initially insecure IWM may become more positive if she encounters a highly nurturant preschool teacher or if his mother develops greater sensitivity (perhaps due to alleviation of her depression or stress). Therefore, researchers who wish to focus on attachment in children have sought to develop new age-appropriate measures.

For preschool and older children, several such measures capitalize on their linguistic and cognitive development. For example, in their **joint storytelling task** (Posada & Waters, 2018), mothers and children are asked to tell a story about a potentially distressful situation (e.g., a child's mother goes away on a trip). Mothers are scored according to how sensitively they encourage their child to think and talk about what emotions would be felt by the story character. In one study that included this measure (Lu, Posada, Trumbell, & Anaya, 2018), mothers' ability to do so was positively associated with their preschool children's **secure base behavior** observed on the playground and in the home (i.e., their willingness to explore the environment while periodically making visual or physical contact with their mothers). Other studies have also indicated that mothers of securely attached children are better at emotion socialization. For example, in a study of fifth and sixth graders in Taiwan, Chen, Lin, and Li (2012) found that mothers who endorsed an emotion-coaching philosophy (i.e., acknowledging children's negative emotions while helping them develop effective coping strategies) were more likely to have children who scored higher in attachment security.

A number of studies have focused more directly on relationships between children's emotional functioning and their attachment status measured concurrently or in infancy (see Kerns & Brumariu, 2016; Parrigon, Kerns, Abtahi, & Koehn, 2015, for narrative reviews). For example, Gilliom,

Shaw, Beck, Schonberg, and Lukon (2002) found that securely attached infant boys (evaluated at 18 months of age) showed less anger and were able to cope more effectively than insecurely attached boys during a frustrating waiting task administered when they were 3½ years old. Abraham and Kerns (2013) found that fourth- to sixth-grade girls who reported greater security in attachment to their mothers also reported experiencing greater positive mood and less negative mood during a 6-day overnight camp experience. They also were reported by their mothers to use more support seeking and problem-focused coping when they became upset. Illustrating the other side of the coin (i.e., attachment insecurity), meta-analytic studies have found that insecure attachments are related to higher levels of emotion-related behavioral problems during childhood (see Fearon, Bakermans-Kranenburg, van IJzendoorn, Lapsley, & Roisman, 2010, for externalizing problems; Madigan, Brumariu, Villani, Atkinson, & Lyons-Ruth, 2016, for both internalizing and externalizing problems).

EMOTION SOCIALIZATION

Outside the domain of attachment research, several models of emotion socialization have been proposed that focus on specifying behaviors through which parents influence their children's emotional development (e.g., Halberstadt, Denham, & Dunsmore, 2001; Gottman, Katz, & Hooven, 1996, 1997). Among these, the model presented by Eisenberg, Cumberland, and Spinrad (1998; Eisenberg, Spinrad, & Cumberland, 1998) has been highly influential, possibly because—if interpreted broadly—it can accommodate a wide range of emotion socialization behaviors. For example, although it was developed to describe the influence of parents on children, the model can easily be extended to apply to other influential figures in the child's social environment, including those who may be encountered via the media (e.g., Scherr, Mares, Bartsch, & Götz, 2018). Furthermore, infants, adolescents, and adults may also be influenced by the processes described within the model. Lastly, if appropriately extended, it can potentially account for cultural as well as individual differences (Raval & Walker, 2019).

Eisenberg's Socialization Model

Eisenberg's model includes four classes of **emotion-related socialization behaviors** (ERSBs): (1) socializers' own expressing of emotion (herein referred to as **demonstrative modeling**), (2) socializers' reactions to the child's emotions (herein referred to as **contingent responding**), (3) socializers' **discussion of emotion** with or in the presence of the child, and (4) socializers' **exposure of the child to emotion-inducing experiences**. In many cases, several types of ERSBs may occur in a single socialization episode. For example, a parent might introduce the child to the aforementioned Great Dane while restraining the dog and smiling. The parent might respond with reassurance if the child shows fear and also explain that the dog is friendly and well trained. These behaviors exemplify *exposure, modeling, contingent responding,* and *discussion,* respectively.

It is also important to emphasize that children's responsiveness to the behavior of a socializer may vary depending upon factors such as the child's temperament, the child's interpretation of the ERSB, the goodness of fit between the socializer's intended outcome and the child's own beliefs, goals, and values, and the child's feelings about or evaluation of the socializer. For example, a temperamentally inhibited child might interpret his parent's effort to have him pet the Great Dane as reflecting naïve optimism about the dog's friendliness and thus steadfastly refuse to approach the animal. Still, as illustrated below, a considerable body of research suggests that the four processes described by Eisenberg and her colleagues have a substantial influence on children's emotional development.

Demonstrative Modeling

With respect to demonstrative modeling, a meta-analytic study conducted by Halberstadt and Eaton (2002) found statistically significant (albeit small to moderate) relationships between parents' and their children's positive and negative expressiveness. Exemplifying this relationship, Valiente and colleagues (2004) found an association between mothers' self-reported negative expressivity and their children's negative facial expressions measured as the children viewed a distressing film. On a larger scale, in a classic study of family interactions, Patterson (1982) showed that parents of aggressive children tended to show more aggressive behavior themselves, thus providing demonstrative models for their offspring.

Supportive and Nonsupportive Contingent Responding

Contingent responding to the child's emotions may take many forms, including approval or disapproval, reward or punishment, ignoring, and/or suggesting an alternative emotional or behavioral response. To investigate contingent responding, Fabes, Poulin, Eisenberg, and Madden-Derdich

(2002) developed the widely used Coping with Children's Negative Emotions Scale (CCNES). The CCNES includes six subscales considered to represent optimal and nonoptimal ways of responding to children's distress or negative emotion. Optimal (or supportive) responses include (1) **expressive encouragement** (i.e., acknowledging and accepting the child's negative emotions), (2) **emotion-focused reactions** (i.e., helping the child feel better), and (3) **problem-focused reactions** (i.e., helping the child solve the problem or cope more effectively with the cause of distress). For example, if a child becomes angry because she is too ill to attend a birthday party, a supportive parent might say "I understand that this upsets you," suggest a future outing with friends, and offer to play a fun game with the child at home. Nonoptimal (or nonsupportive) responses include: (1) **minimization** (i.e., minimizing, devaluing, or dismissing the child's emotion), (2) **punitive reactions** (i.e., punishing or threatening punishment), and (3) **distress reactions** (i.e., parental distress in response to the child's distress). For example, a nonsupportive parent might react in the same scenario by saying "You're acting like a baby," threaten to cancel the child's own birthday party, and/or become almost as upset as the child. Other measures that assess similar sets of behaviors have also been used in socialization research, for example, the Maternal Emotions Style Questionnaire (Lagacé-Séguin & Coplan, 2005), based on Gottman's meta-emotion philosophy framework (Gottman et al., 1996, 1997; Katz, Maliken, & Stettler, 2012).

Presumably, supportive reactions to children's negative emotions should be related to more positive outcomes than nonsupportive reactions. Indeed, this has been found in a number of studies. For example, Fabes et al. (2002) found that mothers' higher scores on the supportive subscales of the CCNES were related to better emotion recognition by their preschool children. Using a similar measure (the Emotions as a Child Scale; Magai, Consedine, Gillespie, O'Neal, & Vilker, 2004), Thompson et al. (2020) found maternal supportive reactions to be associated with fewer child behavior problems as rated by their preschool teachers. Rather than relying on questionnaires, Denham and Grout (1993) observed and coded mothers' contingent responses to their children during a play session and the children's emotional expressivity in their preschool classroom. Mothers who calmly responded to their children's anger had children who showed more positive emotion in preschool. In a meta-analysis of the few studies involving fathers, Rodrigues et al. (2021) found that paternal sensitivity (i.e., supportive responding) was significantly related to better emotion regulation and fewer behavior problems in 3- and 4-year-old children. Regarding nonsupportive reactions, Luebbe, Kiel, and Buss (2011) reported that preschoolers' internalizing symptoms were related to their mothers' minimizing and/or punishing reactions to the child's fear and sadness assessed a year earlier.

At the same time, unexpected results have been reported in a number of cases arguing for a more nuanced view of socializers' contingent responding. For example, Mirabile, Oertwig, and Halberstadt (2018) found that parents' supportive reactions were positively related to 3- and 4-year-old children's social and emotional competence (i.e., better emotion regulation, fewer internalizing or externalizing behaviors) but were negatively related to 5- to 6-year-old children's social emotional competence. Nelson and Boyer (2018) reported that nonsupportive reactions were positively related to externalizing behaviors in 5-year-old children, were unrelated to such behaviors in 6-year-old children, and were negatively related to such behavior problems in 7-year-old children. Castro, Halberstadt, and Garrett-Peters (2018) found that mothers' supportive reactions to their third-grade children were positively related to higher maternal ratings of social competence but were associated with lower ratings by their teachers. As proposed by Castro and Nelson (2018), together these studies suggest that parent reactions designated as supportive on the CCNES may be more appropriate for younger than older children (e.g., reflecting overprotection at older ages).

In addition, not all supportive reactions may be beneficial to the same degree in a particular setting. For example, Nelson et al. (2013) found that African American mothers' expressive encouragement of their kindergarten children was actually related to lower social and academic adjustment as rated by the children's teachers. The authors speculated that expressing distress too openly outside the home may violate cultural norms in these children's communities and thus impede the development of positive relations with teachers and peers. In fact, one can imagine that such open expression of distress when among peers may be problematic for older children from a wide range of ethnic backgrounds (including European American).

Discussion of Emotion

Socializers' reactions to children's emotion often will include some discussion of the emotion being experienced and may accompany both supportive and nonsupportive contingent responding. Emotion-related discussion may take place in various contexts, for example, book reading, observing emotion episodes involving other people, reminiscing about one's own past experiences. Mothers and fathers may both have such emotion discussions with their children, but mothers have been found to be more engaged and elaborative in their discussions and sometimes—but not always—more engaged and elaborative with their daughters than their sons (Zaman & Fivush, 2013).

Emotion-related discussions may include the labeling of emotions, reference to the causes or elicitors of the emotions being discussed, indications about whether emotions are appropriate or inappropriate, and similar references to the appropriateness of particular emotion-related behaviors. Not surprisingly, discussion of emotion has been related to greater emotion understanding. For example, in a naturalistic study of parent–child interactions in the home, Dunn and Brown (1994) found that more family talk about emotion was related to greater emotion understanding in preschool children. Consistent with this result, in a more recent meta-analytic investigation, Tompkins, Benigno, Lee, and Wright (2018) reported that parents' talk about mental states (e.g., thinking, wanting) was also related to greater emotion understanding. In a more detailed analysis of the content of emotion discussions, Knothe and Walle (2018) found that parents (mostly mothers) described storybook images portraying emotion situations differently for different emotions. For example, for fear and disgust episodes, they referred to the object portrayed as eliciting the emotion (e.g., a piece of broccoli), but for anger and sadness episodes, they referred more often to the story character expressing the emotion. The authors suggested that these differences may communicate to children what aspect of each emotion episode merits their greater attention (e.g., the expresser for sadness and anger vs. the expression target for fear and disgust).

Some investigations have found discussion of emotion to be related to measures of socially desirable behaviors. For example, Laible (2004) found that an elaborative style of mother–child reminiscing and story reading (in which emotion episodes are discussed in detail) was positively related to preschoolers' **prosocial behavior** and ability to resist temptation. However, a less rosy picture has emerged in other studies. To illustrate, Garner, Dunsmore, and Southam-Gerrow (2008) found that mothers' explanations of emotion during a story-reading task were positively correlated with both their preschoolers' emotion knowledge and their relational aggression (e.g., taunting, ignoring, or excluding playmates). As acknowledged by the authors, emotion knowledge (like other forms of knowledge) can be harnessed even by preschoolers in the service of either prosocial or antisocial goals.

Exposure to Emotional Experiences

Relatively few studies have focused on exposure to emotion-inducing situations as a socialization strategy. However, in a thought-provoking ethnographic study, Miller and Sperry (1987) described how White working-class mothers used teasing to both incite and socialize their daughters' anger and aggression. Teasing was accompanied by cues (e.g., laughing) that communicated permission for their daughters to respond aggressively and thus gain practice in enacting anger in the context of playful arguments and fighting. Turning to a rather different (and perhaps more comfortable) example of situational exposure, Rothenberg et al. (2017) found that parents who valued gratitude exposed their children to gratitude-inducing situations by choosing activities that provided opportunities for them to learn and express this emotion.

Unintentional socialization via exposure to others' emotions may also influence children's emotional development. Arguably, some studies of family climate illustrate this point. For example, children exposed to high levels of marital conflict have been found to exhibit a number of maladaptive outcomes, including heightened emotional reactivity, stress-related physiological reactivity, and a greater number of emotional and behavioral problems (Cummings, El-Sheikh, Kouros, & Buckhalt, 2009). However, these effects vary depending upon multiple factors, including the child's age and temperament (Leerkes & Bailes, 2019). Such **moderation effects** illustrate the importance of considering child factors when conceptualizing the process of emotion socialization (as noted above and emphasized in Eisenberg's model; Eisenberg, Cumberland, & Spinrad, 1998; Eisenberg, Spinrad, & Cumberland, 1998).

The Influence of Parents' Beliefs, Values, and Goals

Several studies have shown that U.S. parents' beliefs and values regarding emotion are related to their emotion socialization behaviors. For example, Halberstadt, Thompson, Parker, and Dunsmore (2008) found that New York parents who believed more strongly that emotions are important reported that they had discussed the 9/11 terrorist attacks with their children more than did parents with less strong beliefs. In another study, Lozada, Halberstadt, Craig, Dennis, and Dunsmore (2016) found that parents who reported valuing negative emotion (e.g., "It's good for children to feel sad sometimes") were observed to more often verbally validate episodes of their child's negative emotions (e.g., "I felt so bad for you. You were crying so hard"). Other studies that focus on cultural differences in beliefs and values are considered later in the chapter.

When parents' socialization goals conflict with researchers' values, the interpretation of child outcomes becomes complicated. This conundrum was illustrated in Miller and Sperry's (1987) study of White working-class mothers. These mothers described a variety of practices through which they conveyed their view that anger and aggression are desirable because they enable one to survive in the real world. Therefore, their daughters needed to develop a set of aggression-related survival skills—but also an understanding of how and when to deploy them. For example, by means of their contingent responses to their children's aggression, mothers taught them that getting angry and aggressive when provoked by the taunts of peers is justified, but getting angry and aggressive when your parents demand obedience is not. In that way the child was taught about anger-relevant goals (i.e., respect from your peers), impediments to your goals (i.e., being taunted), and appropriate behavioral responses (e.g., aggression).

Moderator Effects

The importance of considering moderator variables was emphasized in a meta-analytic study of relations between parents' socialization and children's conduct problems (e.g., aggression, rule breaking, noncompliance; Johnson, Hawes, Eisenberg, Kohlhoff, & Dudeney, 2017). Although results showed that parents' ERSBs were significantly related to the conduct problems of children and adolescents considered as a group, the effect sizes were small. Interestingly, ERSBs were more closely related to conduct problems in younger rather than older children, perhaps reflecting the shifting influence of parents and peers over the course of development. In addition, ERSBs that involved negative emotions were more strongly related to conduct problems than those focusing on positive emotions. Somewhat surprisingly, neither parent nor child gender were significant moderators in this study.

EMOTION REGULATION

What Is Emotion Regulation?

The distinction between emotion and emotion regulation is rooted in a historical separation of emotion and cognition dating at least as far back as Descartes (Damasio, 1994). Within this perspective, emotion regulation is said to occur when cognitive processes exert control over emotion processes, allowing persons to act in a rational manner. More recently, however, this view has been challenged in light of research that shows the inextricable intertwining of emotion and cognition in both emotion functioning and the brain networks that underlie such functioning (see Gross & Barrett,

2011, for discussion). For example, as previously noted, virtually all contemporary emotion theories acknowledge the importance of cognitive appraisals in the generation of an emotional response. Therefore, some scholars (e.g., Campos, Frankel, & Camras, 2004; Campos, Walle, Dahl, & Main, 2011) have advocated reconceptualizing emotion regulation as a functional form of emotion reorganization that occurs in response to appraisals that may accompany or follow one's initial emotional response (e.g., replacing anger with sympathy when you learn that your friend arrived late because her child had become ill). Still, developmentalists are reluctant to abandon the term *regulation* in part because it has been so widely used in the past literature (including studies in which no evidence for regulation is provided). Adopting a compromise position, herein the term **emotion regulation** is retained but applied primarily to those forms of emotion reorganization that involve deliberate and effortful strategies.

Largely consistent with this compromise position, Thompson (1994, 2014) has defined emotion regulation as "extrinsic and intrinsic processes responsible for monitoring, evaluating, and modifying emotional reactions, especially their intensive and temporal features, to accomplish ones' goals" (Thompson, 1994, pp. 27–28). Extrinsic processes can include behavior by others (e.g., a mother's comforting of her crying baby). Intrinsic processes can include reappraising a situation in a way that leads to a change in emotion (e.g., realizing that your anger is based on a misunderstanding) or leads to a change in your emotion-related actions (e.g., realizing that your shouting is frightening your child). It can also be anticipatory (e.g., avoiding a situation that you know will make you angry). In such cases, regulation may not be observable, making it difficult to measure in children who cannot reliably report their internal processes. In addition, without further assumptions or sources of information, it may not be clear whether a child's emotion-related behavior actually involves any regulation at all. Despite these difficulties, researchers have bravely proceeded to build a picture of children's emotion regulation based on research that often includes reasonable (albeit unproven) assumptions about the processes underlying their observed behavior. Interested readers may wish to consult Cole, Martin, and Dennis (2004) and Campos et al. (2004) for more detailed discussions of both conceptual and methodological issues involved in the study of emotion regulation.

Emotion Regulation Behaviors

As noted in Chapter 2, emotion regulation in infancy is conceptualized as a mutual modification process involving behaviors of both caregivers (who may soothe infants' distress or provoke their excitement) and infants (who may engage in gaze aversion or self-soothing behaviors such as thumb sucking). By early childhood, developments in the areas of cognition, language, and motoric functioning enable children to use a greater variety of self-produced regulatory behaviors. For example, children will become better at "using their words" rather than their fists when they are thwarted by another child. As development further proceeds, children also begin to utilize unobservable cognitive strategies to a greater degree (Levine, Kaplan, & Davis, 2013). For example, older children may mitigate their distress when anticipating an unpleasant medical procedure by thinking about the candy reward that will follow rather than the procedure itself. Therefore, researchers have employed a variety of age-appropriate methods for studying children's emotion regulation.

How Is Emotion Regulation Studied?

Behavioral Observation

Illustrating this method, Grolnick, Bridges, and Connell (1996) observed 2-year-olds as they participated in several procedures designed to elicit mild to moderate frustration or distress, for example, **delay of gratification tasks** that involved waiting for 6 minutes to open a present or to eat a cookie. During the waiting periods, children engaged in a number of behaviors, including (1) active distraction (e.g., playing with an available toy), (2) passive distraction (e.g., looking around the room), (3) symbolic self-soothing (e.g., "I'm a big girl"), (4) physical self-soothing (e.g., thumb sucking), (5) comfort seeking (e.g., climbing onto their mothers' laps), and (6) focusing on the source of frustration (e.g., staring at the forbidden object). Active distraction was the most common behavior and was associated with the least amount of observable distress, whereas focusing on the source of frustration was the next most common behavior but (not surprisingly) was associated with the highest level of distress. In a study that also included older children (1½- to 4½-year-olds), Cole et al. (2011) examined responses in an 8-minute delay of gratification task (i.e., waiting to open a present). Older children shifted their attention from the desired object and engaged in distraction sooner than did younger children and showed less frustration overall. Both older and younger children made bids for help to their mothers (who were instructed to do what they normally would do when the child needed to wait), but older children's bids were accompanied by less frustration than were younger children's bids. Together these two studies suggest that children's ability to select and enact effective strategies for emotion (and behavioral) regulation increase during early childhood and that distraction can be a particularly effective strategy in some situations.

Rating Studies

Other studies have employed parent or teacher ratings of children's emotion regulation based on their experience with the child. For example, the Emotion Regulation Checklist (ERC; Shields & Cicchetti, 1995) includes 24 items assessing emotion modulation (e.g., wild mood swings, recovery from distress), situational appropriateness (e.g., responding positively to friendly overtures), and organization (e.g., expressing feelings verbally). This measure is particularly noteworthy in that it illustrates the conceptual difficulties surrounding emotion regulation. In particular, some items (e.g., responding to friendly overtures) might not necessarily involve monitoring, evaluating, or modifying one's emotions and might instead be considered to measure emotional reactivity. Still, using this scale, Blair et al. (2015) found that mothers' ratings of their children's emotion regulation at 5 and 7 years predicted teacher's ratings of their social skills at 10 years, as well as peer measures of their social acceptance and the children's own ratings of their friendship quality.

Self-Report Studies

Because children increasingly utilize unobservable cognitive strategies for emotion regulation, studies of school-age children often involve their verbal reports. For example, Waters and Thompson (2014) presented 6- and 9-year-old children with stories about situations that elicited anger or sadness in the protagonists (e.g., a sold-out movie, a broken bicycle). For each story, the researcher obtained children's effectiveness ratings for eight potential responses: problem solving (e.g., repairing the bicycle), seeking adult support, seeking peer support, **cognitive reappraisal** (e.g., deciding the bike was old anyway), venting (i.e., expressing their emotion very strongly), aggression, distraction, and doing nothing. Problem-solving strategies were rated as most effective at both ages, followed by the support-seeking strategies for the 6-year-olds and either support-seeking or cognitive reappraisal by the 9-year-olds. Aggression and doing nothing were rated least effective at both ages, although they were rated higher by 6-year-olds than 9-year-olds. Girls rated peer support seeking and venting more highly than did boys. However, as noted by the authors, children's evaluations of regulation strategies do not always translate into behavioral usage.

Developmental Trends

A considerable amount of the research on emotion regulation in children is embedded in the literature on coping with stress. According to Lazarus's seminal model (Lazarus, 1966; Lazarus & Folkman, 1984), coping involves both problem-focused strategies (i.e., those acting on the source of the stress) and emotion-focused strategies (i.e., those acting on one's distressing emotions). Although both types of responses are typically included in studies of children's coping, they often are not clearly distinguished, particularly because the same behavior may often serve both ends (i.e., dealing with the stressor itself and dealing with the emotion it engenders). Still, reviews of the coping literature (Compas et al., 2017; Zimmer-Gembeck & Skinner, 2011) have identified some consistent developmental trends for strategies considered to be emotion-focused. For example, both Compas et al. (2017) and Zimmer-Gembeck and Skinner (2011) reported that seeking support from adults declines from preschool to middle childhood, whereas self-reliance and seeking support from peers increases. In addition, as earlier noted, reliance on cognitive strategies (e.g., evaluating the situation differently or thinking about something else) increases. Furthermore, children become better at identifying those strategies most appropriate for the particular stress-inducing situation. To illustrate, in an interview study with 6-, 9-, and 12-year-old children, Band and Weisz (1988) found that reliance on emotion-focused strategies (e.g., seeking support, thinking about something else) increased with age in response to an unavoidable medical procedure, whereas problem solving increased in response to school failure and conflict with authority.

Expressive Regulation

One interesting form of emotion-related regulation involves the modification of expressive behavior rather than the modification of emotion feelings. Expressive modification has been studied most often using a **disappointing present procedure** in which children are promised a reward and then given a broken toy, an age-inappropriate baby toy, or even just a piece of wood! (Of course, the undesirable reward is exchanged for a desirable gift later in the experiment.) The disappointing present procedure has been used with children ranging from 3 to 11 years of age. In the original study, Saarni (1984) compared 7-, 9-, and 11-year-old children's facial, vocal, and verbal responses to a disappointing present with their responses to a subsequently presented desirable gift. She found that the younger children of both genders responded more negatively to the disappointing present than to the desirable present (e.g., by frowning and saying "This is for babies!"). Younger children responded more negatively than older children, and boys responded more negatively than girls. Additionally, the older girls showed more positive expressions (e.g., smiling) when given the undesirable reward than did older boys, presumably out of politeness. Thus the older children, particularly the girls, appeared to be suppressing and masking their disappointment more than the younger children.

In a subsequent study with 3- to 9-year-olds, Cole (1986) again found that children of both genders increased their negative expressions when disappointed and that girls showed more positive expressions than boys. Somewhat surprisingly, no age differences were observed. Cole (1986) also included a follow-up study with preschool girls in which she introduced a control condition designed to clarify the interpretation of responses to the disappointing versus the desirable gift. In this new condition, the girls opened the disappointing present in private rather than in front of the experimenter. Analysis of covertly recorded videotapes indicated that the girls showed more negative expressions in the private than in the public condition, thus confirming that children are indeed disappointed by the undesirable reward but are modifying their expressive responses when in the presence of an experimenter. Subsequent to these initial studies, several other investigations have found positive associations between measures of children's inhibitory control (a component of EC) and their responses in the disappointing present paradigm (Carlson & Wang, 2007; Hudson & Jacques, 2014; Kieras, Tobin, Graziano, & Rothbart, 2005; Liew, Eisenberg, & Reiser, 2004; Simonds, Kieras, Rueda, & Rothbart, 2007). Age and gender effects corresponding to those found by Saarni (1984) and Cole (1986) are often, but not always, found.

Temperament, Social, and Cognitive Influences on Emotion Regulation

Some children find it easier to regulate (or reorganize) their emotional responses than do others. Two temperamental factors conceptualized within Rothbart's reactivity and regulation model— negative reactivity and EC—might be expected to have a significant influence on children's abilities to regulate their emotion. In particular, high levels of negative emotional reactivity would be expected to create regulation challenges, whereas high levels of EC should facilitate emotion regulation (Eisenberg et al., 1996). Consistent with this proposal, Moran, Lengua, and Zalewski (2013) found that 3-year-old children who were high in negative emotionality showed more externalizing behaviors if they were also low (rather than high) on EC.

Many discussions of emotion regulation focus on the development and influence of EC, perhaps because of its intrinsic regulatory function (e.g., Eisenberg, Hofer, Sulik, & Spinrad, 2014). As previously described, Rothbart and her colleagues conceptualize EC as a component of temperament defined as "the efficiency of executive attention, including the ability to inhibit a dominant response and/or to activate a subdominant response, to plan, and to detect errors" (Rothbart & Bates, 2006, p. 129). The components of EC (e.g., inhibitory control, attentional focusing) emerge during infancy and toddlerhood and further develop throughout childhood (see Eisenberg, Smith, & Spinrad, 2014; Eisenberg, Spinrad, & Eggum, 2010, for reviews). As opposed to involuntary reactivity (e.g., as seen in BI), EC is volitional or at least originates as volitional behavior that may become habitual over time. As applied to emotion, EC supports the child's ability to engage in many emotion regulation behaviors that are necessary for social competence. Accordingly, higher EC has been associated with greater social competence in many studies (see Eisenberg, Hofer, et al., 2014; Eisenberg, Smith, & Spinrad, 2014, for reviews).

The development of emotion regulation is also importantly influenced by social factors including both attachment and parenting. In a meta-analytic study, Cooke et al. (2019) found that secure attachment was associated with better emotion regulation, whereas both avoidant and resistant/ambivalent attachment were related to lower levels of emotion regulation. Although the mechanisms underlying these relationships have not been explicitly demonstrated, mothers of securely attached infants might be expected to use socialization behaviors that would encourage the development of emotion regulation. Indeed, several studies have found that parent socialization is related to children's emotion regulation. For example, Ramsden and Hubbard (2002) found that mothers' acknowledgment of their fourth-grade children's negative emotions (considered a form of supportive response, as described above) was related to higher teacher ratings of their children's emotion regulation.

Cognitive and language development also can support emotion regulation. For example, in a longitudinal study of children from 18 months to 4 years of age, Roben, Cole, and Armstrong (2013) found that better language skills were associated with use of active distraction as a regulation strategy and that children who developed better language skills appeared less frustrated in a delay of gratification task at 4 years. In a study of first-grade children, Ilan, Tamuz, and Sheppes (2019) found that those with low working memory capacity tended to choose distraction over reappraisal as their preferred method for resisting temptation. Still, this less cognitively demanding strategy was associated with fewer behavior problems for these children.

CULTURE AND EMOTION

Emotional Expressivity

Examining children's emotional development across cultures may provide information regarding the influences of socialization and social norms. As noted in Chapter 2, cultures differ in the value placed on emotional expressivity, with expressive restraint being historically valued in many Asian cultures, including China. Consistent with this value, Camras, Chen, Bakeman, Norris, and Cain (2006) found that 3-year-old mainland Chinese girls were significantly less facially expressive than European American girls while watching a set of emotionally evocative slides (e.g., a cute kitten, a giant cockroach) and talking about them with a culturally matched experimenter. Expressivity scores of adopted Chinese girls (raised in European American families for at least 1 year) and Chinese American girls (raised in the United States by Chinese American parents) fell in between the other two groups. Mothers' self-reported affiliation with Chinese cultural values was negatively associated with children's expressivity scores, suggesting an influence of mothers' socialization on children's emotional expression. Similar findings were obtained in Chen and Zhou's (2019) more recent study of Chinese American parents' expressivity and cultural values. Of importance, such cultural differences in expressivity may have consequences for children of immigrant families. Illustrating this possibility, Louie, Wang, Fung, and Lau (2015) found that anger displays by Asian American preschoolers were associated with lower ratings by their teachers on peer acceptance and prosocial behavior; this association was not found for European American children. Possibly the anger displays of Asian American children were deemed more significant by their teachers because they stood out against a background of lower overall expressivity.

Temperament and Parenting

Other research illustrates cultural influences on how parenting and temperament may interact in the development of children's problem behaviors. Providing an example, Tsotsi and colleagues (2019) found that Singaporean mothers' self-reported parenting stress was related to parents' reports of their children's internalizing problems (e.g., symptoms of anxiety and/or depression). This relationship was stronger for children who had shown higher levels of temperamental exuberance (assessed during a bubble-popping procedure taken from the preschool Lab-TAB; Goldsmith, Reilly, Lemery, Longley, & Prescott, 1999). In contrast, studies of Western children (e.g., Nigg, 2006) have found that high exuberance is more typically associated with externalizing problems (e.g., aggression and/or rule breaking). In interpreting their results, Tsotsi et al. (2019) suggested that Singaporean parents may respond more harshly than Western parents to their children's exuberant behavior because they value emotional restraint more highly. In addition, their harsh responding may involve more culturally characteristic punitive responses, such as making unfavorable comparisons between their child and other children (Camras, Sun, Fraumeni, & Li, 2017; Camras, Sun, Li, & Wright, 2012; Fung, 1999). Excessive use of different punitive practices may lead to a different set of adjustment problems for Singaporean and Western children (i.e., internalizing rather than externalizing problems).

Do Western Measures of Emotion Socialization Generalize across Cultures?

Focusing on Eisenberg's model of emotion socialization (Eisenberg, Cumberland, & Spinrad, 1998; Eisenberg, Spinrad, & Cumberland, 1998), Raval and Walker (2019) added several factors designed to more explicitly capture cultural differences. For example, their extended model includes child factors related to children's goals, values, and appraisals that may be derived from exposure to worldviews other than those of their parents (e.g., Asian Indian children's greater valuing of autonomy following exposure to global social media). In addition, the authors noted some important adaptations that have been made (or should be made) when using methodologies developed by Western researchers to study emotion socialization in other cultures (e.g., incorporating culturally relevant vignettes and response options into the CCNES).

In their narrative review of the literature, Raval and Walker (2019) highlighted both similarities and differences across cultures. For example, with respect to parental expressivity, European American mothers report themselves as showing more positive emotional expressivity than mothers from India, as well as from China. Regarding parents' contingent responding, studies generally have shown that nonsupportive reactions are related to maladaptive outcomes across a wide range of cultures, although a few exceptions have been found. In contrast, relations between supportive reactions and adjustment outcomes in studies of non-Western cultures have been mixed. With respect to discussion of emotion, the majority of studies have focused on Chinese or Chinese American mothers, who have been found to be less elaborative in their emotion language than European American mothers and to focus more on social norms and behaviors rather than mental states (e.g., feelings).

In an interesting program of research, Raval and his colleagues (e.g., McCord & Raval, 2016) have studied families in India, as well as Asian Indian families that have immigrated to the United States. Based on qualitative interviews, the researchers modified the CCNES to include contingent responses found to be commonly described by Asian Indian parents that are not represented in the original version of the measure (e.g., providing an explanation to help the child understand the emotion episode). Using the modified instrument, McCord and Raval (2016) found that Asian Indian immigrant parents of 8- to 16-year-old children reported using nonsupportive responses more often than European American parents. However, in contrast to the findings for European American families, there was no relationship between Asian Indian parents' use of nonsupportive responses and their children's behavioral adjustment. This finding suggests that European American and Asian Indian children may have different interpretations of the behaviors categorized as nonsupportive on the CCNES. The importance of children's interpretations of their parents' behaviors has also been found in studies of mainland Chinese and European American children (Camras, Sun, et al., 2017; Camras et al., 2012).

Parents' Intentions, Beliefs, Goals, and Behaviors

Research by Cole and Tamang (1998) provides an example of cultural differences in emotion socialization that may exist within the boundaries of a single nation. In their study, mothers from two ethnic groups within Nepal (i.e., Brahmin and Tamang) reported responding very differently to children's anger directed toward themselves. Tamang mothers said they would try to modify the child's emotion (i.e., make the child happy) by cajoling the child or acceding to the child's demand. In contrast, Brahmin mothers appeared to accept the child's anger but emphasized that they would instruct the child about how to control it. The researchers speculated that Brahmins' higher social status within Nepal was a factor underlying their greater acceptance of anger as an appropriate emotion to experience, albeit an emotion that must also be kept under control. At the same time, Cole, Tamang, and Shrestha (2006) subsequently observed that Brahmin adults often relented in the face of children's demands in real life (e.g., demands for extra portions at the dinner table). As anyone who has ever broken a New Year's resolution knows, intentions and goals do not always translate to actual behaviors. In any particular situation, socialization goals may sometimes conflict with other goals (e.g., keeping the peace at dinner) and be subordinated to those other goals. Still, studies of parents' emotion-related beliefs, goals, and values can provide important information regarding the motivations underlying differences in socialization behaviors observed both between and within cultures.

Further extending the study of parental beliefs and values across cultures, Halberstadt and her colleagues (Parker et al., 2012) interviewed mothers from three different ethnic groups within the United States: European American, African American and Lumbee Native Americans. Both similarities and differences among the groups were found. For example, mothers from all groups believed that emotional connections with children were important. At the same time, only European American mothers thought it was appropriate for children to process their emotions in private before sharing them with parents.

When considering cultural differences in beliefs, values, and behaviors regarding emotion, scholars have often focused on the dimension of **individualism/collectivism** or the related dimension of **independence/interdependence** (to be described further in Chapter 5). However, Halberstadt and Lozada (2011) identified a number of other factors that may be particularly relevant to children's emotion socialization. These include cultural differences in the value placed on children, beliefs about the importance of respect for authority or emotional closeness, and beliefs about when, how, and from whom children learn (e.g., in early or later childhood, by observation or from explicit instruction, from adults and/or other children). These considerations merit more systematic examination in future studies.

GENDER AND EMOTION

What Differences Have Been Found for Children?

Gender differences in emotion-related temperament variables are similar in infancy (as described in Chapter 2) and childhood (as described here; see Else-Quest et al., 2006). At both ages, girls are rated slightly higher in fearfulness, whereas boys are rated slightly higher in difficulty and emotional intensity. Boys in both infancy and childhood are rated higher in high-intensity pleasure, whereas girls are rated higher in less intense positive approach. Of note, these temperament variables are typically assessed via ratings by parents or teachers.

In contrast to these findings of age-related consistency, Chaplin and Aldao (2013) reported that new gender differences emerged during early childhood based on their meta-analysis of studies involving objectively coded emotional behaviors. Although infant boys and girls had not differed in how often they were scored as showing anger, disgust, and contempt, preschool boys now showed more of these "externalizing" emotions than did girls. In both infancy and early childhood, girls were found to display more "internalizing" emotions (i.e., sadness, fear, and anxiety) than boys. Findings for older children (6–12 years) showed that the gender differences seen in early childhood were maintained. In addition, girls were found to show more positive emotion and less negative emotion overall than did boys. Thus further differences in expressivity consistent with gender stereotypes appeared to emerge during childhood—although the effect sizes for these differences would be considered small or even trivial.

Where Do Gender Differences Come From?

Research on parents' emotion socialization has pinpointed some behaviors directed to boys versus girls that would seem to encourage gender differences. For example, Fivush and her colleagues have found that parents of preschoolers engage in more elaborate emotion conversations with their daughters than with their sons (Adams, Kuebli, Boyle, & Fivush, 1995; Fivush, 1991). With respect to specific emotions, parents talk about sadness more with daughters but talk about anger more with sons (e.g., Fivush, 1991). In a study in which parents read their 2- and 4-year-old children a picture book in which gender-ambiguous characters showed different emotions (van der Pol et al., 2015), mothers talked about emotions more than fathers. However, both mothers and fathers tended to refer to angry characters as boys (e.g., using the pronoun *he*) and sad or happy characters as girls (e.g., using the pronoun *she*). Fathers may encourage adherence to some gender stereotypes more than mothers. For example, Cassano, Perry-Parrish, and Zeman (2007) found that fathers reported themselves to be more dismissive than mothers of sadness in boys. Beyond the meta-analyses described earlier, other research suggests that children are responsive to the gender stereotyping to which they have been exposed. For example, as noted previously in this chapter, girls have been found to mask their disappointment with smiles more than boys in some (although not all) studies.

Is There a Female Advantage in Emotion Understanding?

As noted in Chapter 2, McClure's (2000) meta-analysis of gender differences in emotional expression processing included studies of emotion recognition and labeling by children and adolescents. Studies of these older age groups were considered together and (as for infants) a small but significant difference was obtained in favor of girls. Moderator analyses indicated that this difference held across studies using different tests of emotion recognition. In interpreting her data, McClure (2000) attributed this **female advantage** to social norms consistent with research on gender differences in emotion socialization, as described above.

NEUROBIOLOGICAL UNDERPINNINGS

Because children's nervous systems cannot be directly manipulated, it sometimes is difficult for researchers to infer causality when associations between behavioral and neurobiological processes are found. Still, uncovering these associations in typical children will eventually enable researchers to compare their neurobiological functioning to that of children with various types of emotional and behavioral problems and thus better understand the nature of those problems (see also Chapter 8).

Brain Functioning

Emotion-related brain development during childhood is most notably characterized by rapid synaptic development in the prefrontal cortex (PFC) during early childhood (around 2–4-years) followed by synaptic pruning during the years up to adolescence (Huttenlocher, 1994; Webb, Monk, & Nelson, 2001). Simultaneously, amygdala volume increases throughout childhood, albeit at a slower rate than during infancy. Amygdala responsiveness to emotion stimuli is greater in childhood and adolescence than in adulthood (Morales & Fox, 2019). At the same time, the amygdala and PFC interact with each other during emotion responding, with the PFC exerting increasing influence on the amygdala as childhood proceeds.

Brain Functioning during Emotion Processing

Different brain areas within the PFC are thought to be involved in different forms of emotion processing, as distinguished by a number of prominent researchers (e.g., Braunstein, Gross, & Ochner, 2017; Moreira & Silvers, 2018). These different forms of processing may involve either implicit/nonconscious or explicit/conscious goals and either automatic/involuntary or controlled/voluntary cognitive control. Although most studies relevant to these distinctions have been conducted with adults, a few have involved children and may shed light on the neurobiological underpinnings of their emotional development.

For example, Gee et al. (2013) investigated implicit controlled emotion processing by obtaining functional magnetic resonance imaging (fMRI) scans of participants ranging from 4 to 22 years of age while they viewed happy, fearful, and neutral facial expressions and pressed a button when they saw a neutral face. Results showed age-related changes in coactivation of the amygdala and PFC: Activation of both the amygdala and the medial PFC were positively associated in children younger than 10 years of age but became negatively associated in older participants. Because the PFC continues to develop structurally throughout childhood, its dampening influence on the amygdala may emerge only as childhood proceeds (Morales & Fox, 2019). Of note, this pattern of developmental change in the relation of the amygdala and PFC is consistent with Tottenham and Gabard-Durnam's (2017) model presented in Chapter 2.

An example of explicit controlled processing is **cognitive reappraisal**, a regulation strategy that involves changing one's thinking about an emotional event. Reappraisal is considered to be developmentally mature and has been widely studied in adults (see Chapter 5). In fMRI studies with children, reappraisal is often assessed by comparing their neural reactions while viewing unpleasant pictures to their neural reactions while being guided to appraise the pictures in a more positive (or at least a less negative) manner. For example, they may be shown a picture of a wounded person but then told that the wound is a fake. Meta-analyses of adult fMRI studies (e.g., Buhle et al., 2014) have pointed to several brain areas that are consistently activated during cognitive reappraisal (i.e., the posterior dorsal medial PFC, bilateral dorsal lateral PFC, ventral lateral PFC, posterior parietal cortex, and left posterior temporal cortex), while amygdala responses are reduced. Meta-analyses are particularly important for evaluating fMRI studies, as their reliability and replicability may be questionable in some cases (Elliott et al., 2020; Kragel, Han, Kraynak, Gianaros, & Wager, 2021; Elliott, Knodt, Caspi, Moffitt, & Hariri, 2021). Although relatively few investigations have been conducted with children, Moreira and Silvers (2018) identified some tentative developmental trends that include decreasing amygdala and lateral PFC reactivity but increasing dorsal medial PFC activity.

Turning to studies of reappraisal utilizing electroencephalography (EEG), DeCicco, O'Toole, and Dennis (2014) measured the late positive potential (LPP; an EEG measure thought to be related to heightened attention) in 5- to 7-year-old children while they viewed emotionally unpleasant images and simultaneously listened to either a negative or a reappraisal statement (e.g., "This snake is dangerous" vs. "This snake is harmless"). A reduced LPP response during the reappraisal condition was interpreted as indicating a lesser focus on the unpleasant image and more successful reappraisal. Older children were found to reduce their LPP more than younger children, suggesting that the 7-year-olds were more responsive to the regulatory priming statements than were the 5-year-old children. Relating these findings to real-world functioning, Babkirk, Rios, and Dennis (2015) showed that children with lower LPP used more adaptive strategies in both a disappointing present task and a delay of gratification task administered both concurrently and 2 years later. Together, these studies suggest that control of attention is an important contributor to children's ability to regulate (or reorganize) their emotion processing in a more adaptive manner.

Brain Functioning and Facial Behavior

Few studies of brain functioning have attempted to incorporate measures of children's facial behavior into their procedures. However, Grabell et al. (2018) recorded both facial expressions and cortical functioning in 3- to 7-year-old children as they engaged in a computer game that included both positive (win) and negative (lose) trials. Cortical functioning was assessed using functional near-infrared spectroscopy (fNIRS), a relatively new technology that measures neural activity in cortical areas of the brain. Like fMRI, fNIRS measures changes in blood flow in different areas of the cerebral cortex (albeit without the same degree of spatial resolution as fMRI). Like EEG, fNIRS is child-friendly in that measures are obtained via sensors on a flexible headcap, and lying still in a scanner is not required. In Grabell et al.'s (2018) study, children's facial behavior during the win and lose trials was comprehensively coded using Ekman et al.'s (2002) anatomically based Facial Action Coding System (FACS). Investigators identified facial actions considered to be components of negative facial expressions and recorded whether or not they co-occurred with contraction of *orbicularis oculi* (i.e., the eye muscle movement hypothesized to be an expressive intensifier, as described in Chapter 2; Messinger et al., 2012). Children who produced intense negative expressions (i.e., expressions that included both a negative facial movement—typically a brow contraction—and the intensifier eye movement) were rated lower by their parents in their emotion regulation (i.e., ability to recover from intense distress, excitement, or arousal). Additionally, the researchers found that these intense negative expressions were associated with lower activation of the lateral prefrontal cortex (lPFC) during loss episodes of the computer game. In light of previous research showing that higher lPFC activation is related to lower levels of frustration (Perlman, Luna, Hein, & Huppert, 2014), Grabell and colleagues (2018) interpreted their results as suggesting that they had identified a type of facial expression (i.e., negative movement accompanied by an intensifier) that might potentially serve as an observable indicator of emotion regulation difficulties when produced in the context of a frustration episode.

Autonomic Nervous System (ANS)

Substantial changes in ANS activity occur during childhood (Hastings & Kahle, 2019; Dollar et al., 2020). Much of the research on ANS functioning involves respiratory sinus arrythmia (RSA), a measure generally indicating greater parasympathetic control (see Chapter 2). Resting RSA increases across childhood, keeping the heart rate low but variable. In contrast, RSA reactivity in response to emotion stimuli decreases across early childhood before increasing again through middle childhood until children reach adolescence (Dollar et al., 2020). In this case, RSA reactivity involves releasing the "vagal brake" and thus allowing increased activation of the sympathetic nervous system (SNS) to support active coping with the stimulus. In terms of individual differences, rank ordering of children's resting RSA scores tends to be moderately stable across childhood, whereas rank ordering of reactive RSA scores tends to be more variable.

Relations between ANS activity and measures of emotion regulation have been studied and (perhaps not surprisingly) have been found to be complex (Hastings & Kahle, 2019). Measures such as RSA relate to activity of the SNS and the PNS (parasympathetic nervous system), but activation of these systems may enhance or impair appropriate emotion functioning depending upon both the emotion and the requirements of the particular situation. For example, when appropriate regulation requires an active response, then RSA suppression might be desirable, but when restraint would be preferred, then the opposite would be true. Therefore, the findings in emotion regulation studies must be interpreted with this in mind.

Illustrating this complex relationship are studies of children's responses to induction of sadness. For example, Miller, Nuselovici, and Hastings (2016) presented 4- to 6-year-old children with brief videos portraying episodes of sadness (e.g., a child's grandfather is very ill) and analyzed dynamical changes in RSA across each episode. Results showed a U-shaped pattern of decreasing RSA followed by increasing RSA across each episode. The authors interpreted this pattern as reflecting an initial orientation to the sadness induction (reflected in the RSA decrease) followed by recovery (i.e., increased RSA and restoration of PNS control), because no active coping was required in the experimental setting. Greater conformity to this situationally adaptive pattern of physiological responding was positively related to the children's self-reported empathic response to the induction (i.e., their own feelings of sadness) and also to their prosocial behavior measured in the laboratory (e.g., comforting an adult who feigned injury). Applying this approach to a different emotion, Miller et al. (2013) found a similar U-shaped pattern of dynamic RSA response during a laboratory procedure that induced anger rather than sadness. In this case, greater conformity to the pattern was negatively related to the children's self-reported tendency to respond aggressively to provocations. Highlighting the importance of considering situational appropriateness, the U-shaped pattern of responding to the laboratory induction was related to rather different forms of adaptive responses in the case of sadness versus anger (i.e., active prosocial helping for sadness vs. behavioral restraint for anger). This observation supports the investigators' proposal that the dynamic RSA patterning found in the laboratory exemplified situationally appropriate flexibility.

Hypothalamic–Pituitary–Adrenal (HPA) System

Childhood is generally considered to be a period of HPA hyporesponsivity. As noted in Chapter 2, responsiveness to physical stressors decreases substantially after the first year. For example, medical procedures that evoke cortisol increases in infants (e.g., inoculation, heel pricks) do not appear to do so for children. HPA reactivity to negative emotion elicitors also is difficult to elicit throughout childhood up to early adolescence (Adam, 2012). For example, a number of studies in which fear/wariness or anger/frustration are presumed to be evoked in preschool and school-age children have found no average increases in cortisol responding (see Gunnar, Talge, & Herrera, 2009, for a general review). However, as noted by Gunnar and colleagues, many of these studies involve rather low-intensity elicitors that may not be strong enough to evoke HPA reactivity.

Another possibility is that fear/wariness and anger/frustration are the wrong negative emotions to study. According to Dickerson and Kemeny (2004), the HPA system responds most strongly to negative social evaluations or self-evaluations that are accompanied by shame and embarrassment. Consistent with this interpretation, Lewis and Ramsay (2002) found that cortisol did increase for 4-year-old children who showed signs of shame or embarrassment after failing a (rigged) color-matching laboratory task. Also consistent with this interpretation, starting at 7 years of age, cortisol increases are consistently found in response to public speaking tasks, tasks that might well elicit shame and embarrassment but cannot be used with younger children (Gunnar, Talge, & Herrera, 2009). Lastly, Gunnar, Sebanc,

Tout, Donzella, and van Dulmen (2003) found that preschool children who were rejected by their classmates had higher cortisol levels than their non-rejected peers. The emotion elicitors in these studies embody key stimulus characteristics proposed by Dickerson and Kemeny (2004) as being critical for evoking HPA reactivity based on the results of studies with adults—that is, social evaluation, uncontrollability, and unpredictability. Their results suggest that these characteristics also evoke HPA reactivity in children.

According to the social buffering hypothesis, the support of sensitive caregivers should be able to mitigate the potential effects of adverse experiences on the HPA system (Gunnar, 2017). To shed light on this question, Hackman, O'Brien, and Zalewski (2018) conducted a set of meta-analyses that examined the relationship between parental warmth and children's HPA functioning. Analyses showed that the relationship between parental warmth and cortisol reactivity depended on both stressor type and child age. At younger ages and for tasks involving elicitation of negative emotions (e.g., wariness/fear, frustration/anger), the relationship between warmth and cortisol reactivity was negative, whereas at older ages and for tasks involving public speaking or threats to social relationships, the relationship was positive. These findings suggest that parents may not serve as adequate social buffers as children grow older, perhaps because of the increasing significance of extrafamilial relationships and social evaluations at older ages.

EMOTION RECOGNITION AND KNOWLEDGE

Evidence from Children's Emotion Language

As children make significant strides in language development after their second birthdays, researchers correspondingly begin to rely on language-based measures to assess their emotion recognition and knowledge. Potentially, one source of information about children's emotion understanding is their spontaneous production of emotion-related language during social interactions with their caregivers and siblings. Indeed, a number of studies have assessed the growth of emotion vocabulary during early childhood and beyond. For example, Ridgeway, Waters, and Kuczaj (1985) provided parents of children between 18 and 71 months of age with a list of 126 emotion-related adjectives (e.g., *happy, sad, mad, friendly, bored, healthy, gloomy*) and asked them to report the age at which their child first understood and then first produced the emotion terms. Regarding the names for some basic emotions, they found that 50% or more parents reported that their child understood the words *happy* and *sad* by 24 months, *afraid, scared, angry,* and *mad* by 29 months, *surprise* by 35 months, and *disgusted* by 59 months. As is typical in language development, comprehension preceded production. Still, 50% or more of the children were reported to actively use the terms *happy, sad, afraid, mad,* and *scared* by 29 months, *angry* by 35 months, and *surprise* by 41 months of age. Of course, one limitation of this study was that children's understanding could not be independently confirmed.

In part to remedy this problem, Dunn, Bretherton, and Munn (1987) conducted extensive home observations of 18- to 32-month-old children and recorded their conversations about feeling states and emotions (e.g., fatigue, fear). They reported that by 2 years of age, most of the children explicitly referred to feelings, as well as the causes or consequences of the affective states being discussed (e.g., "No like peas. No eat"). However, specific emotion terms were rarely used. Children's references to feelings and emotions increased further between 24 and 32 months and were related to the amount of emotion-related talk they had heard from mothers and siblings at earlier ages. Girls both heard and produced more emotion-related language than did boys.

Dunn and her colleagues also systematically assessed relationships between family talk about feelings and emotions and children's emotion understanding. In a study of 3-year-old children, Dunn, Brown, and Beardsall (1991) found that emotion-related talk by both the children and their mothers was positively related to children's performance on an emotion recognition task, the Rothenberg Test of Social Sensitivity—a test that requires children to match pictures of happy, sad, angry, and fearful facial expressions to each of these emotions as portrayed in audiotaped verbal statements. In a subsequent study of children at 33 and 40 months of age, Dunn and Brown (1994) also assessed their families' more general emotional climate via measures of nonverbal positive and negative emotional expression and conflict episodes. Emotion recognition was assessed at 40 months using a procedure that involved matching facial expressions for happiness, sadness, anger, and fear to verbal labels and to emotion situations enacted during the course of a puppet show (as developed by Denham, 1986). Results showed that children from families having higher overall levels of conflict and negative expressivity performed more poorly on the test of emotion recognition. Mothers in these families also were less likely to engage in emotion-related discussion when their children were expressing negative emotion. Thus, although children in these families had opportunities to observe and potentially learn about negative emotion, they appeared less able to do so in the context of a highly charged negative family environment. As suggested by the researchers, discussion of negative emotion in the context of a lower level of overall negativity seems most conducive to emotion learning.

Emotion Concepts

Parents' reports of their young children's emotion vocabulary (i.e., Ridgeway et al., 1985) might seem to imply an adult-like concept of various specific emotions. However, some laboratory studies suggest that this may not, in fact, be the case. Based on an extensive body of research, Sherri Widen, Jim Russell, and their colleagues have hypothesized that children's emotion concepts develop substantially throughout childhood via a process of differentiation. These studies have involved a number of procedures, including asking children to provide verbal labels (i.e., to name the associated feelings) for photographs showing prototypic emotional facial expressions or asking children to similarly label a set of stories that adults identify as eliciting particular emotions (e.g., a birthday party, losing a toy, being chased by a big dog). Russell and his colleagues (e.g., DiGirolamo & Russell, 2017; Nelson et al., 2018) have argued that requiring children to provide verbal labels is a more valid method for assessing emotion understanding than multiple-choice procedures that may artificially inflate recognition scores if participants employ a process of elimination.

According to Widen's **broad-to-differentiated hypothesis** (Widen, 2016; Widen & Nelson, 2022), children move through six levels in their labeling of facial expressions and stories representing the Big Six emotions of happiness, anger, sadness, fear, surprise, and disgust. At Level 1 (at approximately 2½ years of age), children use only one verbal label (*happy*). At Level 2 (at a little over 3 years), children use two labels: *happy* plus one label that is applied to any of several negative emotions (i.e., *angry* for negative facial expressions, *sad* for negative stories). At Level 3 (at a little over 3½ years), they now use two negative labels: *angry* for anger and disgust stories or faces and *sad* for sad and fearful faces and stories. At Level 4 (at approximately 4 years), they now add either *scared* or *surprised* to their emotion label repertoire. Only at Level 6 (starting at approximately 6 years) do children come to use all six emotion labels in the same way as do adults. Although there is some variability among children in the rate at which they move through these levels and there are some minor differences in the age at which they reach each level with respect to emotion faces versus stories, the sequence of development is consistent.

These studies raise questions about 2½-year-old children's understanding of negative emotion words as reported by their parents. Still, by 4 years of age, most children are able to provide verbal labels for happiness, sadness, fear, and anger when they are shown dynamic emotion cues rather than still photos—that is, video clips of actors portraying these emotions via facial expressions, body postures, or a combination of facial, postural, and vocal cues (Nelson & Russell, 2011). However, identification of vocal expressions alone appears to lag behind. Perhaps unexpectedly, these investigators do not consistently find gender differences in preschool children's emotion labeling (Widen & Russell, 2002).

Widen and Russell also have conducted studies that systematically examine children's understanding of (or beliefs about) the causes and consequences of emotions. For example, Russell and Widen (2002) presented 3- and 4-year-old children with either an emotion label (*happy, surprised, scared, disgusted, angry,* or *sad*) or a facial expression corresponding to one of the emotions and asked the children to explain why someone might feel that way. Children's responses were presented to raters who first guessed which emotion was being described and then rated the plausibility of the response for that particular emotion. Results showed that more than half of the children at both ages were able to produce plausible causes for happiness, fear, and sadness. The 4-year-old children were also able to produce plausible causes for anger. Overall, children produced more plausible causes in response to the emotion words than in response to the emotion faces. In a subsequent study, Widen and Russell (2004) used the same procedure but omitted the emotion of happiness and added a condition in which 3- to- 5-year-olds were presented with behavioral consequences associated with each of the other five emotions (e.g., "he ran away" for fear, "he looked around and tried to figure out what [happened]" for surprise). Results showed that over half of the children were able to generate plausible causes for fear, sadness, anger, and disgust when presented with behavioral consequences associated with the emotion, and 48% of children were also able to do so for surprise.

In summary, by about 4 years of age, most children are able to verbally label multimodal expressions of happiness, fear, sadness, and anger. They also can think of plausible causes for these emotions and recognize plausible behavioral consequences. Understanding of surprise and disgust appears to develop during the next several years.

Harris and Pons's Stage Theory

One key aspect of emotion knowledge is the understanding that emotions are mental states (i.e., feelings) and may operate differently across individuals, situations, and ages. Based on an extensive body of research, Paul Harris and Francisco Pons (Harris, de Rosnay, & Pons, 2016; Pons & Harris, 2019; Pons, Harris, & de Rosnay, 2004) have presented a three-stage model to describe this development from early childhood to the beginning of adolescence.

In the external stage (from 1–2 years to 4–5 years), children begin to label and identify some of the basic emotions and can associate them with plausible eliciting causes and consequences. They also begin to understand that different people may have different emotional responses to the same situation (e.g., being given a glass of milk) depending on whether they like it or not (Harris, Johnson, Hutton, Andrews, & Cooke, 1989). Other factors such as ownership may also influence their emotional response. For example, Pesowski and Friedman (2015) showed that 3-year-olds predicted that a child would become upset at the loss of her own toy but not that of another child. Importantly, this suggests an initial implicit understanding that emotions are responses to one's *appraisal* of a situation rather than to the situation itself. Similarly, it represents an initial implicit understanding that emotions are internal mental states that mediate between experiential input and expressive or behavioral output.

In the mental stage (from 4–5 years to 7–8 years), children develop a better understanding of how beliefs and memory can influence one's emotional response. For example, during this stage, they begin to develop an understanding that memories of past experiences can evoke an emotional response and that such memories can be evoked by present experiences (Lagattuta & Wellman, 2001; Lagattuta & Kramer, 2021). In addition, they understand that a person's expectations will influence his or her emotional response to an event. For example, unexpected success in a bowling game will generate greater happiness than success that was expected (Asaba, Ong, & Gweon, 2019). By the end of this stage, children also realize that someone's emotional response in a situation will depend on the person's beliefs about it, irrespective of whether those beliefs are accurate. For example, if Little Red Riding Hood does not know that the wolf is inside her grandmother's cottage, she will not be afraid when she knocks on the door (Harris, de Rosnay, & Ronfard, 2013). In addition, children come to understand that a person can (and sometimes will) simulate or hide his or her emotion (e.g., to avoid a bully, to avoid hurting another person's feelings; Saarni, 1979; Wu & Schulz, 2020). Lastly, they begin to understand what types of strategies might be most effectively used to regulate (i.e., influence) other persons' emotions (e.g., cheering them up when they feel sad; López-Pérez & Pacella, 2021).

In the reflexive stage (from 7–8 years to 10–11 years), children come to understand that one may experience mixed emotions (Peng, Johnson, Pollock, Glasspool, & Harris, 1992). For example, one may feel happy about winning a prize but also sad that his or her best friend did not. Children also understand emotional responses related to some moral transgressions (e.g., that a rule breaker might feel bad about breaking the rule but also good about achieving a forbidden goal; Lagattuta, 2005). Lastly, children begin to understand strategies for controlling one's emotions. For example, when confronted with the death of a favorite pet, one can try to feel better by seeking social support (Quiñones-Camacho & Davis, 2020).

Pons and Harris have developed a measurement instrument to capture both developmental and individual differences in the features of emotion understanding described in their model (i.e., Test of Emotion Comprehension [TEC]; Pons & Harris, 2000). However, theirs is only one of many measures that have been used by researchers. In fact, in their review of the literature, Castro and colleagues (2016) identified 56 methods for measuring emotion understanding, although only a few (including the TEC) assessed a broad range of emotion-related proficiencies.

Many of these various measures have been used in studies that examined relations between emotion understanding and academic, social, and/or behavioral adjustment. For example, Ursache et al. (2020) found that greater emotion knowledge predicted higher math and reading scores for Black and Latinx kindergarteners living in low-income neighborhoods. In a set of meta-analyses, Voltmer and von Salisch (2017) found small to medium effect sizes for associations between emotion recognition of faces or causes and children's academic performance, peer acceptance, and school adjustment. In a meta-analysis of studies that could include children and/or adolescents, Trentacosta and Fine (2010) found significant negative associations between measures of emotion recognition and children's externalizing and/or internalizing problems. In contrast, a significant positive association was found between emotion recognition and social competence. Still, as pointed out by several researchers (e.g., Harris et al., 2016), emotional understanding does not always lead to social competence. For example, in one widely cited study of school-age children, Sutton, Smith, and Swettenham (1999) reported that ringleader bullies scored higher on a test of emotion understanding than did their followers or the victims of their bullying. Thus emotion knowledge—like other forms of knowledge—can be deployed for nefarious as well as praiseworthy purposes.

SUMMARY AND FINAL THOUGHTS

Because of the important role they played in the revival of emotion theory and research at the end of the 20th century, prototypic facial expressions have received considerable research attention. Ironically, this research has shown that initial assumptions about their role in real-life social communication are not entirely warranted. Further research is needed to understand the factors that determine when prototypic emotional facial expressions (or their components) are or are not produced in an episode of emotion. In the meantime, the use of multimodal scoring systems that assess both facial and nonfacial emotion cues are recommended, and this approach indeed has been adopted by many developmental researchers.

Children's emotional expressivity varies across individuals, social contexts, and cultures. Positive expressivity is related to greater social acceptance, whereas negative expressivity (particularly anger) is related to less acceptance. Expressivity may decline across childhood, but more research is needed on this question.

Research conducted within the framework of Rothbart's model of temperament has focused on both emotional reactivity (including negative reactivity and positive exuberance) and regulation (i.e., EC). These interact to generate behaviors that may be adaptive or maladaptive. Recent studies suggest that maladaptive fear may be identified by looking at contexts in which fear is shown in nonthreatening circumstances rather than merely measuring fear intensity in contexts that induce fear in most children. Temperament can be modified by parenting. For example, research on behaviorally inhibited children indicates that overprotective and/or intrusive control by parents encourages the maintenance of inhibited behaviors, whereas supportive parenting may help mitigate BI.

As assessed via age-appropriate measures, attachment continues to be related to better emotion functioning throughout childhood. One means through which such effects are produced may be parents' emotion socialization behaviors. The model proposed several decades ago by Eisenberg and her colleagues (Eisenberg, Cumberland, & Spinrad, 1998; Eisenberg, Spinrad, & Cumberland, 1998) continues to provide a useful framework for conceptualizing emotion socialization. However, the effects of specific socialization behaviors may differ depending upon a number of factors, for example, child age, fit between the goals of parents and children, and cultural context.

The distinction between emotion and emotion regulation continues to be debated. Many studies have focused on the range of strategies that children may use in a deliberate effort to modify their emotional responses. As children advance in age, their tendency to use cognitive rather than behavioral strategies increases (e.g., cognitive reappraisal rather than thumb sucking). However, in some situations, distraction (a behavioral response) can still be a useful strategy. Expression regulation can be considered conceptually distinct from emotion regulation, although—as is discussed in a later chapter—this distinction is not always made in the adult literature. Both temperament and socialization influence children's emotion regulation.

Commensurate with traditional cultural valuing of emotional restraint, Asian children are less expressive than children from Western societies. Other research illustrates how differing values may lead to cultural differences in parents' use of various emotion socialization practices. Association of specific parenting practices with child outcomes may also differ across cultures.

Gender differences in temperament and emotional expression are notably small but tend to be consistent with gender stereotypes. A female advantage is seen in children's emotion recognition and labeling. Observed differences in parents' socialization of boys versus girls is thought to be primarily responsible for gender differences in behavior and understanding.

Findings regarding the neurobiological correlates of emotion functioning in typically developing children can provide benchmarks against which atypically developing children might later be compared. Toward this end, many studies of children have focused on their neural activity during emotion regulation procedures measured using fMRI, EEG, and fNIRS. Studies of ANS functioning have demonstrated that the adaptive value of increasing or decreasing RSA can vary with the particular demands of an emotion episode. HPA reactivity in children is low in response to laboratory elicitors of negative emotions such as anger/frustration and fear/wariness. However, procedures that elicit shame or embarrassment can lead to cortisol increases in children (as they do for adults).

Emotion recognition is multifaceted and includes the processes of linking together causes, expressions, behavioral actions, and verbal emotion labels. Although young children use emotion words in their everyday language, their use may not reflect an adult-like understanding of these associations. However, by about 4 years of age, most children can produce plausible causes for happiness, fear, sadness, and anger. Children can also recognize plausible behavioral actions for these emotions, plus disgust. Development of emotion knowledge is captured within Harris and Pons's three-stage model and includes understanding that different people can have different emotional reactions to the same situation, that a person's beliefs and memories can influence his or her emotional responses, that a person can experience mixed emotions, and that it is possible to modify one's emotions or one's emotional expressions.

CHAPTER 4

Adolescence

10–17 Years

Historically, adolescence has been viewed as a period of emotional turmoil or "storm and stress" (Hall, 1904, p. 306). Without contradicting this description in its entirety, contemporary research has led to a more nuanced view of this developmental time period. Factors identified as importantly influencing children's emotional development continue to play a role in adolescence (e.g., temperament, attachment relations, culture, gender). Although conflicts with parents and risk-taking behaviors increase, so does adolescents' ability to regulate their own emotions and understand the emotions of others. This overall picture of development during adolescence is elaborated in this chapter.

HOW OLD ARE ADOLESCENTS?

Perusal of various sources reveals a notable lack of consensus about the ages at which adolescence should be considered to begin and end. According to a reference cited by the National Institutes of Health, "Adolescence begins with the onset of physiologically normal puberty, and ends when an adult identity and behaviour are accepted" (Sacks, 2003, p. 577). However, both the onset of puberty and the age at which individuals make the transition to adult roles are highly variable, and thus any designation of a standard age range is obviously somewhat arbitrary. Both Sacks (2003) and the World

Health Organization (WHO; 2020) consider 10 years and 19 years to be the lower and upper limits of adolescence. Yet one popular textbook on adolescence (Steinberg, 2020) considers this developmental period to extend into the early 20s. At the same time, many studies of emotion in adults involve college students who may be as young as 18 years old, and most self-identified studies of adolescents do not include participants older than high school age. As a compromise, herein the age range of 10–17 years has been designated as adolescence. However, readers will find that some of the investigations to be reported do not fit precisely in this age range.

EMOTIONAL EXPERIENCE

Adolescence is characterized by less emotional turbulence than previously believed (Arnett, 1999; Rutter, Graham, Chadwick, & Yule, 1976). Much of the research leading to this current view has involved studies in which adolescents document their emotional experiences in their daily lives. New technologies have emerged that enable individuals to record their feelings at frequent intervals during the day (e.g., smartphones). These have provided researchers with a more intimate window into adolescents' emotions.

Positive and Negative Affect

Illustrating this type of **experience sampling methodology (ESM)**, Reed Larson and his colleagues (Larson, Moneta, Richards, & Wilson, 2002) provided 220 fifth- to eighth-grade working-class and middle-class children and adolescents with pagers and signaled them once every 2 hours throughout the day and evening for 1 week. When signaled, the participants used a paper diary book to rate their current emotional states (i.e., happy–unhappy, cheerful–irritable, friendly–angry) on 7-point scales. Responses were averaged to create an overall affect score ranging from +3 for "highly positive" to –3 for "highly negative." At the end of the week, the adolescents also completed brief measures of depression and self-esteem, while their parents completed the Child Behavior Checklist (CBCL; Achenbach, 1991) as a measure of their behavioral adjustment. The children and parents subsequently participated in a second week of data collection that took place 4 years after the first (i.e., when they were in 9th–12th grades). Results showed that adolescents' ratings of their affect declined between 5th grade (i.e., 10–11 years) and 10th grade (15–16 years). Still, average scores remained in the positive

range and leveled off after 10th grade. More specifically, the average proportion of positive ratings (i.e., scores > 0) declined only slightly (i.e., from
approximately 74% to approximately 71%) over the 4-year interval between
each participant's two ratings. During the same time period, the average
proportion of negative ratings (i.e., scores < 0) increased from approximately
13% to approximately 20%. Adolescents' ratings of their affect were positively related to their self-esteem but negatively related to reports of stressful
life events, depression, and behavior problems at both assessments.

Other studies have obtained similar results (see Bailen, Green, &
Thompson, 2019, for a review). For example, in an earlier investigation using a
methodology similar to that described above, Larson and Lampman-Petraitis
(1989) found that average affect scores decreased across age in a sample that
included 9- to 15-year-old participants. In a study that compared high school
students with working adults, Larson, Csikszentmihalyi, and Graef (1980)
found that adults also reported higher average affect scores than did the high
school students. However, countering the stereotype portraying adolescent
affect as primarily negative, average affect scores for the adolescent participants remained within the positive range (i.e., > 0) in both studies.

Moodiness

Another stereotypical feature attributed to adolescence is moodiness. Interestingly, studies that have compared adolescents' moodiness with that of
children and adults have produced mixed results, possibly due to differences
in how the construct is operationalized. To illustrate, Larson et al. (1980)
found that high school students scored higher than adults on several measures of moodiness, for example, use of the extreme positive or negative affect
ratings (i.e., +3 or –3) or size of the change in their affect ratings between
one paging event and the next. However, Larson and Lampman-Petraitis
(1989) operationalized moodiness as the size of each participant's standard
deviation for affect rating scores at a given age and found no increase in this
measure for boys and only a slight increase for girls between 9 and 15 years.
A similar result was reported by Larson et al. (2002) in their study of 5th-
to 12th-grade students. In one of the very few studies to examine different
specific emotions, Maciejewski, van Lier, Branje, Meeus, and Koot (2015)
separately examined ratings for happiness, anger, sadness, and anxiety and
operationalized moodiness as the size of the change in rating scores between
one rating event and the next. Using this measure, the researchers found a
decrease in moodiness scores for happiness, anger, and sadness from 13 to

18 years of age. In contrast, moodiness scores for anxiety first increased, then decreased, and then increased again in the course of their longitudinal study. To summarize, it appears that adolescents may indeed be more moody than adults. However, further research is needed to clarify its trajectory from preadolescence though adolescence itself.

Negative Self-Consciousness

Another feature of the adolescent stereotype is self-consciousness. Although self-consciousness has not been the focus of ESM studies, it has been investigated in some laboratory experiments. For example, Somerville et al. (2013) led 8- to 23-year-old participants to believe that they were being watched by a peer as they passively viewed a video monitor in preparation for an experimental procedure. Participants then rated their level of embarrassment and several other emotions. Embarrassment ratings increased from 8 to 17 years of age before subsequently declining. Other studies have utilized the Trier Social Stress Test (TSST; Kirschbaum, Pirke, & Hellhammer, 1993), a procedure that involves preparing and giving a short speech in front of a potentially critical audience. In a meta-analytic investigation, Seddon and colleagues (2020) found that this procedure effectively elicited self-reported negative affect and anxiety in 7- to 17-year-old participants and increases in several neurobiological stress responses. However, there was no evidence that adolescents were affected more than the younger children in this study. Thus it appears that adolescents are indeed self-conscious when under public scrutiny but that they are not always more self-conscious than 7- to 9-year-old children.

Affect and Context

Although identifying normative trends in affect development is important, it is equally important to remember that emotion does not occur in a vacuum. That is, affective experience also depends upon the varying circumstances encountered by different individuals. With this in mind, some ESM studies have collected more detailed data on the contexts surrounding adolescents' experiences of affect and emotions in daily life. For example, Rogers et al. (2018) studied older adolescents' daily experiences before and during their first semester in college. Students were sent a text message twice weekly signaling them to complete a survey in which they separately rated their positive and negative affect and reported the types of interactions they had with family and friends on that day. Consistent with findings by Larson et al. (2002), the data in Rogers et al.'s (2018) study showed that positive affect was rated higher than negative affect overall. Reflecting the stress of entering college, average positive affect decreased, although negative affect remained stable over the time period of the study. Further regarding the contextual embedding of emotion, positive affect was related to more satisfying interactions with family and friends, and negative affect was related to greater conflict.

How Important Are Hormonal Influences?

The storm-and-stress view of adolescents attributed most of their emotional turmoil to biological changes associated with puberty (Arnett, 1999). In contrast, Rogers et al.'s (2018) findings suggest that the trajectory of adolescents' affect may reflect their experience of emotion elicitors as much as any changes in biologically related emotional reactivity. In a systematic review of the literature, Buchanan, Eccles, and Becker (1992) concluded that there is some evidence for relatively weak hormonal influences on adolescents' mood and behavior. Similarly, Van Den Akker et al. (2021) concluded that hormonal influences on personality development during adolescence are present but weak. Instead, developmental challenges and environmental circumstances appear to have a stronger influence (see also Steinberg, 2020; Steinberg & Morris, 2001).

Adolescents in Western cultures are tasked with developing stronger relationships with peers, including both friendships and romantic relationships, and with achieving a greater level of autonomy and academic success (Klimes-Dougan & Zeman, 2007; Steinberg, 2020). Exemplifying common responses to these challenges, high school students are notoriously reluctant to be seen in public with their parents rather than their peers and may become increasingly anxious as decisions about college loom ever nearer. Thus the challenges of adolescence can be experienced as stressful and indeed are associated with lower affect ratings in ESM studies. For example, Henker, Whalen, Jamner, and Delfino (2002) found that 9th-grade adolescents who scored higher on a measure of anxiety reported being more stressed and "hassled" than less anxious adolescents and also reported experiencing more anger, more sadness, and less happiness in their ESM diaries. Like children and adults, adolescents may use various regulation strategies to cope with their negative emotions, as is described in a later section of this chapter.

TEMPERAMENT

Individual differences between adolescents in their experienced emotions are also influenced by their temperament. At the same time, this is a reciprocal relationship, since (as previously emphasized) temperament itself may be modified over the course of development as a result of life experiences. Following Rothbart's reactivity and regulation model (see Chapter 2), investigators have found associations between adolescent's temperament and their social and emotional adjustment.

Emotional Reactivity and Effortful Control (EC)

Oldehinkel, Hartman, Ferdinand, Verhulst, and Ormel (2007) examined relations between temperament and behavioral adjustment in 11-year-olds (considered to be preadolescents in this study) and 13- to 14-year-olds using the Revised Early Adolescent Temperament Questionnaire (EATQ-R; Putnam, Ellis, & Rothbart, 2001). Results showed that higher levels of EC mitigated the effect of temperamental fearfulness on internalizing behaviors and the effect of temperamental frustration on externalizing behaviors for both age groups. Youssef et al. (2016) investigated relations between temperament and self-reported risk taking by 16-year-old adolescents using the EATQ-R, along with two laboratory measures of cognitive control. Results showed that the EATQ-R surgency factor (consisting of items representing low fear, low shyness, and greater high-intensity pleasure) predicted greater risk taking. In addition, higher EATQ-R scores on frustration were related to greater risk taking for those adolescents who also scored low on control. The results of this study mesh well with the neurobiological models of adolescent risk taking presented later in the chapter. Using a wider range of outcome measures, Snyder et al. (2015) examined the relationship between 8- to 19-year-olds' scores on the EATQ-R and their depression, anxiety, symptoms of hyperactivity and impulsivity, antisocial behavior, victimization by peers, and school performance. Differentiated relationships were found between some of the specific negative emotionality subscales of the EATQ-R and some specific outcomes. For example, scores on the fear-related subscale were associated with higher anxiety, whereas scores on the aggression-related subscale were associated with more antisocial behavior. The authors concluded that meaningful differences among subscales may often be obscured when they are combined to form a general measure of negative emotionality. Still, consistent with results of previous studies, higher EATQ-R scores on EC and lower scores on overall negative emotionality were generally associated with better scores on all measures of psychosocial functioning.

Temperament in Context

Other studies have investigated interactions between life circumstances and temperament in order to develop a more nuanced picture of contributors to behavioral adjustment in adolescence. Together, these investigations confirm that stressful life events exacerbate the effect of negative emotionality on adjustment, whereas higher control can attenuate this effect (e.g., R. Ellis et al., 2017; Gulley, Hankin, & Young, 2016; Laceulle, Nederhof, Karreman, Ormel, & van Aken, 2012). In one study, Jeronimus, Riese, Oldehinkel, and Ormel (2017) identified three different pathways that could lead from high levels of temperamental frustration (assessed at 16 years via the EATQ-R) to externalizing problems assessed at 19 years. To identify and characterize these pathways, the investigators conducted a detailed interview that focused on stressors experienced by adolescents in the 3-year interval. Three pathways from frustration to externalizing problems were identified: (1) selection (whereby the adolescent gravitated to or generated stressors), (2) carryover (whereby the adolescent was involuntarily exposed to the same stressors across the time interval), and (3) direct vulnerability (whereby the adolescent was particularly sensitive to encountered stressors). Interestingly, the first pathway accounted for very little of frustration's effect on externalizing problems (about 5%), whereas the latter two pathways were approximately equal in their contribution (50% and 45%, respectively).

Turning to behavioral inhibition (BI), the relationship between this temperamental disposition and later adjustment problems has also been investigated. Reflecting the importance of peer relationships in adolescence, social involvement during this age period might be expected to moderate the relationship between BI in childhood and later development of anxiety problems. Frenkel et al. (2015) investigated this possibility in a 20-year longitudinal study of children who had been evaluated for BI at multiple time points. Social involvement data were acquired when participants were 14–16 years of age, and scoring reflected the adolescents' self-reported number of friends and time spent with these friends in social activities. At 18–21 years of age, psychopathology was evaluated via both clinical interviews and questionnaire measures. Results showed that BI predicted anxiety scores for those individuals who had little social involvement during adolescence, but early inhibition did not predict later anxiety for those who had greater social engagement during those years. This finding paves the way for future research to identify factors that determine different levels of social involvement for adolescents who had been identified as behaviorally inhibited children. For example, it will be important to determine whether greater social involvement during adolescence results from increased social opportunities, a spontaneous decline in the adolescents' inhibitory tendencies, and/or an effort by adolescents to overcome those tendencies.

ATTACHMENT

As adolescents' social focus shifts increasingly from the family to the outside world, their attachment status comes to influence their extrafamilial social relationships and their psychological adjustment within those relationships. As previously noted, throughout development, the individual's internal working model (IWM) of attachment is continually modified based on accumulated experiences with significant figures both within and outside of the family (Bowlby, 1969; Sroufe, Coffino, & Carlson, 2010). Thus understanding attachment in adolescence requires contemporaneous assessment rather than exclusive reliance on measurements obtained during childhood or infancy.

Measuring Attachment in Adolescence

Although many attachment measures for adolescents are available (see Jewell et al., 2019, for a review), the Adult Attachment Interview (AAI; Hesse, 2016) is arguably the most strongly grounded in Bowlby's attachment theory and can be used with adolescents as well as adults. The AAI is an interview procedure that focuses on the individual's attachment-related *state of mind*, conceptualized as a more mature version of his or her IWM. During the interview, individuals are asked to recall their early upbringing with specific references to positive and negative interactions with their parents. Classification of an individual as having a secure state of mind does not primarily depend upon his or her recalling a predominance of positive experiences (although this is often the case). Rather, the most important factor is whether the person has a coherent understanding of his or her past and—irrespective of any difficulties—still places a high value on attachment relationships. To illustrate, a securely attached adolescent might describe her father as neglectful but understand that it was due to his depression and might have hope for a better relationship in the future.

Are Adolescents Still Attached to Their Parents?

Adolescents' original attachment figures (typically their parents) continue to play a role in their lives, still serving as sources of security under conditions of stress (Allen & Tan, 2016; Rosenthal & Kobak, 2010). At the same time, adolescents (at least in Western cultures) are seeking greater independence, including emotional self-sufficiency (Allen & Tan, 2016). As every parent knows, balancing adolescents' needs for autonomy, relatedness, and competence (La Guardia, Ryan, Couchman, & Deci, 2000) can be difficult, requiring a great deal of negotiation and a certain amount of conflict regarding rules and behaviors. Nonetheless, the security of the attachment relationship itself need not be threatened.

Just as maternal sensitivity is related to attachment security in infancy, Allen et al. (2003) found that maternal supportiveness was related to attachment security in adolescence. In this study, several other contributing factors also were identified. One was the mother's attunement to her adolescent's self-perception, that is, her understanding of the adolescent's beliefs about his or her competence in areas such as academics, athletics, romantic appeal, social acceptance, and close friendships. Another contributing factor to secure attachment was the ability of the dyad to engage with each other in an empathic and respectful manner while discussing a topic on which they strongly disagreed. Of course, not all parent–adolescent attachments are secure. In a study that focused on emotional expressivity during discussions in which adolescents and their mothers were asked to resolve their disagreement, Kobak, Cole, Ferenz-Gillies, Fleming, and Gamble (1993) found that insecurely attached adolescents tended to express higher levels of anger and/or to disengage altogether from the discussion in comparison with more securely attached adolescents. Further research on parent–adolescent conflict discussions is described later in this chapter.

Attachment and Peer Relations

As adolescents develop more extensive ties to peers, some of their stronger bonds with friends or romantic partners may be considered attachment relationships, that is, potentially important sources of security. These deep relationships (especially romantic ones) may be characterized as either secure or insecure in ways that are similar to secure and insecure relationships between parents and children (Hazan & Shaver, 1987; Zeifman & Hazan, 2016). In point of fact, according to Bowlby's theory, secure parent–child attachments set the stage for secure romantic relationships through their influence on the adolescent's (and later the adult's) IWM. However, as opposed to parent–child attachments, romantic and peer attachments operate within relationships that are egalitarian rather than hierarchical.

In general, adolescent attachment security has been consistently related to a number of desirable social and emotional outcomes involving peers. For example, securely attached adolescents are better liked by their peers (Allen, Moore, Kuperminc, & Bell, 1998), behave more prosocially (Dykas, Ziv, & Cassidy, 2008), and have better friendship and romantic relations (Dykas, Woodhouse, Cassidy, & Waters, 2006; Zimmermann, 2004) than insecurely attached adolescents. Differences in their emotion functioning also have been found. For example, Zimmermann, Maier, Winter, and Grossmann (2001) coded the behavior of pairs of adolescent friends as they cooperatively played a difficult computer game and also obtained self-reports of their experienced emotions at several points during the game. The researchers observed that securely attached adolescents showed less disruptive behavior than did insecurely attached adolescents at those points in the game when they experienced intense negative emotion. Securely attached adolescents also appear to be at less risk overall for a variety of behavioral and emotional adjustment problems compared with insecurely attached adolescents (see Allen & Tan, 2016, for a detailed review).

Do Early Attachments Still Influence Adolescents?

Early attachment has sometimes been found to predict significant emotion-related aspects of adolescent development. For example, Boldt, Goffin, and Kochanska (2020) proposed that secure early attachment sets children on a path leading to the development of better emotion regulation, which in turn is related to better social functioning. They obtained evidence for this proposal in a longitudinal study in which infants' attachment security to both mother and father was assessed at 2 years of age, regulation was assessed in early childhood, and social functioning was assessed in early adolescence (i.e., at 10 and 12 years). Regulation in early childhood was operationalized as responding without anger or defiance in tasks that might potentially evoke those emotions (e.g., delay of gratification tasks, being prohibited from touching an attractive toy, being asked to stop playing and clean up a set of toys). Parents also provided ratings of the young child's temperamental anger/frustration using Rothbart, Ahadi, Hershey, and Fisher's (2001) Children's Behavior Questionnaire (CBQ). At 10 and 12 years of age, regulation was operationalized as showing low levels of negative emotion during discussions with their parents. Parents also rated their young adolescents on symptoms of defiance (e.g., opposition, disregard for rules, conflicts with others, hostility, and aggression). Lastly, the young adolescents completed a questionnaire measure that assessed their adherence to adult rules and values (e.g., not texting in class). Data analyses revealed significant paths leading from early security with each parent to better emotional functioning as assessed in early childhood. Furthermore, associations were also obtained between early childhood functioning and early adolescent social and emotional functioning. For example, children who showed better ability to delay gratification subsequently showed greater adherence to adult rules and values in adolescence. Children who showed greater temperamental anger later showed more defiance.

SOCIAL INTERACTIONS

How Significant Are Parent–Adolescent Conflicts?

Although their attachment ties remain strong, adolescents' conflicts with their parents increase during early through mid-adolescence before declining in later adolescence (Arnett, 1999; Hadiwijaya, Klimstra, Vermunt, Branje, & Meeus, 2017). Interestingly, the increase in conflict appears tied to the onset of puberty rather than age per se (Buchanan et al., 1992). However, some researchers suggest that this increase is not directly due to the hormonal changes that puberty brings (e.g., Smetana, Crean, & Campione-Barr, 2005). Instead, they propose that adolescents see their more mature adult-like bodies as an indication that they should be given greater autonomy than their parents are willing to extend to them. Consistent with this proposal, parent–child conflicts often involve disagreements about which decisions should be considered a matter of personal choice (and thus left to the adolescent) and which decisions may have serious implications for the future of the adolescent or the family (and thus should be left to the parents). In any case, studies suggest that parent–adolescent conflicts are less common and less serious than they often are portrayed in popular culture (Steinberg, 2020).

Still, some parent–adolescent pairs come into conflict more often than others. In a meta-analytic investigation, Weymouth, Buehler, Zhou, and Henson (2016) found that greater conflict between adolescents and parents is associated with more adolescent internalizing problems, externalizing problems, and academic problems. Conflicts with mothers are more common than conflicts with fathers (Shek, 2007; Steinberg, 2020). Partly for this reason, many studies of parent–adolescent conflicts focus on mothers and daughters. One common strategy for studying conflicts is to ask parents and children to discuss a topic on which they disagree. For adolescents and their parents, these topics often include daily chores, showing manners and respect (e.g., not swearing), doing homework, and leisure activities. Moed and colleagues (2015) videotaped 11- to 16-year-old adolescents (both boys and girls) discussing (and trying to resolve) two such topics with their primary caregivers (usually their mothers). Nonverbal expressions of anger and distress/sadness by each participant were coded based on facial, vocal, and body actions. Within the discussion, episodes of conflict were identified when an expression of either anger or distress/sadness by one participant was reciprocated by an expression of anger or distress/sadness by the other. Reciprocal exchanges of negative affect continued until the conflict was considered to end when one participant failed to respond with anger or distress/sadness. Results showed that conflicts ended by the adolescent went on for a longer time than those ended by the parent. That is, when parents persisted in reciprocating their adolescents' negative affect, then adolescents also persisted for longer before they backed down. Not surprisingly, participants reported less satisfaction with discussion outcomes for these longer, more negative interactions. In addition, adolescents who engaged in these longer discussions were rated higher in oppositional defiance by their teachers. These findings suggest that parents who persist in reciprocating negative affect are not engaging in effective emotion socialization strategies.

Subsequent studies have examined other features of successful versus problematic conflict discussions. For example, Main, Paxton, and Dale (2016) examined synchrony (e.g., co-occurrence) in 13- to 18-year-olds' and their mothers' expressions of positive affect, negative affect, and interest during a conflict discussion. Participants' affect and interest were coded based on facial, vocal, body, and verbal cues. Higher satisfaction with the discussion was associated with lower levels of mutual negative affect. In contrast, a turn-taking pattern for the emotion of interest (rather than a pattern of co-occurrence) also was associated with higher satisfaction, probably because interest by one interactant requires co-occurring interest-eliciting behavior by the other rather than co-occurring interest itself.

Beyond Parent–Adolescent Conflicts

Extending the study of conflict discussions to include significant nonfamilial relationships, Lougheed et al. (2016) compared 16- to 17-year-old girls' discussions with a close friend to discussions with their mothers. Supportive responses to both positive and negative affect were identified. These included expressions of reassurance, empathy, approval, or validation (e.g., "You should feel proud of yourself"), as well as encouragement of **reappraisal** (e.g., encouraging the adolescent to reinterpret a negative event in a more positive light). The adolescents also provided self-ratings of their depressive symptoms. Results showed that girls who reported more symptoms of depression received less support from their close friends after expressing positive affect. They also received less support from their mothers after expressing both positive and negative affect. Thus both peers and parents appear to play an influential role in adolescent girls' emotional adjustment.

Extending the study of mother–daughter discussions beyond a focus on conflict, Lougheed and Hollenstein (2016) utilized an **emotional roller coaster task** to elicit episodes of conversation about times when they felt (1) happy/excited, (2) worried/sad, (3) proud, (4) frustrated/annoyed, and (5) grateful. Participants' positive affect, interest, neutral affect, negative externalizing affect (e.g., anger, contempt), and negative internalizing affect (e.g., sadness, fear) were coded. All instances of each possible combination of mother affect–adolescent affect codes were identified (e.g., mother proud–daughter neutral, mother proud–daughter worried/sad). The data were analyzed in light of the investigators' hypothesis that higher relationship satisfaction would be associated with greater affective flexibility (i.e., tending to move among varying emotional states rather than being "stuck" in one). Results indeed showed that greater flexibility within each of the five emotion discussion episodes was related to higher levels of relationship satisfaction.

Social Media and Texting

The central role that social media play in the lives of contemporary adolescents makes it important to consider the role of these media in their emotional development and functioning. According to some estimates, more than 90% of adolescents use social media and text messaging daily (Lenhart, 2015). Although representations in the popular press tend to emphasize the negative aspects of social media usage (e.g., cyberbullying), positive effects also have been documented. For example, in a survey study by Lenhart, Madden, Smith, Purcell, and Zickuhr (2011), approximately 69% of adolescents said that their peers are "mostly kind" to each other on the Internet, and approximately 60% reported that some things they had seen on social media made them feel better about themselves and closer to other people. At the same time, 88% said that they had witnessed cruel or mean behavior, and 15% reported that they themselves had been the target of harassment. Clearly, social media use is a two-edged sword.

Although adolescents make use of many social media platforms, as of 2015, Facebook was still their most favored site (Lenhart, 2015). In a now-infamous study, Kramer, Guillory, and Hancock (2014) manipulated Facebook users' news feeds so that they saw either fewer negative or fewer positive items. Results showed that users correspondingly produced fewer negative or positive messages themselves for a short time following the news feed manipulation, a phenomenon labeled *digital emotion contagion*. As noted by Goldenberg and Gross (2020), perhaps even better evidence for such contagion was the outrage expressed by Facebook users that became increasingly intense as news of the study spread across the Internet.

Kramer et al.'s (2014) study is not alone in demonstrating the effect of media content on viewers' emotions. However, studies involving adolescents typically focus on other means of emotion dissemination rather than emotion contagion. For example, in a study of deliberate emotion sharing, Vermeulen and her colleagues (Vermeulen, Vandebosch, & Heirman, 2018a, 2018b) conducted in-depth interviews with 22 adolescents (ages 14–18 years) in which they asked participants to describe recent events during which they experienced an emotion, which emotion(s) were experienced, whether they had shared their experience, and, if so, why, where, and with whom. Participants reported sharing almost all of their emotional experiences, most often with their close friend(s), who were perceived as being best able to understand and help the participant if needed and to be most trustworthy. Family members were second choices, but events were not shared if the adolescent thought there would be negative consequences (e.g., embarrassment, punishment). Only 5 of the 22 participants reported sharing their emotions with strangers (via Twitter, Tumblr, or a professional helpline). All participants shared their emotions both face-to-face and by texting. About half used Twitter; fewer used Snapchat or Instagram or posted a status message on Facebook. Reasons for preferring face-to-face sharing of emotion were its richness of cues, opportunities for feedback, and privacy. Reasons for texting were primarily its ease, cost-effectiveness, and popularity, as well as privacy. Social media sites that reached a broader audience were used more carefully with impression management and social norms in mind; typically, only positive emotions were shared.

How Do Social Media Affect Adolescents' Emotional Well-Being?

The bias toward publicly posting only positive information is understandable and also has predictable effects on those who view such postings. However, not everyone is similarly affected. In one experimental study (Weinstein,

2017), adolescents viewed a simulated Instagram feed of a highly attractive teen model (for female participants) or athlete (for male participants). Depending on the experimental condition, the Instagram feed included (1) only positive posts, (2) both positive posts and those in which the poster admitted to having a bad day, and (3) only positive posts but also a message reminding viewers that Instagram users typically avoid posting items about having a bad day. Participants reported their positive and negative affect both before and after reviewing the Instagram feed and also indicated whether they perceived the model or athlete to be happier or better off than themselves. Results showed that those who compared themselves most negatively to the model or athlete reported a greater increase in negative affect after viewing the posting. However, this effect was lessened in the conditions that involved mixed positive and negative postings or the cautionary message.

As opposed to sharing emotions by texting or face-to-face communication, expressing one's emotions on public social media sites has been linked to problematic social media use (e.g., preoccupation, withdrawal symptoms, concern expressed by parents). In a study of adolescents in Italy, Marino, Gini, Angelini, Vieno, and Spada (2020) surveyed high school students about their frequency of social media use, their perceptions of their peers' use, their self-perceived difficulties with emotion regulation, their tendency to express their emotions online, their belief that perceiving others' emotions online helps them function better in real life, and symptoms of social media addiction (e.g., neglecting homework and other signs of extreme preoccupation). Results showed that adolescents' self-reported difficulties with emotion regulation were associated with a greater tendency to express emotions on social media sites, with a belief that perceiving others' emotions on such sites is helpful, with greater overall Internet use, and with more symptoms of social media addiction.

Problematic Internet usage is also associated with **fear of missing out (FOMO)**. In a study again with adolescents in Italy, Fabris, Marengo, Longobardi, and Settanni (2020) surveyed 11- to 19-year-olds about their symptoms of FOMO (e.g., "I get anxious when I don't know what my friends are up to"), their sensitivity to neglect or negative reactions to their online posts (e.g., "I would feel stressed if my posts did not receive comments"; "I would feel stressed if my posts received negative comments"), their symptoms of Internet addiction (e.g., extreme preoccupation), and their experiences of distress (e.g., "I worry a lot"; "I am often unhappy"). Data analyses showed a pathway from greater FOMO to great sensitivity about neglect by online peers to more symptoms of Internet addiction to greater emotional distress. Similarly, Lee et al. (2020) found that receiving fewer "likes" on social media was related to greater depressive symptomology and that this relationship was particularly strong for adolescents subjected to peer victimization at school. In summary, these studies suggest that problematic Internet use can be both a cause and a consequence of emotional difficulties.

EMOTION REGULATION

Reactivity versus Regulation

From a conceptual point of view, disentangling emotion from emotion regulation can be challenging in studies of adolescents as well as children. For example, when adolescents face a challenge with apparent equanimity, is it because they are able to control their distress or because they are not upset in the first place? Some laboratory investigations have attempted to distinguish reactivity and regulation via instructions given to participants. Perhaps surprisingly, these studies have not always shown that emotional reactivity increases in adolescence, as might be predicted given stereotypes about adolescent emotionality. For example, Silvers et al. (2012) presented neutral and negative emotion pictures to 10- to 23-year-old participants and asked them to rate their own negative affect on a 4-point scale. In one condition (i.e., the reactivity condition), participants were told to react naturally to the pictures, whereas in the second condition (i.e., the regulation condition), they were told to tell themselves a story that would make them feel better about what they were viewing. No age differences were found in participants' ratings in the reactivity condition. However, in the regulation condition, negative affect ratings declined from 10 to 16 years of age before leveling off, indicating increasing success in emotion regulation.

In a second part of their study, Silvers et al. (2012) examined differences in participants' responses to negative pictures that depicted social versus nonsocial stimuli (e.g., a hospital patient hooked up with numerous tubes vs. a rattlesnake). Participants were instructed to either distance themselves from the pictured stimuli (i.e., to regulate by focusing on concrete features rather than emotional details) or remain close (i.e., allow themselves to fully experience their emotion). Participants also completed a self-report measure of their sensitivity to social rejection. Again, no age differences were found in the reactivity (i.e., remaining close) condition. In the regulation condition, negative affect ratings again decreased with age, indicating an overall age-related increase in emotion regulation. Taken together, findings from Silvers et al.'s (2012) study suggest that adolescents may be increasingly capable of regulating emotion when they are instructed to do so in low-stakes situations (e.g., in a laboratory study). However, whether they spontaneously do so in more stressful situations and/or real-world contexts is a separate question.

Effortful Control (EC)

The types of regulation investigated by Silvers et al. (2012) emerge in the child's repertoire as deliberate, highly controlled processes, although some may become more automatic after habitual use. This is not true of all forms of emotion regulation described in current adult-oriented models (Braunstein et al., 2017; see also Chapter 5 in this volume). Still, most developmental studies do focus on strategies that involve some degree of deliberate effort. For this reason, the development of EC is considered to undergird the development of emotion regulation in adolescence as well as childhood.

Although there is wide agreement that EC continuously improves through childhood into early adolescence, consensus breaks down when adolescence itself is considered. This is especially true for studies in which EC is assessed via ratings by parents, teachers, or even adolescents themselves. As noted by Atherton, Lawson, and Robins (2020), some studies have reported increases in EC across adolescence (e.g., Williams, Ponesse, Schachar, Logan, & Tannock, 1999), whereas others have reported decreases or nonlinear trajectories (e.g., a self-regulatory "dip"; Soto & Tackett, 2015). In Atherton et al.'s (2020) own longitudinal investigation, Mexican American adolescents (and their parents) were studied from 10 to 19 years of age. Child- and mother-report measures of EC were obtained at several ages. In addition, data were gathered on potential family and neighborhood influences on EC, including parental warmth, parental hostility, parental monitoring, school and neighborhood violence, and the adolescent's association with deviant peers. Results showed a U-shaped trajectory of EC development with a dip at around 14 years of age. In addition, hostile parenting, deviant peers, and neighborhood violence were associated with a greater dip in EC. Although neighborhood characteristics related to EC have not been widely studied, parental influences have received considerable attention. In a meta-analysis of almost 200 studies, Li et al. (2019) confirmed that negative parenting (e.g., **neglect**, rejection, harshness) is related to lower levels of adolescents' self-control, whereas positive parenting (e.g., warmth and support) and good attachment relationships are related to higher levels of self-control.

Although EC is most often treated as a unitary construct, some investigators have examined several different subtypes of control: inhibitory control, updating, and shifting. In their narrative review of these studies, Schweizer, Gotlib, and Blakemore (2020) argued that these forms of control may have different developmental trajectories and may be associated with different forms of emotion regulation. *Inhibitory control* involves resisting a response impulse and is often measured in an **emotional go/no-go task**. This task involves presenting participants with a series of facial expressions and instructing them to press a button as quickly as possible after seeing a particular emotional expression but to refrain from pressing the button when any other expression is presented. *Updating* involves comparing past and present information and revising one's thinking accordingly. In updating tasks, participants also are presented with a series of stimuli (e.g., facial expressions). In each trial, they are required to compare the current stimulus with one that was presented in a previous trial (e.g., the stimulus presented one or two trials before) while ignoring irrelevant features (e.g., the gender of the poser). *Shifting* involves changing the focus of one's cognitive efforts. In shifting tasks, participants are required to sort stimuli according to criteria that change during the course of the procedure (e.g., from gender to emotional expressions). Although research results have been somewhat mixed, Schweizer et al. (2020) conclude that adolescents are not significantly impaired compared with adults in their ability to exert these three forms of control. However, individual differences do exist among both adults and adolescents. With respect to such differences, Schweizer et al. (2020) suggested that poorer inhibitory control is related to higher levels of nonproductive rumination in adolescents, whereas better updating and shifting are respectively related to less use of expressive suppression and more use of reappraisal.

Reappraisal and Expressive Suppression

Reappraisal and expressive suppression are two strategies for emotion regulation (or reorganization) that have been studied widely in the adult literature and to a lesser extent in developmental investigations. Reappraisal involves thinking about a situation in a way that changes its emotional impact (Gross & John, 2003). For example, reappraisal might lead to a decrease in one's anger at a tardy friend after one learns she was in a minor car accident. Although reappraisal can result in either an increase or a decrease in experienced emotion, most studies have focused on its effectiveness in decreasing negative emotion. Several meta-analyses have consistently shown reappraisal to be effective in influencing emotional experience (e.g., Webb, Miles, & Sheeran, 2012). However, it must be noted that almost all studies included in these meta-analyses have focused on adults due to the dearth of developmental investigations that met inclusion criteria. Still, self-reported use of reappraisal as a regulation strategy appears to increase across the period of adolescence (Williams & McGillicuddy-De Lisi, 1999) and into adulthood (Garnefski, Legerstee, Kraaij, van den Kommer, & Teerds, 2002). Correspondingly, its effectiveness in terms of altering emotional experience also appears to increase with age (Silvers et al., 2012). Greater use of reappraisal also has been associated with positive adjustment outcomes in adolescence (e.g., lower levels of depression; Garnefski et al., 2002; Lougheed & Hollenstein, 2012).

Expressive suppression involves the inhibition of overt observable behavior reflecting an experienced emotion (Gross & John, 2003). For example, one might mask one's anger at a tardy friend in order not to jeopardize the friendship. Expressive suppression has been widely studied in adults, and a developmental literature is also emerging (see Gross & Cassidy, 2019, for a conceptual review). For adults, habitual expressive suppression is generally considered to be associated with negative consequences (e.g., greater sympathetic nervous system [SNS] reactivity, increased inflammation, memory impairment, less positive responding by social partners; Gross, 2013; Gross & Levenson, 1993). However, these effects may depend upon a number of factors. For example, in cultures in which emotional control is highly valued (e.g., China), expressive suppression is not always associated with depressed mood and poorer life satisfaction (Soto, Perez, Kim, Lee, & Minnick, 2011; Yeh, Bedford, Wu, Wang, & Yen, 2017; but see also Sai, Luo, Ward, & Sang, 2016).

As described in Chapter 3, studies using the disappointing present paradigm show that children are capable of suppressing their expressive behavior and have some understanding about when and why a person might do so (e.g., Saarni, 1979). However, the developmental course of expressive suppression across adolescence is unclear, with some studies reporting a decrease in its usage across adolescence (e.g., Gullone, Hughes, King, & Tonge, 2010) and other studies finding no change (e.g., Zimmermann & Iwanski, 2014). Interestingly, in many (though not all) studies, male adolescents report using suppression more than females, perhaps in conformity to gender-related expression norms of male stoicism (e.g., Gullone et al., 2010; Zimmerman & Iwanski, 2014).

Regarding the effectiveness of suppression, in their meta-analysis of primarily adult studies, Webb et al. (2012) found that suppressing one's emotional expression had no overall effect on emotional experience and only a minimal negative effect on physiological measures. Still, at least two meta-analyses have found higher levels of expression suppression to be related to higher levels of depressive symptoms in children and/or adolescents (Compas et al., 2017; Schäfer, Naumann, Holmes, Tuschen-Caffier, & Samson, 2017). At the same time, suppression may be considered appropriate in some situations (e.g., when receiving a disappointing present from a well-meaning relative) but not in others (e.g., when your friend breaks a promise). Further research would seem necessary to clarify the costs and benefits of expressive suppression within specific situational and relationship contexts.

Other Regulation Strategies

Of course, reappraisal and suppression are not the only responses to emotion-eliciting events seen in adolescents, children, or adults. Based on a review of the extant literature, De France and Hollenstein (2017) identified six common response strategies that have been studied: (1) distraction (e.g., keeping busy), (2) rumination (e.g., continually thinking about the event), (3) reappraisal (e.g., taking a different perspective), (4) suppression (e.g., pretending not to be upset), (5) engagement (e.g., showing what one is feeling), and (6) relaxation/arousal control (e.g., taking deep breaths). Of note, some of these responses (e.g., rumination, engagement) might not be expected to effectively down-regulate one's negative emotions. In their own investigation, De France and Hollenstein (2019) asked adolescents (12- to 15-year-olds), young adults (20- to 25-year-olds), and middle-aged adults (40- to 60-year-olds) to rate how often they used each strategy in response to their negative emotions using a scale of 1–7. The investigators found that utilization of these strategies (considered together as a group) increased between early adolescence and young adulthood and between young adulthood and middle adulthood. However, when the investigators examined participants' relative reliance on each one, they found that adolescents used more distraction, more relaxation, and less rumination than did the young adults. Adolescents also used more relaxation and suppression and less rumination than did the middle-aged adult participants.

In a subsequent investigation, Lennarz, Hollenstein, Lichtwarck-Aschoff, Kuntsche, and Granic (2019) used ESM to study adolescents' use of a somewhat different set of response strategies by asking them how they coped with the events that elicited a negative emotion. For each negative situation that they recorded, participants indicated whether or not they used distraction, rumination, reappraisal, suppression, problem solving (i.e., attempting to alter the situation), avoidance (i.e., leaving the situation), social support (i.e., sharing emotions, asking for advice), and acceptance (i.e., accepting that the situation happened). Again, some of these responses would be expected to decrease one's initial negative reaction (e.g., reappraisal), whereas others might actually be expected to increase or maintain it (rumination). Results showed that acceptance was reported to be the most frequent response, followed by problem solving, rumination, distraction, avoidance, reappraisal, social support, and suppression. However, strategy use also differed depending on whether the eliciting event had evoked a high-intensity or low-intensity level of negative affect. For low-intensity levels, acceptance was more likely to be used, whereas for high-intensity levels, suppression, problem solving, distraction, avoidance, social support, and rumination were more likely. Regarding their success in down-regulating negative affect, problem solving, reappraisal, and acceptance were more successful than rumination. These interesting results raise further questions about the specific situational circumstances and specific negative emotions associated with each strategy.

Depending on the situational circumstances, some regulation strategies may be preferred over others. For example, distraction may be a desirable strategy for a person undergoing a necessary but unpleasant medical procedure, whereas problem solving would be more desirable when one is attempting to complete a frustrating task. According to James Gross's process model of emotion regulation, developed in the adult literature (English, Lee, John, & Gross, 2017; Gross, 2015a, 2015b; see Chapter 5 for further description), a key factor influencing one's emotional response to any situation is one's situation-related goals (e.g., to win the game, to maintain a friendship). Within the developmental literature, the importance of relational goals is also emphasized in functional theories of emotion (Barrett & Campos, 1987). Because different strategies may be optimal under different circumstances depending on one's goals, having a range of strategies available for deployment would seem beneficial. Indeed, Lougheed and Hollenstein (2012) found that adolescents who used a wider range of emotion regulation strategies in their daily lives scored lower on measures of internalizing problems (e.g., depression, anxiety, social anxiety). After an initial decline from early adolescence (i.e., around 11 years) to middle adolescence (i.e., around 15 years of age), strategy repertoires appear to increase in size (Zimmerman & Iwanski, 2014).

Do Good Things Come to Those Who Wait?

As described in previous chapters, tasks involving delay of gratification have been included in many developmental studies of emotion regulation. An important inspiration for including such tasks has been the research of Walter Mischel and his colleagues, who began their work with studies of children attending an elite preschool on the Stanford University campus (e.g., Mischel, Shoda, & Peake, 1988; Mischel, Shoda, & Rodriguez, 1989; Shoda, Mischel, & Peake, 1990). These children participated in the **marshmallow task**, a procedure that has gained considerable renown since numerous parents and celebrities began attempting informal replications with their own children and posting the results on social media. In its simplest and most "diagnostic" form (Shoda et al., 1990), the child is confronted with a single marshmallow and is left to contemplate it while the experimenter leaves the room. Children are told that if they wait until the experimenter returns, then they will receive two marshmallows instead of one. However, if they wish, they can ring a bell and the experimenter will return and give them the single marshmallow. Mischel and his colleagues found that children's ability to delay gratification (and presumably tolerate or regulate the frustration it engendered) was related to a number of positive outcomes assessed over a decade later, most notably higher SAT scores and parents' ratings of their adolescents' self-confidence and ability to cope with stress. However, more recently, these results have become controversial.

In a conceptual replication with children of less educated mothers, Watts, Duncan, and Quan (2018) reported that the relationship between delay of gratification in preschool and adolescent achievement was substantially lower than that reported by Mischel and his colleagues. Furthermore, when the data analyses controlled for factors such as socioeconomic status (SES), early cognitive ability, and home environment, most relationships became statistically nonsignificant. Not surprisingly, Watts et al.'s study itself has generated considerable pushback. For example, Falk, Kosse, and Pinger (2020) critiqued Watts and colleagues' statistical procedures, used different statistical techniques to analyze the data, and reported results that more closely mirrored those originally reported by Mischel and his colleagues. Doebel, Michaelson, and Munakata (2020) argued that Watts and colleagues' (2018) inclusion of statistical controls was inappropriate in that the effect of children's ability to delay gratification was overwhelmed by the very "control" factors that support its development. Others (e.g., B. J. Ellis, Bianchi, Griskevicius, & Frankenhuis, 2017) have argued that delaying gratification actually is not adaptive for children from poorer backgrounds considering that one may not be able to reasonably expect that a reward will still be available at a later time. As such, parents from these backgrounds may socialize their children to opt for rewards that may be smaller but are more immediate and certain. Consistent with this latter proposal, Duran and Grissmer (2020) reported that opting for immediate rewards was related to better executive functioning and teacher ratings of behavior in low-income kindergarten children. Both executive functioning and choosing immediate gratification predicted teacher ratings to an equivalent degree. Executive functioning rather than gratification choice was related to academic achievement. These findings are important in that they affect the practical implications of the marshmallow task. That is, if the benefits of gratification delay depend on one's ecological context and/or can be better explained by other factors (e.g., executive functioning), then universal intervention efforts that merely involve training children to wait longer for two marshmallows might seem misdirected. Rather, intervention efforts should target those factors that operate most directly within each ecological context to support behavioral and academic functioning (e.g., adaptive coping with frustration, executive functioning). As debates over the marshmallow task continue, they highlight the need for scholars to be cautious when they consider what any particular study reveals about causal relationships and practical applications.

ACCULTURATION AND EMOTION

Adolescents growing up in immigrant families face special challenges as they negotiate a culture that differs from that of their parents (Cervantes & Cordova, 2011). For example, immigrant parents who do not speak English may expect their adolescents to assume more family responsibilities than is typical for adolescents in nonimmigrant families. Nonetheless, despite such acculturation-related stress, some studies have reported adolescents from immigrant families to have fewer behavior problems and higher academic achievement than those from families with U.S.-born parents, a phenomenon known as the "immigrant paradox" (Marks, Ejesi, & Coll, 2014). At the same time, a more nuanced picture regarding immigrant adolescents' emotional adjustment has emerged in a recent meta-analysis that separately examined their internalizing and externalizing problems (Tilley, Huey, Farver, Lai, & Wang, 2021). Although adolescents were found to indeed score lower for externalizing problems (e.g., aggression, delinquency) than their nonimmigrant peers, they scored higher on measures of internalizing problems (e.g., anxiety, depression).

Emotion processing by adolescents from immigrant families is virtually uncharted territory. One possibility is that these adolescents will adjust their emotions when interacting with their parents versus their American-born peers and teachers. Such **code-switching** with respect to emotion has been studied in adults, although not yet in adolescents. In an illustrative investigation, De Leersnyder, Kim, and Mesquita (2020) asked immigrant Korean American and immigrant Turkish Belgian adults to rate how they would feel when interacting with a member of their heritage culture or someone from their adopted country using a number of emotion-related scales (e.g., *interested, proud, worthless, afraid, irritable, bored*). Participants from both immigrant groups differed significantly in their emotional responses to the two types of co-interactants. Additional research has shown that Turkish Belgian adolescents' greater exposure to Belgian culture predicted greater similarity to non-immigrant Belgian adolescents when asked about their emotions experienced when interacting with peers (Jasini, De Leersnyder, Phalet, & Mesquita, 2019). Together, these studies point to a novel path for future research that examines immigrant adolescents' emotional experiences and behaviors and the potential relationship of these to their adjustment both at school and in the home.

GENDER AND EMOTION

Do Gender Differences Increase in Adolescence?

As reported in earlier chapters, Else-Quest and colleagues' (2006) meta-analysis of gender differences in temperament indicated that girls were rated slightly higher than boys on both fearfulness and positive approach, whereas boys were rated slightly higher on emotional intensity, difficulty, and surgency (a higher order factor that includes high-intensity pleasure). Moderation analysis failed to yield a significant age effect. Thus, presumably, these gender differences held for the young adolescents (up through 13 years of age) who participated in the studies that were included in their meta-analysis.

In contrast, Chaplin and Aldao (2013) found that gender differences in emotional expressivity were not always consistent across childhood and adolescence. In their meta-analytic investigation, boys showed slightly more anger, disgust, and contempt than girls in childhood (considered to extend from 6 to 12 years), but girls showed slightly more of these emotions than boys during adolescence (i.e., from 13 to 17 years). Although girls showed more expressions of sadness, fear, and anxiety than boys during childhood, no significant gender differences were found for adolescents. Results for adolescents' negative emotions appear to be counter-stereotypical, as males are often thought to show more anger than females and females are often thought to show more sadness than males. However, moderation analyses shed some light on Chaplin and Aldao's (2013) findings in that the pattern of gender effects differed across different social contexts. Boys expressed more anger, disgust, and contempt than did girls in interactional contexts involving peers. Girls expressed more sadness, fear, and anxiety when inter-acting with adults. Thus conformity to gender stereotypes regarding nega-tive emotions did occur, but only in particular contexts. In addition, the overall results suggested that conformity to one existing gender stereotype did increase in adolescence, with girls now being somewhat more emotion-ally expressive than boys overall.

Socialization and Stereotyping

Although a substantial number of studies have examined gender differences in adolescent emotional expressivity, research on emotion socialization of adolescents is almost nonexistent. Several studies have analyzed retrospec-tive reports by adolescents of their socialization experiences at younger ages but not contemporaneously. For example, Klimes-Dougan and colleagues (2007) asked 11- to 16-year-old adolescents to rate the extent to which their parents had responded to their sadness, fear, or anger with each of four socialization strategies: (1) reward (e.g., comforting, empathy, problem solv-ing), (2) punishment (e.g., mocking or disapproval), (3) overriding (i.e., dis-missing or distraction) or neglect (i.e., ignoring), and (4) magnifying (i.e., expressing the same emotion). Few differences were found in the socializa-tion of girls versus boys. Girls reported that their parents tried to override their fears more than did boys. Boys reported that their parents punished their anger more than did girls. Boys reported that their anger was punished by their fathers somewhat more than by their mothers. Parents themselves were also asked about their emotion socialization strategies, and again few differences were obtained. However, both mothers and fathers reported punishing anger in sons more than daughters. Considered in conjunction with the findings for anger expression described above, it appears that par-ents' punishment of sons' anger may result in boys' controlling of their anger when interacting with adults but not necessarily with peers.

The disjunction between parents' punishing responses to sons' anger and their sons' greater expression of anger with peers suggests that adoles-cents may become increasingly influenced by extrafamilial experiences. As adolescents become increasingly invested in peer-group relations, they may encounter behavioral norms that are more consistent with gender stereo-types and seek conformity to those norms, at least when they are operating outside the family. Research relevant to this proposal is sparse, but some studies do suggest that adolescents are cognizant of and influenced by the stereotypes to which they have been exposed. For example, Morelen, Zeman, Perry-Parrish, and Anderson (2012) found that 11- to 15-year-old girls from

Kenya and Ghana, as well as the United States, reported exerting more control over their expressions of anger than did boys, while boys reported more control over their sadness. Furthermore, adolescents may socialize each other via their responses to their peers' emotional expressions. Consistent with this proposal, Perry-Parrish and Zeman (2011) found that 12- to 13-year-old boys who were perceived as exerting greater control of their sadness expressions were more accepted by their classmates. No relationship was found between sadness expression and peer acceptance for girls. In general, peer socialization of emotion is a sadly understudied topic that merits increased research attention.

Is the Female Advantage in Emotion Understanding Maintained?

As described in Chapters 2 and 3, McClure (2000) found a small but significant female advantage in her meta-analytic investigation of facial expression processing in infants, children, and adolescents up to 18 years of age. The size of this advantage did not significantly differ across her age groups. A small female advantage also was obtained by Rivers et al. (2012), who examined additional aspects of emotion understanding within the conceptual framework of **emotional intelligence (EI)**, a framework described in more detail later in the chapter.

NEUROBIOLOGICAL UNDERPINNINGS

Although the brain reaches 95% of its adult size by the end of childhood, structural and functional changes are seen during adolescence and young adulthood (Somerville, 2016). In particular, increases in the volume of the amygdala continue (Morales & Fox, 2019). At the same time, the prefrontal cortex (PFC) also continues to develop, and its functional connectivity to the amygdala increases. However, the PFC's limited influence on behavior during adolescence is widely considered (in both the research literature and popular discourse) to be at least partly responsible for an upsurge in sensation seeking and risky behavior during this age period.

Brain Functioning and Risk Taking

Risk taking provides the focus of much current research on the adolescent brain. Currently two competing models have been proposed to present a more detailed picture of its neural underpinnings. The first is the **dual** systems model that was advanced by Laurence Steinberg over a decade ago (Steinberg, 2008). In its most recent iteration (Shulman et al., 2016), the model posits the presence of two relatively independent systems (i.e., the socioemotional control system and the cognitive control system) that follow different developmental trajectories during adolescence and into young adulthood. Whereas the influence of the cognitive control system increases linearly during this period, the socioemotional system develops according to an inverted U-shaped function, peaking in early to middle adolescence and declining in influence thereafter. Until the socioemotional system reaches a certain point in its decline, its influence overshadows that of the cognitive control system, enhancing the probability of adolescent risk taking. On the neurobiological level, the socioemotional system is importantly rooted in the functioning of the **reward system** that includes a number of anatomical structures, for example, the subcortical ventral striatum (which itself includes the nucleus accumbens). Reward system functioning is thought to be enhanced at the onset of puberty due to the release of puberty-related hormones. At this point, the reward system becomes sensitized, and the person becomes more focused on and responsive to rewards. These rewards can include the varied, complex, novel, and intense sensation levels that are often the goal of risk-taking behaviors (Zuckerman, 1994). However, according to the dual process model, after some time, the brain becomes somewhat desensitized to hormonal input (as represented by the declining tail of the socioemotional system's inverted U-shaped function). In the meantime, the PFC continues to mature, including the lateral portion of the PFC that is considered to be most involved in response inhibition. As indicated above, toward the end of adolescence, its influence may overpower that of the reward-seeking system, leading to the prediction that risk taking will spontaneously decline.

The **imbalance model** (Casey, 2015; Casey, Heller, Gee, & Cohen, 2019) is more elaborate but shares some key features with the dual systems model. Both highlight age-related shifts in interactions between cortical and subcortical areas of the brain. However, the imbalance model also focuses on developments within each region and direct effects that the subcortical and cortical areas have on each other and on the individual's behavior. Consistent with the model of brain development presented in Chapter 2 (Tottenham & Gabard-Durnam, 2017), functional connectivity between the areas is proposed to run principally from subcortical areas to the cortex during infancy and childhood, but this directionality reverses itself over the course of adolescence. This reverse in directionality is posited to involve a cascade of changes beginning with early strengthening and refinement of subcortical circuits (e.g., through myelination, pruning), leading to subcortical signaling to cortical areas that then stimulate the strengthening of cortical projections running in the reverse direction. Another difference between the two models is the greater emphasis placed on the role of the amygdala in the imbalance model. In this model, the amygdala's role is to attend to environmental cues so that their emotional significance can be determined (including their reward value). Therefore, connectivity between the amygdala and the ventral striatum (part of the reward system) is particularly important.

Evidence for both models comes from functional magnetic resonance imaging (fMRI) studies that map relationships between brain functioning and performance on tasks designed to tap the proposed underlying processes. For example, the emotional go/no-go task is a procedure often used to assess the balance between reward seeking and inhibitory control. As described earlier, in this task, participants are shown a sequence of emotion expressions one at a time and instructed to press a *go* button only when a particular target expression appears (e.g., the happy expression). In the sequence, target expressions predominate, so the challenge is to withhold responding when another expression is displayed. Using this procedure, Somerville, Hare, and Casey (2011) conducted a study with children (6- to 12-year-olds), adolescents (13- to 17-year-olds), and young adults (18- to 29-year-olds) using neutral expressions as the target and paired them with happy expressions. Results showed that adolescents performed more poorly than either the children or adults when required to withhold responding to a happy expression. In addition, analysis of fMRI data collected during the procedure indicated that activation of the ventral striatum (representing the reward system) was stronger for adolescents than for either of the other two age groups. Thus the findings suggest that the reward-seeking system outweighed inhibitory control at that age, as would be predicted by both models. Consistent with this emphasis on the reward system's importance, Telzer, Jorgensen, Prinstein, and Lindquist (2021) found that adolescents with greater ventral striatum reactivity were more susceptible to the influence of peer norms encouraging risky behavior.

One challenge to both models and their supporting research is the question of **ecological validity.** That is, both models would predict risk taking in the real world to decline after adolescence when, in fact, statistics show that risk-taking behaviors actually are more common in young adulthood than during adolescence (Willoughby, Good, Adachi, Hamza, & Tavernier, 2013). Addressing this apparent paradox, Shulman et al. (2016) point out that real-world risk taking is facilitated or constrained by additional factors that are important—but unrelated to brain functioning. More specifically, they note that most adolescents are constrained within their families and school environments and thus have many fewer opportunities to engage in risky behaviors compared with young adults. In addition, Do, Sharp, and Telzer (2020) have argued that when adolescents do take risks, it is not always due to their neurobiological immaturity but instead can reflect the result of a deliberate cognitive calculation of potential costs and benefits of engaging in the risky behavior. For example, an adolescent might determine that the reputational benefit of drinking at a party outweighs the possible cost of getting caught by his parents.

Autonomic Nervous System (ANS)

Having peaked at around 10 years of age, normative levels of resting respiratory sinus arrythmia (i.e., RSA, a measure of parasympathetic [PNS] control) do not appear to change significantly as children enter and proceed through adolescence (Dollar et al., 2020). Similarly, RSA reactivity to age-appropriate frustration tasks administered in the laboratory is not significantly altered.

Some studies of RSA function in adolescence have revealed an interesting pattern of dynamic changes over the course of an emotion episode. For example, Cui et al. (2015) measured adolescents' RSA activity as they engaged in a discussion with their primary caregivers (typically their mothers) about an anger episode that occurred when the caregivers had not been present. Adolescent participants also completed questionnaires on which they rated their ability to regulate sadness and anger, their prosocial behavior, and their aggressive behavior. Results showed that a U-shaped pattern (i.e., decreasing RSA followed by increasing RSA across the discussion time period) was associated with adolescents' higher ratings of their ability to regulate anger and sadness and with more prosocial behavior. The researchers interpreted this U-shaped pattern as reflecting an initial increase in arousal when recalling the angry event (reflected in the RSA decrease) followed by a rebound (i.e., increased RSA and restoration of PNS control) as the adolescent engaged in calmer discussion with his or her parent. Of particular note, this U-shaped pattern of RSA responding is similar to that obtained in a study of younger participants described in Chapter 3 (Miller et al., 2016) and can be considered to reflect a situationally appropriate reorganization of emotion responding.

Other studies have explored the question of whether differences in RSA activation may underlie individual differences in relations between family functioning and adolescents' problem behaviors. For example, Li,

Sturge-Apple, Martin, and Davies (2019) measured 12- to 14-year-old adolescents' RSA reactivity during a discussion with both parents on a topic of disagreement. Parents also completed a questionnaire measuring family instability (e.g., job loss, relationship dissolution, death, serious illness, residential changes). Adolescents completed a measure of internalizing and externalizing behaviors both at the initial visit and also 1 year later. Results showed that RSA reactivity moderated the relationship between family instability and externalizing problems—that is, only adolescents with higher RSA reactivity responded to greater family instability with increased externalizing problems between the two measurement time points.

Hypothalamic–Pituitary–Adrenal (HPA) System

Following a period of apparent HPA hyporesponsivity during childhood, cortisol levels increase during adolescence in conjunction with pubertal development (Gunnar, Wewerka, Frenn, Long, & Griggs, 2009). In addition, cortisol reactivity to at least some social stressors also increases, partly because parents no longer provide a buffering effect as they did during childhood (Hackman et al., 2018; Hostinar, Johnson, & Gunnar, 2015).

Reflecting the growing prominence of peer relations during adolescence, cortisol responding might also be associated with emotion-related peer problems or poor social adjustment (Murray-Close, 2013). One problem that has received some attention is peer victimization. Because cortisol reactivity is related to the perception of social-evaluative threat (Dickerson & Kemeny, 2004), one might expect that peer victimization would be associated with higher cortisol levels. Countering this expectation, the opposite pattern of results has been found in many studies. To illustrate, Knack, Jensen-Campbell, and Baum (2011) found a difference between victimized and nonvictimized adolescents in their cortical awakening response (CAR; i.e., the increase in cortisol level measured shortly after awakening). Victimized adolescents showed a blunted response, that is, less of an increase than their nonvictimized peers. In contrast, Kliewer (2006) found no difference in CAR between victimized and nonvictimized adolescents in a study of urban youth living in violence-prone neighborhoods. However, victims' overall cortisol levels were lower than those of nonvictimized peers. Focusing on relational aggression, Calhoun et al. (2014) reported blunted cortisol reactivity to a social stressor (i.e., the TSST) in a sample of relationally victimized adolescent girls. One possible explanation for these unexpected findings is that peer victimization is a form of chronic stress. In many individuals, chronic stress eventually produces blunted cortisol reactivity and lower overall cortisol levels (i.e., "burnout") because the HPA system ultimately responds to consistently higher cortisol by overregulating itself via a negative feedback loop (Gunnar & Adam, 2012). However, in some individuals, the system instead appears to reset itself such that higher levels are simply tolerated. The factors determining one or the other response to chronic stress are unclear.

EMOTION UNDERSTANDING

Normative development of emotion understanding during adolescence and beyond has received relatively little attention. For example, as described in Chapter 3, Harris and Pons's three-stage model does not extend into adolescence, and children are assumed to have achieved basic competence in emotion recognition and knowledge by 10 or 11 years of age. Perhaps for this reason, rather than focusing on normative development, some researchers have turned to investigating individual differences among adolescents as encompassed by the concept of **emotional intelligence (EI).**

What Is Emotional Intelligence (EI)?

The idea of emotion understanding as a form of intelligence was introduced in the early 1990s by Salovey and Mayer (1990), who developed a model and measurement system that they first applied to adults. Over the years, both model and measures have been modified so as to be applicable to younger ages. Still, the bulk of the research to date has involved adult participants and has examined relationships between **emotional intelligence (EI)** and successful adaptation primarily in domains of adult functioning (e.g., work, marriage). This research is reviewed in the next chapter. At the same time, there has also been interest in relations between EI and both socioemotional adjustment and academic success during adolescence. Therefore, an outline of the general model is presented here, along with related research involving adolescents.

The Ability EI Model

Salovey, Mayer, and their colleagues (e.g., Brackett, Rivers, Bertoli, & Salovey, 2016; Mayer, Caruso, & Salovey, 2016) conceive of EI as a set of abilities (e.g., ability to accurately perceive others' emotions) rather than a set of dispositional traits (e.g., one's inclination to be sociable or optimistic).

Furthermore, they argue that EI should be measured objectively rather than by participants' self-ratings of their own abilities. In these two ways, their model of **ability EI** is distinguished from other EI models and measures that have been subsequently proposed and used in some research (e.g., Bar-On, 2000). Within Mayer and Salovey's model, EI abilities are organized into four overarching *branches*, each encompassing a number of specific types of reasoning. To provide some examples (see Rivers et al., 2012), the first branch of abilities (i.e., *perceiving emotion*) includes identifying one's own emotions, perceiving others' emotions through their facial, vocal, verbal, and behavioral cues, and understanding that emotional displays may vary across cultures and contexts. For example, an emotionally intelligent person would understand that persons from some cultures might raise their voices and speak faster when angry, whereas persons from other cultures might lower their voices and speak very, very slowly. The second branch (i.e., *facilitating thought using emotion*) includes knowing what type of thinking would be facilitated by different types of emotion (e.g., happiness vs. anger). For example, an emotionally intelligent person would know that an appropriate level of anger (i.e., not too much and not too little) could help one formulate more effective strategies for addressing social injustice. The third branch (i.e., *understanding emotions*) includes understanding which situations are likely to elicit certain emotions, recognizing cultural differences in the value placed on certain emotions, and understanding how a person might feel in the future if circumstances were to change. For example, an emotionally intelligent person could understand that his or her partner would likely become less irritable if he or she were able to find less stressful employment. The fourth branch (i.e., *managing emotions*) includes understanding how one might most effectively manage one's own and others' emotions to achieve a desired outcome, monitoring one's emotional reactions to determine their reasonableness, and staying open to both pleasant and unpleasant feelings as needed. For example, an emotionally intelligent person would know when to use distraction as a regulation strategy and when to use reappraisal.

Measuring Ability EI

In order to assess individual differences in emotion-related abilities, the Mayer–Salovey–Caruso Emotional Intelligence Test (MSCEIT; Mayer, Salovey, Caruso, & Sitarenios, 2003) was developed for use with adults, followed by an age-appropriate Youth Version to be used with adolescents (MSCEIT-YV; Rivers et al., 2012). Items include rating the emotions portrayed in pictures, predicting what emotion would be felt in particular situational circumstances, indicating what emotion might help someone function most effectively or appropriately in a particular situation, and evaluating possible strategies for maintaining or changing one's emotions. Notably, there is considerable (but not complete) overlap between the set of abilities assessed in the MSCEIT or MSCEIT-YV and Harris and Pons's Test of Emotion Comprehension (TEC) described in Chapter 3. Both evaluate recognition of emotional cues, understanding of the causes of emotion, and understanding how emotions might be regulated; however, the particular cues, causes, and regulation strategies that are considered do differ substantially. For example, the TEC assumes that most prototypic facial expressions should be recognized by 5 years of age; thus it is not surprising that more complex and/or subtle expressive cues are used in the MSCEIT and MSCEIT-YV.

Is Ability EI Related to Adolescent Adjustment?

EI as measured by the MSCEIT or MSCEIT-YV has been related to measures of social and emotional adjustment in several studies of adolescents. To illustrate, Wols, Scholte, and Qualter (2015) found that lower scores predicted higher levels of loneliness in young adolescents. Lopes, Mestre, Guil, Kremenitzer, and Salovey (2012) found that lower scores were related to higher levels of disruptive behavior in high school students. Similarly, an association between lower MSCEIT-YV scores and higher levels of **callous unemotionality (CU;** i.e., lack of concern for others) was found in adolescents who were incarcerated in a juvenile detention center (Kahn, Ermer, Salovey, & Kiehl, 2016). In a meta-analysis of studies conducted in English or Spanish, Resurrección, Salguero, and Ruiz-Aranda (2014) reported negative associations between ability EI and adolescents' internalizing problems, depression, and anxiety.

A number of studies have examined EI and academic performance. In these studies, *trait EI* as well as ability EI may be measured. For example, Qualter, Gardner, Pope, Hutchinson, and Whiteley (2012) measured young British adolescents' ability EI (using the MSCEIT-YV) and trait EI (using the Emotional Quotient Inventory–Youth Version [EQi-YV]; Bar-On, 2000) and related these measures to the adolescents' school performance 4 years later. The EQi-YV asks participants to rate their own social and emotional abilities and dispositions (e.g., **emotional self-awareness**, social responsibility, optimism; Bar-On, 2000) and was considered by Qualter et al. (2012) to be a measure of emotional self-efficacy. Adolescents' cognitive abilities (i.e., verbal, quantitative, and nonverbal reasoning) were also measured at the start of the study. Results showed that higher ability EI predicted better academic performance for adolescents of both genders who had scored high on the cognitive ability measures at the beginning of the study. Higher ability EI also predicted higher academic performance for boys who had scored low on cognitive ability, although not for low-scoring girls. Trait EI made a smaller (but significant) contribution to academic performance, but only for boys. In a more recent meta-analytic study, MacCann et al. (2020) also found that ability EI contributed to academic performance more than trait EI, with scores on the understanding and management branches being most important.

The Female Advantage in EI

The female advantage in EI appears to increase across early adolescence. In Rivers et al.'s (2012) study, total MSCEIT-YV scores for girls and boys differed by only 2 points at 10 years of age. However, whereas scores for girls were progressively higher at 11, 12, and 13 years of age, scores for boys did not show a significant increase. When the ability branches were examined individually, girls scored higher than boys for each of the four branches. Thus the female gender advantage found for EI parallels findings for other measures of emotion understanding, for example those included in McClure's (2000) meta-analysis.

SUMMARY AND FINAL THOUGHTS

Adolescence is no longer considered to be typically characterized by "storm and stress." Still, adolescents do seem to experience somewhat more negative and less positive affect than reported by preadolescents and adults. By some measures, they also appear to be moodier than adults. However, it is important to emphasize that adolescents' average affect ratings typically remain in the positive range throughout this developmental period.

Adolescent temperament (i.e., dispositional tendencies) is associated with behavioral adjustment. In particular, high levels of negative emotionality and low EC are associated with a range of maladaptive outcomes (e.g., risk taking, depression, anxiety, hyperactivity, antisocial behavior). Investigations that distinguish among different negative emotions may lead to a better understanding of the relationship between temperament and particular forms of maladjustment. Investigations of contextual variables (e.g., exposure to stressors) that may mediate or moderate relations between temperament and adjustment are also important. For example, social involvement during adolescence may mitigate the relationship between early BI and later anxiety.

Adolescents' attachment status is conceptualized in terms of their current state of mind regarding attachment relations in general (i.e., not only with their parents). Securely attached adolescents place a high value on attachment relations, even if their own past experiences may have been somewhat troubled. Still, parental supportiveness during adolescence also is associated with a secure state of mind. Attachment security has been associated with several measures of positive social and emotional adjustment.

Parent–child conflicts peak in the earlier years of adolescence and often involve disagreements about what decisions should be left to the young person's personal choice. Not surprisingly, higher levels of negative affect during such discussions are associated with lower levels of mutual satisfaction with the outcome of the discussion. Higher levels of conflict are related to adjustment difficulties (e.g., internalizing problems, externalizing problems, academic difficulties), especially when the adolescent does not receive support for the emotions he or she expresses.

The advent of social media and texting technologies have revolutionized young persons' interactions with their peers. Adolescents report both positive and negative experiences with these forms of social communication. Importantly, negative effects appear to be stronger for those who have a poor self-image or difficulties with emotion regulation or who have been victimized by peers.

Regarding emotion regulation, laboratory studies generally find that adolescents' ability to deliberately down-regulate their negative affect when instructed to do so increases across this developmental period. Theoretically, this is presumably tied to an increase in EC. However, studies of EC outside the laboratory suggest that the development of EC across adolescence may not follow a linear trajectory. This may be partly because a variety of factors can determine whether adolescents actually apply their control capabilities in their daily lives. Reappraisal is generally considered to be an effective method for down-regulating negative affect, and its use appears to increase across adolescence. In contrast, habitual suppression of emotional expression is considered to be maladaptive but may be desirable in some circumstances. Other response strategies have also been identified (e.g., distraction, trying to relax). Considered together as a group, the use of these strategies appears to increase across adolescence. Adolescents also increase the number of different response strategies in their repertoires. A larger response repertoire allows for greater flexibility in choosing the strategy most appropriate for one's particular circumstances and emotion goals. Delay of gratification may be an index of emotion regulation that predicts adaptive functioning by adolescents in some (but not all) environmental contexts.

Adolescents from immigrant families often show fewer externalizing problems (e.g., aggression, delinquency) and higher academic achievement than those from nonimmigrant families. However, they also may experience more internalizing problems (e.g., symptoms of anxiety or depression). Exploring their emotion processing (including emotion code-switching) would provide a profitable avenue for future research.

Adolescent girls are slightly more expressive than adolescent boys. At the same time, gender differences reflecting conformity to gender stereotypes may be context dependent, for example, greater expression of anger by boys when interacting with their peers rather than with their parents. Peers may play an increasingly important role as socializing agents. A small female advantage in emotion understanding is seen in adolescents.

Two models of brain functioning have been proposed to explain adolescent risk-taking behavior. Further research will be necessary to adjudicate between them. However, studies comparing adolescents and young adults suggest that risk-taking behavior in adolescence is (fortunately) limited by fewer risk-taking opportunities afforded within most adolescents' environments. Studies of dynamic changes in RSA across emotion episodes illustrate the close relationship between ANS functioning and the body's preparation for physical action. Emotions are not always accompanied by the same pattern of physical action or any necessary action at all. Perhaps for this reason, as discussed in the next chapter, investigations seeking to pinpoint unique emotion-specific patterns of ANS activity have been largely unsuccessful. The HPA system continues to be responsive to social stressors, particularly those involving social evaluation. However, chronic stress is thought to often result in blunted cortisol responding. Studies that find such blunted responding in peer-victimized adolescents are consistent with this expectation.

Studies of EI dominate the literature on emotion understanding in adolescence. Ability measures of EI focus exclusively on the person's ability to recognize emotions, understand their causes and consequences, and understand how to utilize and manage them. Higher ability EI has been related to better academic performance and better behavioral and emotional adjustment in adolescence.

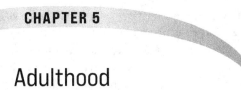

CHAPTER 5

Adulthood
18–65 Years

As noted in Chapter 1, there has been limited interaction between scholars who focus on adult emotion and those who focus on development. Many have bemoaned this estrangement, but efforts to bridge the divide have been few and far between. This chapter constitutes an attempt to represent current approaches to studying adult emotion and findings in areas that roughly correspond to topics addressed in previous chapters (e.g., emotional experience, temperament/personality, emotion regulation, attachment, emotion understanding). Adults' functioning in these areas builds upon their experiences earlier in development. Considering both developmental and adult-oriented approaches to the same emotion-related topics hopefully will constitute a positive step toward closing the gap between them in the minds of readers.

EMOTIONAL EXPERIENCE

One of the most exciting developments in recent decades has been the advent of world surveys that provide a window into the daily emotional experiences of persons across the globe. These surveys assess three components of **subjective well-being (SWB)**: positive affect, negative affect, and life satisfaction (Diener, 1984). Affect is typically measured by asking participants to indicate whether or not they experienced each of four positive and six negative emotion-related states or behaviors on the previous day, for example, happiness, enjoyment, worry, sadness, stress, fear, depression. Life satisfaction is measured by asking participants to simply rate their satisfaction with their current lives on an 11-point scale. The simplicity of this methodology makes it possible to recruit large numbers of participants of varying ages and from varied backgrounds, including those who might otherwise be unwilling or unable to participate due to competing demands on their time, limited education, or limited availability of or facility with technology. Of course, there are tradeoffs in that such surveys include minimal information on the contextual circumstances surrounding affective experiences. Still, they offer a unique opportunity to extend the participant pool well beyond the WEIRD (i.e., Western, educated, industrialized, rich, and democratic) populations that have been most often studied in the past.

Are Most People Happy?

The Gallup Organization has instituted worldwide surveys that have provided a database for researchers studying SWB. For example, Jebb, Morrison, Tay, and Diener (2020) analyzed data from participants living in 166 countries and ranging in age from 15 to 99 years. The countries themselves were grouped into 10 regional/cultural categories: Anglo (e.g., United Kingdom, United States, Australia, Canada, New Zealand), Latin Europe (e.g., France, Italy, Portugal, Israel), Germanic Europe (e.g., Austria, Belgium, Switzerland, Germany), Nordic Europe (e.g., Norway, Estonia, Lithuania), Eastern Europe (e.g., Russia, Kazakhstan, Greece, Poland), Latin America, Confucian Asia (e.g., China, Japan, Mongolia, Singapore), Southern Asia (e.g., India, Afghanistan, Philippines, Thailand), Arab (e.g., Turkey, Egypt, Palestinian territories, Iraq), and sub-Saharan Africa. In order to maximize the representativeness of participant samples within each country, in-person interviews were conducted in areas where access by phone was minimal; otherwise, surveys were conducted over the phone.

Of particular relevance to emotional development, Jebb et al. (2020) analyzed the affect and life satisfaction data for each regional/cultural category separately and for all regional/cultural categories combined to investigate age differences within their sample. Collapsing across regions, the investigators observed minimal differences across their age range for either life satisfaction or negative affect. In contrast, global positive affect declined with age. Still, at all ages, scores for positive affect were higher than scores for negative affect in all regions. In fact, both life satisfaction and positive affect were above the neutral point for all regions but one (Eastern Europe), and negative affect was below the neutral point for all regions. Readers should note that positive affect rather than life satisfaction served as their best measure of happiness, as the two measures are sometimes confused in the popular press.

Focusing specifically on results for the Anglo region (the region that includes the United States), Jebb et al. (2020) reported that life satisfaction and positive affect were stable across age and higher than those for the entire set of regions considered as a single group (i.e., the global scores). Negative affect scores declined for respondents between 40 and 80 years. This pattern of decline is generally similar to that found in several studies of aging, reviewed in the next chapter.

The results obtained by Jebb et al. (2020) are consistent with those from other related studies (e.g., Diener, Diener, Choi, & Oishi, 2018) and suggest that SWB is relatively strong and stable across ages and cultures. In interpreting these findings, Diener, Diener, et al. (2018) proposed that SWB (particularly positive affect) may be a default state that most people experience as long as their basic needs are being met. From an evolutionary perspective, this predisposition could be advantageous in that it promotes sociability and the accrual of social capital. That is, people who are happy and satisfied are more congenial social partners and thus develop a wider circle of friends and relations who can provide help and support when needed. At the same time, additional analyses of the Gallup data (Diener, Seligman, Choi, & Oishi, 2018) demonstrated boundary conditions for experiencing SWB. High positive affect was not maintained for individuals in circumstances of extreme stress (e.g., food shortages, homelessness, health problems, criminal victimization).

EMOTIONAL FACIAL EXPRESSIONS

As emphasized in several previous chapters, the relationship between facial expressions and emotion remains the subject of vigorous debate. Relevant studies of infants and children have already been described (see Chapters 2 and 3), but much of the research on this topic has involved investigations of adults in both Western and non-Western cultures that address the question of universality—that is, are there indeed universal facial expressions of emotion and, if so, how many are there? Research involving participants from Western cultures is described here, and research involving participants from non-Western cultures is reviewed later in the chapter.

Expression Recognition Studies

The bulk of this research involves studying observers' recognition of facial expressions posed by models who may be instructed on how to express an emotion (e.g., to reproduce the prototypic expressions described by discrete emotion theorists). Alternatively, models—especially trained actors—may be asked to portray emotions as they see fit. In this case, their posed expressions are sometimes curated by asking naïve observers to identify the intended emotion; those expressions that are identified as intended by a majority of judges are used in further research. A smaller body of research involves studying expressions that are spontaneously produced during laboratory procedures or "in the wild" (i.e., outside the laboratory).

When recognition studies utilize prototypic facial expressions and ask participants to choose among a set of emotion labels (i.e., emotion names), then participants typically achieve high levels of "accuracy"; that is, they make choices that conform to predictions derived from basic emotion theories. For example, in a meta-analysis in which 95% of the studies used this **forced-choice** methodology, Elfenbein and Ambady (2002) found recognition rates exceeding 70% for expressions of the Big Six emotions (i.e., happiness, surprise, anger, sadness, fear, and disgust) when the expressions were judged by members of the poser's own culture. Recognition rates exceeded 55% (still well over chance) when the expressions were judged by members of a different culture. However, critics have argued that emotion identification in real life does not involve making a forced choice among emotions (e.g., Barrett et al., 2019; Nelson & Russell, 2013; Russell, 1994) and that research participants may use procedure-specific strategies to generate correct guesses about expressions that they do not actually recognize (e.g., a process of elimination among the emotion options; DiGirolamo & Russell, 2017; Nelson et al., 2018). Recognition studies that require participants to generate their own labels for posed facial expressions produce lower rates of recognition, even when researchers are generous in their scoring of responses (e.g., counting *pity* as a correct identification for the sadness expression). For example, Izard (1971) reported an average recognition rate of 84.95% using a forced-choice procedure and an average rate of 68.85% using free labeling. (See Russell, 1994, for a detailed review of recognition studies.)

One significant limitation of recognition studies is their potential lack of **ecological validity**. This means that the studies lack evidence that the expressions presented to participants are actually produced in real life episodes of their presumed corresponding emotions. Studies of spontaneous expressions produced in response to real emotion elicitors are arguably more ecologically valid but have their own set of serious challenges. For example, laboratory studies that attempt to elicit genuine emotions may not be able to present sufficiently powerful stimuli (e.g., for anger or fear) because of legitimate ethical constraints. In addition, elicitors may evoke different emotions and/or intensities of emotion across individuals, and this must be considered when interpreting results. Although self-reports of emotion experience can be obtained in laboratory studies, this may not be possible when studying expressive behavior produced in the natural environment. Furthermore, if social or personal norms of expression are operating in a particular situation, then expressive suppression or masking may occur. Lastly, interpreting the results of such studies may be difficult if the spontaneous expressions have not been objectively coded so that their morphology can be compared across studies and with the prototypes commonly used in recognition research. Still, studies of naturally occurring spontaneous expressions have made a significant contribution, especially in pointing to important directions for future research.

Studies of Spontaneous Expressions

In one of the first modern studies of spontaneous facial expressions, Kraut and Johnston (1979) observed bowlers' responses after scoring a strike, presumably a happy event. Their findings showed that smiles rarely occurred unless the bowler was socially engaged (i.e., looking at their fellow players), suggesting that smiles were serving as social signals rather than purely spontaneous expressions of experienced emotion. Kraut and Johnston's study set the stage for further investigations of naturally occurring responses during episodes of presumably positive emotion (i.e., during successes or wins) and negative emotions (i.e., during failures or losses) in sporting events (e.g., soccer, judo, tennis). For example, Ruiz-Belda, Fernández-Dols, Carrera, and Barchard (2003) took Kraut and Johnston's study a step further by interviewing bowlers and soccer fans to obtain self-reports of their emotional experiences to be compared with their smiling behavior. Results confirmed the original findings in that happy bowlers and soccer fans were significantly more likely to smile when socially engaged than when not attending to their companions. These findings are consistent with the conclusion that smiling is a behavior determined by multiple factors, only one of which is the corresponding experience of emotion.

Other research on emotional expression in natural settings has shown that adults (as well as children; see Chapter 3) produce very similar expressions at moments of high-intensity positive or negative affect (e.g., Aviezer,

Trope, & Todorov, 2012; Israelashvili, Hassin, & Aviezer, 2019). These expressions (mostly grimaces) typically include brows lowered, eyes squeezed shut, mouth stretched wide either horizontally or vertically, and sometimes a slight smile. They can often be seen in pictures appearing in the popular press (e.g., winners or losers in tennis matches). Observers who are asked to rate such expressions on affect scales are unable to distinguish between those occurring during positive or negative events. However, when the facial expressions are accompanied by contextual cues (e.g., body postures or the emotion-eliciting stimulus), then such discriminations are made more readily, demonstrating the utility of providing multimodal emotion cues in studies of emotion perception.

Spontaneous emotional expressions have also been studied in laboratory settings that provide more control over the emotion stimulus and the opportunity to obtain self-reports of participants' emotional experience (Reisenzein, Studtmann, & Horstmann, 2013). In these studies, films are often used to evoke emotional responses in participants. For example, Jakobs, Manstead, and Fischer (2001) and Gross, John, and Richards (2000) both analyzed the facial expressions of college-age students who viewed film clip episodes designed to elicit sadness (e.g., showing a dying mother or a distraught mother at a funeral). Facial expressions of sadness were coded by Jakobs and colleagues (2001), whereas Gross and colleagues (2000) used a more global multimodal measure of sadness expression. Participants provided self-reports of their sadness feelings in both studies. Data analyses showed a significant relationship between sadness expression and sadness experience in the study by Gross et al. (2000) but not in that by Jakobs et al. (2001). These findings are again consistent with the emerging consensus that emotional expression does not always or exclusively involve facial behavior. Confirming this consensus, in a set of meta-analyses that included both naturalistic and laboratory studies of the Big Six emotions, Durán, Reisenzein, and Fernández-Dols (2017) reported that the average correlation between facial expression and self-reported experience was .35 (a moderate relationship) and the average proportion of participants who showed the predicted expression was .23.

One interesting additional finding in Jakobs et al.'s (2001) study of sadness facial expressions involved differences in expressive behavior across experimental conditions that varied in terms of social engagement. In particular, participants showed more facial sadness when viewing the film alone than when in the presence of a fellow viewer (either a friend or a stranger). This finding for sadness stands in contrast to Kraut and Johnston's (1979) study in which smiling occurred most often during social engagement. In interpreting their results, Jakobs et al. (2001) suggested that social display rules regarding public expressions of sadness might have mitigated their expression by participants in their study. Considered together, these studies of smiling and sadness illustrate the importance of exercising caution when generalizing from studies that include only one type of emotional expression or one situational context.

As noted earlier, another implication of the above studies is that non-facial behaviors (e.g., body movements and postures, vocalizations) may also serve as important cues for communicating emotion. Due to the histori-cal emphasis on facial expression in emotion research, systematic investiga-tion of these has lagged considerably. An additional impediment to broad-ening the field of investigation to include nonfacial activity has been the lack of systems for objectively describing and coding such actions (i.e., a system that would correspond to Ekman et al.'s [2002] anatomically based Facial Action Coding System [FACS]). Still, research on vocal expression is emerging as a promising area of research within which the familiar debates about universality are currently taking place (e.g., Barrett & Gendron, 2016; Cordaro, Keltner, Tshering, Wangchuk, & Flynn, 2016; Cowen, Elfenbein, Laukka, & Keltner, 2019; Cowen, Laukka, Elfenbein, Liu, & Keltner, 2019; Hoemann et al., 2019; Laukka & Elfenbein, 2021).

FROM TEMPERAMENT TO PERSONALITY

Temperament and personality are distinct but overlapping areas of schol-arship from both a historical and a conceptual perspective. Both seek to explain individual differences in dispositional traits that include emotion-related characteristics. Both seek to apply their theoretical frameworks to a broad age range. However, historically, they originated in the study of differ-ent points in the lifespan (infancy for temperament, adulthood for person-ality) and consequently differ to some degree in how they characterize the individual differences they investigate. Still, consistency between the two approaches is impressive.

How Are Temperament and Personality Constructs Related?

In attempting to bridge the conceptual gap between temperament and personality, Rothbart and her colleagues (e.g., Rothbart, Ahadi, & Evans, 2000) have made a number of age-appropriate adaptations to tempera-ment measures designed to capture the developmental emergence of new temperamental features. At the adult level, the result is an age-appropriate measure (Adult Temperament Questionnaire; ATQ) that maps well onto the most predominant personality framework currently in use, that is, the **Big Five/Five-Factor model** (McCrae & Costa, 2003; McCrae & John, 1992).

The Big Five factors include *Conscientiousness, Intellect/Openness to Experience, Extraversion, Agreeableness,* and *Neuroticism* (McCrae & John, 1992). To illustrate, a person who is efficient and reliable, curious and imaginative, enthusiastic and outgoing, as well as sympathetic and trusting, would score high on the first four factors. A person who is anxious and touchy would score high on Neuroticism. The Big Five factors are both conceptually and statistically related to the ATQ factors of *Effortful Control* (EC), *Orienting Sensitivity, Extraversion, Affiliativeness,* and *Aggressive and Nonaggressive Negative Affect,* respectively (Evans & Rothbart, 2007). Each Big Five factor includes a number of constituent traits (termed *facets*), some of which are emotional in nature (McCrae & John, 1992). For example, Extraversion includes positive emotion, as well as warmth, gregariousness, assertiveness, activity, and excitement seeking. Neuroticism includes anxiety, angry hostility, and depression, as well as impulsivity, self-consciousness, and vulnerability.

Individual Differences and Normative Changes

Personality appears to be relatively stable over time in terms of the rank ordering of individuals within a study sample. To illustrate, a person who scores higher than the average score for Agreeableness at Time 1 is likely to score higher than average for Agreeableness at Time 2 even if the average score itself increases or decreases over time. In a meta-analytic modeling study, Anusic and Schimmack (2016) reported correlations of approximately .60 for scores assessed at intervals that could range from approximately 4 years to 15 years. Intervals shorter than 4 years generated even higher correlations. However, there is some controversy about the age at which significant stability begins to be seen and whether stability dips, peaks, or plateaus within certain age ranges (see Costa, McCrae, & Löckenhoff, 2019, for discussion). Regarding the normative trajectory of development, Costa et al. (2019) reported a general consensus across studies that the average score for Neuroticism declines throughout adulthood while Conscientiousness and Agreeableness increase. Although there is less agreement regarding Openness and Extraversion, studies using the NEO Personality Inventory developed by Costa and McCrae (1992) show that both decline across adulthood.

Several proposals have been advanced to account for both rank-order stability across individuals and normative developmental changes within individuals, although none have garnered incontrovertible support. These include genetic factors and niche selection (i.e., choosing environments compatible with one's personality) for rank-order stability and social investment for normative changes across development. According to the social investment principle (Roberts & Nickel, 2017), as individuals assume progressively more adult responsibilities, they correspondingly become more inclined to develop dispositions that facilitate their success, for example, Agreeableness and Conscientiousness rather than Neuroticism. Costa et al. (2019) favor more evolutionary and biologically based explanations, although these are not necessarily incompatible with functional explanations such as social investment.

Personality and Emotional Experience

The inclusion of emotion-related facets within several of the Big Five factors implies that personality should be related to emotion experience in daily life. Although this possibility has not been extensively studied, several investigations have indeed examined relations between personality and emotional experiences. Perhaps surprisingly, these studies generally focus on the higher order personality factors rather than the emotion-related facets themselves. Still, some interesting findings have been obtained. For example, Leger, Charles, Turiano, and Almeida (2016) analyzed daily diary data from more than 2,000 adults (ages 30–84 years) who rated their positive and negative affect for the day along with the occurrence of stressors (e.g., having an argument, something bad happening to a friend or relative, a stressful event at work). In addition, participants completed a personality measure assessing the Big Five factors. Among their complex results, the investigators found that Neuroticism was related to a greater number of reported stressors and more daily negative affect. In a subsequent part of the study, the investigators also obtained participants' appraisals of how much control they had over each stressor, as well as their appraisal of how much risk the stressor posed for various aspects of their lives (e.g., finances, relations with others, personal health). Data analyses suggested that the influence of Neuroticism on stressor-related negative affect was partially mediated by the person's appraisal of the stressor's significance (i.e., the risk it imposed) and her or his perceived control over the stressor.

ADULT ATTACHMENT

According to attachment theory, adults' state of mind regarding attachment relations should continue to influence their emotional and social functioning. However, investigating this proposal using the Adult Attachment

Interview (AAI) can be challenging, because conducting and coding interviews is highly labor intensive and requires special training and certification. Consequently, many researchers have turned to alternative measures (Mikulincer & Shaver, 2016).

One widely used instrument is a self-report questionnaire that assesses participants' levels of attachment security, avoidance, and anxiety: the Experiences in Close Relationships (ECR) scale (Brennan, Clark, & Shaver, 1998) and its revised version (Fraley, Waller, & Brennan, 2000). Using this measure, participants rate their level of agreement with a number of statements representing secure, insecure–avoidant, or insecure–anxious attachment (e.g., "It helps to turn to my partner in times of need"; "I try to avoid getting too close to my partner"; "I need a lot of reassurance that I am loved by my partner"). Findings in studies using this questionnaire are generally consistent with predictions made based on attachment theory. For example, adults with insecure attachment styles are found to be less able than secure adults to effectively seek and utilize emotional support when stressed or distressed (Mikulincer & Shaver, 2016).

Other research has shown that adults' attachment status also is related to some aspects of emotion processing. To illustrate, in a study of emotion regulation, Pereg and Mikulincer (2004) measured Israeli college students' attachment status via a questionnaire similar to the ECR and later primed them for either negative or neutral affect by having them read a neutral or tragic news story. Following priming, participants were shown a set of positive, neutral, and negative news headlines and then—unexpectedly—were asked to recall them. Results showed that students who had scored higher on attachment security remembered more positive than neutral headlines in both priming conditions, whereas participants who scored higher on attachment anxiety remembered fewer positive than neutral headlines. The researchers interpreted these findings as suggesting that securely attached adults are more able to engage in mood repair strategies after experiencing negative affect.

As noted earlier, adult attachment is conceptualized as resulting from the accumulation of life experiences with ones' parents, as well as other persons with whom one has significant emotional relationships. Still, the role of sensitive parenting is deemed of particular importance, and this raises questions about the origins of sensitive parenting. One plausible hypothesis is embedded in the research on **intergenerational transmission** of attachment and parenting, that is, the hypothesis that parents' own adult attachment status influences their parenting sensitivity, which in turn influences their offspring's attachment (Main, Kaplan, & Cassidy, 1985; van IJzendoorn & Bakermans-Kranenburg, 2019). Yet systematic evaluation of the intergenerational transmission hypothesis suggests that sensitivity is only part of the attachment story. To illustrate, Verhage et al. (2016) conducted a meta-analytic study that demonstrated significant associations between parents' adult attachment status and the attachment status of their offspring. One piece of good news was that transmission of security was more likely than transmission of insecurity; a substantial number of insecure parents were able to develop a secure relationship with their own children. However, a path analysis showed only partial mediation of intergenerational transmission by parental sensitivity. That is, parental sensitivity could not completely account for the relationship between parents' and offspring's attachment status. This **transmission gap** has led some researchers to suggest that parenting factors other than sensitivity (e.g., autonomy support and warmth) must also serve as mediators of intergenerational attachment transmission and should be considered in future research (van IJzendoorn & Bakermans-Kranenburg, 2019).

SOCIALIZATION OF EMOTION-RELATED PARENTING BEHAVIORS

Sensitive Parenting

Although sensitivity may not fully account for the attachment transmission gap, it nonetheless is an important parenting factor influencing infants' emotional development (see Chapter 2). Thus investigating possible intergenerational origins of sensitive parenting is itself of interest. Toward this end, Leerkes, Bailes, and Augustine (2020) conducted a three-wave study in which both African American and European American expectant mothers recalled how their own mothers had responded to their distress during childhood in Wave 1. For Wave 2, when their infants were 6 months old, mothers viewed video recordings of their infants' distress and were assigned scores representing both sensitive infant-oriented responses (e.g., acknowledgment of baby's distress, empathy) and insensitive mother-oriented responses (e.g., annoyance at the crying, minimizing its importance). For Wave 3, when the infants were 14 months old, mothers were assigned a score representing their level of sensitive parenting based on researchers' observations of how they responded to their toddlers' distress during a laboratory visit and also their scores on the Coping with Toddlers' Negative Emotions Scale (Spinrad et al., 2007), an age-appropriate version of the CCNES (described in Chapter 3). Path analyses showed that higher levels of remembered insensitive responding (Wave 1) were related to higher levels of insensitive mother-oriented responding to their own infant's distress (Wave 2), which were negatively related to sensitive parenting in Wave 3. Thus it appeared that insensitive parenting recalled (and presumably experienced) by the mother engendered her own insensitive behaviors, exemplifying the emotion socialization process of demonstrative modeling (see Chapter 3). This pattern held for both the African American and European American mothers.

Other Measures of Parenting Quality

A number of investigations have examined intergenerational transmission of other aspects of parenting associated with better or worse child outcomes. For example, Shaffer, Burt, Obradović, Herbers, and Masten (2009) studied two generations of the same families to assess associations between first-generation (G1) and second-generation (G2) parenting quality and possible mediation of the association by G2's social competencies assessed at 10 and 20 years of age. Parenting quality was evaluated by raters who conducted interviews with participants and focused on expression of positive feelings, as well as age-appropriate disciplinary techniques. Social competence was assessed via both interviews with the G2 participants and peer ratings of qualities such as friendliness and ability to get along with others. Results of path analyses indicated that higher quality G1 parenting was related to greater social competence by their children (i.e., G2), whose social competence was significantly related to the higher quality of their own (i.e., G2) parenting.

Providing another example, Campbell and Gilmore (2007) studied the relationship between both mothers' and fathers' self-reported parenting styles and their recollections of the styles used by their own parents. Participants completed appropriately worded versions of the Parental Authority Questionnaire (PAQ; Buri, 1991; Reitman, Rhode, Hupp, & Altobello, 2002) to represent their own parenting styles and those of their mothers and their fathers. The PAQ includes subscales for authoritative, authoritarian, and permissive parenting. As conceptualized by Baumrind (1971), **authoritative** parents are emotionally warm but also exert appropriate control over their children, **authoritarian** parents are controlling but not warm, and **permissive** parents are warm but exert little control. Discussion of these well-known parenting styles (including contemporary conceptual extensions, newer measures, and debates about their cultural applicability) is beyond the scope of this volume. However, research has generally shown that authoritative parenting leads to the best outcomes for European American children, followed by authoritarian and, finally, permissive parenting. The latter two are associated with behavioral and emotional difficulties. In their own study, Campbell and Gilmore (2007) found significant intergenerational transmission of both authoritarian and permissive parenting; that is, parents who themselves adopted each of these styles also reported predominant use of the same style by their own parents. However, parents who utilized authoritative parenting were not significantly likely to have had authoritative parents themselves. The authors suggest that the latter findings may reflect a decline over the years in the acceptability of authoritarian parenting (at least in Australia, where the study took place). It appears that a substantial number of adults who experienced authoritarian or permissive parenting themselves rejected those styles in favor of one that affords the gratification of a warmer parent–child relationship. However, one limitation of Campbell and Gilmore's study was the fact that parenting styles for both generations were reported by the same person. Thus **common method variance** across measures could artificially increase the likelihood of finding a statistical relationship between them.

This limitation was circumvented by Neppl, Conger, Scaramella, and Ontai (2009), who objectively measured harsh parenting in two generations of parents (G1 and G2) and examined possible mediation of their association by G2s' externalizing behaviors. When G2s were adolescents, they and their parents (i.e., G1s) were videotaped while engaging in a family interaction task. Observers rated G1 parents on three features of harsh parenting having emotional overtones: (1) hostility (hostile, critical, rejecting behavior), (2) antisocial behavior (signs of socially irresponsible behavior), and (3) angry coercion (threats, angry attempts to control the other person). Adolescents' (G2s) externalizing behavior was assessed via a self-report questionnaire with items pertaining to rule breaking, criminal activity, unsafe driving, and substance use. When G2s were young adults, they participated with their own children in a difficult puzzle task, and their own parenting behavior was scored for hostility, antisocial tendencies, and angry coercion. At the same time, they also reported on their current levels of criminal activity, unsafe driving, and substance use. Data analyses showed that G1 harsh parenting directed toward G2 during adolescence was significantly associated with G2 harsh parenting at a later date. In addition, this relationship was shown to be mediated by the G2s' own externalizing behavior. Presumably, one generation's harsh parenting generates a similar suite of behavioral tendencies in their children that may be manifested in their children's own future parenting behaviors.

In summary, a number of studies have demonstrated significant intergenerational transmission of negative parenting styles, and some mediating factors have been identified. However, moderating factors that enable adults to break the chain of transmission merit further research attention.

EMOTION REGULATION

Emotion regulation has been an important theme running through the developmental literature reviewed in earlier chapters. At several points, James Gross's process model of emotion regulation was referenced, but a more complete description has not yet been provided. Because the bulk of the research by Gross, his colleagues, and many other scholars has focused on adult functioning, that more complete description has been reserved for this chapter.

As noted in Chapter 3, making a conceptual distinction between emotion and emotion regulation has long been problematic. Indeed, as Gross's model has been revised over the years, the difference between regulated and unregulated emotion has become increasingly blurred (see Braunstein et al., 2017). However, descriptions of the model often present a somewhat simplified version in which a clear distinction can be easily made by focusing on strategies that are deliberate and require some degree of EC. This approach is followed here. However, readers inclined to wrestle with the nuanced concept of implicit emotion regulation (and to consider whether it implies that regulation should be conceptualized as reorganization) are directed to Braunstein et al. (2017) for further details.

James Gross's Model

The process model of emotion regulation is best described by first presenting Gross's model of the emotion process itself (Gross, 2015a, 2015b; McRae & Gross, 2020). Consistent with the current views of many researchers, the emotion process is considered to involve four steps: (1) encountering a situation, (2) attending to various features of that situation, (3) appraising how the situation relates to one's own goals, and (4) responding to the situation with emotional feelings, physiological responses, and/or observable behaviors. Emotion regulation is defined as "activation of a goal to modify the unfolding emotional [process]" (Gross, 2015a, p. 11). This activation can take place during any of the four steps and even before an emotion-eliciting situation is physically encountered (e.g., by avoiding a situation that is expected to elicit unwanted emotions). In this last case, presumably one is encountering the situation in one's mind and engaging in anticipatory emotion regulation.

Five categories (or **families**) of **emotion regulation strategies** are outlined in Gross's model, and specific strategies within each family are identified (Gross, 2015a, 2015b; McRae & Gross, 2020). First, **situation selection** refers to a family of strategies that enable one to control (at least in part) the emotion-eliciting situations to which one is exposed. For example, you may choose to attend or to avoid your cousin's wedding after learning that a particularly disliked uncle will be there. Second, **situation modification** refers to a family of strategies that involve altering some feature of the situation so as to modulate your expected emotional response. For example, you might ask your cousin to seat you at a different table from your narcissistic uncle. Third, **attentional deployment** refers to a family of strategies that involve modulating your emotion by attending or disattending to particular features of the situation. For example, you might focus on talking to your beloved grandmother rather than your disliked uncle. If he traps you in a corner, you might distract yourself by thinking about something else while he bloviates. Fourth, **cognitive change** refers to a family of strategies that involve accepting, reinterpreting, or reevaluating the situation. For example, you might resign yourself to having to listen to your uncle's bloviating for some period of time but remember that this is an infrequent necessity. **Cognitive reappraisal** is a specific strategy within this family that involves reinterpreting or reevaluating the emotion elicitor. For example, you may find that your uncle occasionally has something interesting to say and thus become less distressed when he attempts to engage you. The fifth family of regulation strategies is **response modulation,** which involves suppressing or altering responses that you might be spontaneously inclined to make. For example, you might refrain from expressing contempt as you listen to your uncle and/ or slow your breathing in an attempt to remain calm.

In previous chapters, developmental research focusing on one or more of these types of strategies has been described (e.g., reappraisal, suppression, distraction). In addition, the role of EC and other factors influencing the deployment and effectiveness of various strategies by children and adolescents were considered. However, the bulk of the research exploring Gross's (2015a, 2015b) regulation model has involved adults (often college-age young adults) and has focused particularly on cognitive reappraisal. Some of this research is described below.

Strategy Use and Effectiveness

Gross's (2015a, 2015b) model recognizes that emotion regulation strategies are not always implemented. In addition, people do not always choose the most effective or appropriate strategies for a particular situation. In part, this may occur because the person has developed strong tendencies to rely on a limited number of regulation strategies. Such inflexibility is maladaptive because one's habitual strategies may be ineffective in some situations, or they may be effective in the short run (i.e., by engendering immediate changes in your own emotions) but have undesirable side effects or long-term consequences.

Grommisch et al. (2019) explored these possibilities in an experience sampling study in which participants were signaled on multiple occasions daily and reported on their use of nine types of responses considered by the authors to be emotion regulation strategies—situation selection, situation modification, distraction, rumination, reappraisal, suppression, social sharing, ignoring the emotion, and accepting the emotion. Participants also rated their positive and negative affect after using each response. Both before and after the experience sampling time period, participants completed surveys that included several measures of well-being (i.e., life satisfaction, anxiety, depression, and stress). The researchers identified nine profiles that captured both the frequency with which participants produced any of the responses at all and whether they favored certain responses over others. Their data analyses showed that participants who used a variety of active responses (e.g., situation selection, situation modification, social sharing) generally rated themselves highest on the measures of well-being, whereas those who tended to use suppression rated themselves lowest. Thus well-being was related to the flexible use of responses that are typically considered most effective. Similar results have been found in other studies of variability in the use of emotion regulation strategies (e.g., Blanke et al., 2020).

Recall that EC is considered to play an important role in children's and adolescents' emotion regulation because it enables them to effectively implement more cognitively demanding regulation strategies such as cognitive reappraisal. Similarly, cognitive control (i.e., executive control) is considered to play an important role in adults' emotion regulation, enabling greater flexibility in strategy choice, as well as more successful implementation of the chosen strategy (e.g., Hendricks & Buchanan, 2016; Pruessner, Barnow, Holt, Joormann, & Schulze, 2020). Reappraisal efforts may be used less often and be less successful in high-intensity emotion situations than in low-intensity situations (Shafir, Schwartz, Blechert, & Sheppes, 2015), presumably because more cognitive control is required in high-intensity situations. In contrast, distraction or suppression may be used more often in high-intensity situations (Sheppes, Scheibe, Suri, & Gross, 2011) because these latter strategies require fewer cognitive resources.

Other factors also may influence the selection and implementation of particular regulation strategies. For example, reappraisal may be used more often in situations that lend themselves more readily to reinterpretation

(Sheppes et al., 2014; Suri et al., 2018). To illustrate, it may be easier to reappraise a curable illness in a more favorable light than an incurable illness. In addition, a person's emotion-related goals must be considered. Emotion regulation in any form may be used less often in situations during which one actually desires to experience the elicited emotion (e.g., to mourn a loved one).

Irrespective of their short-term success in modifying a person's emotions, regulation strategies sometimes may have maladaptive long-term consequences. For example, distraction may be effective in the short run in that it lessens the experience of negative affect; however, protracted distraction might also have long-term costs if it precludes eventual processing of the emotional event and possible problem solving (Sheppes et al., 2014). Even cognitive reappraisal, a regulation strategy that has been "widely acclaimed" in the adult literature, can incur costs for similar reasons (Ford & Troy, 2019). For example, forgiving an abusive partner by reappraising the person's motives (e.g., in terms of his or her unfortunate childhood) may result in perpetuating the abuse unless it is accompanied by self-protective and other remediating measures. At the same time, in some situations over which a person has no control (e.g., an incurable illness), reappraisal—no matter how difficult—may be associated with better well-being (e.g., Haines et al., 2016).

Does Personality Influence Emotion Regulation?

Personality appears to influence a preference for some regulation strategies more than others. In her meta-analytic study, Barańczuk (2019) found that people who scored high in Neuroticism were more likely to use avoidance (a situation selection strategy) and less likely to use problem solving (a situation modification strategy) or reappraisal (a cognitive change strategy). In contrast, those scoring high on the four other personality factors (i.e., Extraversion, Openness, Agreeableness, and Conscientiousness) were more likely to use both problem solving and cognitive appraisal and were less likely to use avoidance. Thought suppression (a response strategy) was positively related to Neuroticism, whereas expressive suppression (another response strategy) was negatively related to Extraversion, Openness, and Agreeableness.

Other studies have examined relations between personality and emotion regulation goals. For example, Eldesouky and English (2019) found significant associations between Neuroticism and impression management goals (i.e., wanting to appear a certain way to others) and between Agreeableness and both pro-hedonic goals (i.e., wanting to feel happy) and prosocial goals (i.e., wanting to promote positive social interactions and relationships).

Openness to Experience was associated with performance goals (i.e., wanting to perform a particular activity). Counter-hedonic goals (i.e., wanting to experience a negative emotion such as anger) were negatively associated with Conscientiousness and Agreeableness.

Emotion Regulation within Relationships

Social relationships also influence the utilization of emotion regulation strategies (Lindsey, 2020). Adults make distinctions among social partners and regulate emotional expression in the presence of some people more than others. For example, in a study of emotion display rules in 32 countries (Matsumoto, Yoo, Fontaine, et al., 2008), participants reported significantly lower levels of spontaneous expressivity with acquaintances in comparison with close friends.

Emotion regulation also may take place within close relationships, and regulation of some emotions may be more important than others. Of relevance to this possibility, John Gottman and his colleagues (Gottman & Gottman, 2017; Gottman & Levenson, 2002; Madhyastha, Hamaker, & Gottman, 2011) have conducted longitudinal studies in which they examine the emotions expressed by married couples during conversations about day-to-day activities, areas of disagreement, and more positive topics. Based on analyses of these conversations, the investigators identified patterns of emotion communication that predicted the subsequent maintenance or dissolution of the marriage. One pattern involves the relative proportion of positive to negative affect expressed (verbally and/or nonverbally) during conflict discussions. Couples who maintained happy marriages expressed more positive than negative affect with about a 5:1 ratio. Couples headed for divorce expressed more negative affect, in particular the **Four Horsemen** (i.e., *criticism, defensiveness, contempt, stonewalling*). Stonewalling involves the virtually complete suppression of emotional expression, and findings here are consistent with other studies of this regulation strategy. Interestingly, expression of anger (at least during videotaped conversation) is not a fifth horseman. Instead, contempt appears to be a particularly toxic emotion that would best be regulated, presumably by transforming it into a less toxic emotion, possibly via a process of reappraisal. In addition, showing interest or even just attention to one's partner is considered to be a positive expression within Gottman's framework. Thus to promote a happy marriage, a person need not smile continuously at his or her spouse during the course of their daily interactions—but one should do one's spouse the courtesy of showing interest and attention. Presumably, this advice also applies to many other types of socioemotional relationships.

Emotion Regulation in the Workplace

Emotion regulation may differ across settings as well as across relationships. The importance of setting is illustrated in many studies of emotion in the workplace that have focused on **emotional labor** (i.e., the regulation of one's emotions to meet workplace demands; Hochschild, 1983). Emotional labor may take several forms. *Surface acting* involves suppressing, masking, or faking an emotional expression, such as one might do when talking to a dissatisfied employer or customer. As another example, in some family restaurants, waiters might try to act enthusiastic and cheerful irrespective of how they feel, whereas in haute cuisine restaurants, they might try to act haughty. *Deep acting* involves modifying the emotion itself in order to make it easier to express oneself in the manner appropriate for the job. For example, via a process of cognitive reappraisal, waiters in haute cuisine restaurants might convince themselves that their patrons really know little about fine dining, and thus waiters' haughtiness becomes a genuine expression of their feelings. The concept of *emotion-rule dissonance* has been used to describe incongruity between one's felt emotion and either the emotion or the expression required by the job.

In a meta-analytic study, Hülsheger and Schewe (2011) evaluated relationships between the three forms of emotional labor and several categories of dependent variables related to: (1) employees' job performance (e.g., customer satisfaction ratings, employer ratings of task performance, observer ratings of employees' appropriate emotional behavior), (2) employees' well-being (i.e., job satisfaction, organizational commitment), and (3) employees' ill-being (e.g., self-ratings of exhaustion, depersonalization, lack of personal accomplishment, psychological stress, physical complaints). Results showed that surface acting and emotion-rule dissonance were positively related to employee ill-being measures (with moderate effect sizes) and negatively related to employee well-being (with small effect sizes). Deep acting was positively related to two measures of job performance (appropriate emotional behavior, customer satisfaction) but not the third (task performance). Deep acting was also related to one measure of employee well-being (job satisfaction) and one measure of ill-being (physical symptoms). Not surprisingly, the positive relationship that was found between emotion-rule dissonance and ill-being was partially mediated by surface acting. In another study, Mérida-López, Extremera, Quintana-Orts, and Rey (2019) investigated relationships between emotion regulation ability, workplace social support, job satisfaction, and happiness ratings. Emotion regulation ability and social support were both associated with higher levels of happiness and job satisfaction. Additionally, when emotion regulation ability was low, then high social support mitigated the relationship between poor emotion regulation and low job satisfaction.

CULTURE AND EMOTION

Are the Prototypic Expressions Universal in Non-Western Cultures?

Proposals regarding the existence of facial expression prototypes for basic emotions were originally based on the early cross-cultural research by Ekman and Izard (e.g., Ekman & Friesen, 1971; Izard, 1971; see Chapter 1). However, some recent studies of remote non-Western societies (e.g., the Himba of Nambia, Tobriand Islanders of New Guinea) have produced mixed results, thus raising questions about expression universality (see Barrett et al., 2019, for review). In one such study, Gendron et al. (2020) presented participants from the United States and also from the Hazda tribe in Tanzania with culturally appropriate emotion stories (e.g., "He is faced with a dangerous animal that looks ready to bite and he feels afraid") accompanied by two pictures of different facial expressions. Four types of expression pairing were examined: (1) pairs that differed in both valence and arousal (e.g., happy and sad), (2) pairs that differed in valence but were similar in arousal (e.g., anger and surprise), (3) pairs that differed in arousal but were similar in valence (e.g., anger and sadness), and (4) pairs that were matched for both valence and arousal (e.g., fear and disgust). Both the U.S. and Hazda participants were able to choose the predicted expression with significant accuracy. However, correct identification rates by Hazda participants were substantially lower than those of U.S. participants for expression pairs that were matched for valence (i.e., both negative or both positive). Furthermore, performance of Hazda participants with minimal formal schooling or exposure to Western cultures was not significantly above chance when anger and disgust expressions were presented together. These findings suggest that past cross-cultural studies that used only random expression pairings may have been misleading because an accurate choice could often be made by focusing on differences in valence or arousal between the two stimuli rather than on their specific emotion meaning.

Nonetheless, other investigators have found evidence for at least some degree of universality in a range of emotions that even exceeds the Big Six that have dominated so much of the literature. Importantly, these studies typically go beyond facial expressions to include head movements, postures, gestures, and/or vocalizations. For example, Cordaro et al. (2018) videotaped college students from the United States, mainland China, India, Japan, and South Korea who were asked to portray how they would respond in situations exemplifying each of 22 emotions, including amusement, awe, coyness, boredom, embarrassment, and shame. The 2,640 expressions produced by participants were coded using an expanded version of Ekman et al.'s (2002) FACS that included gaze direction, head movements, arm movements, and visible respiratory movements. For each emotion, the researchers then identified those facial and nonfacial behaviors that were produced with significant frequency by the students in all four cultures. These empirically derived **international core patterns (ICPs)** were then compared with hypothetical prototypes for the 22 emotions derived by the researchers on the basis of descriptions found in the literature. The investigators then calculated a percentage score representing the degree of overlap between their empirically derived ICPs and the previous descriptions. Results showed considerable variability among the emotions. For example, overlap between the hypothesized prototype for surprise and the ICP for surprise was 89%. The overlap scores for fear, anger, happiness, sadness, and disgust were 71%, 67%, 44%, 33%, and 18%, respectively. Although overlap was considerable for a few emotions (e.g., surprise), the investigators concluded that overall "participants did *not* express emotion in terms of prototypical displays" (Cordaro et al., 2018, p. 87). In a separate set of analyses, the researchers calculated how much of each participant's expressive behavior corresponded to the empirically derived ICPs (i.e., the subset of expressive movements that were common across cultures). Averaging across participants, scores ranged from 76% (for amusement) to 21% (for interest). The scores for the Big Six emotions were 72%, 69%, 54%, 52%, 39%, and 23% for happiness, surprise, fear, disgust, sadness, and anger, respectively. Based on these figures, Cordaro et al. (2018) concluded that "emotional expression is not limited to rigid, fixed action patterns, but rather is more fluid, and emerges in more dynamically varying expressions" (p. 87). Taken together, the picture that emerges is one of both universality and variability in emotional expression and illustrates the importance of going beyond the traditional set of Big Six emotions.

Cordaro et al.'s (2018) findings also provide support for a **dialect theory of emotion expression** proposed by Hillary Elfenbein (2017). In her own research, Elfenbein and her colleagues also observed both similarities and differences across the cultures that they studied. For example, Elfenbein, Beaupré, Lévesque, and Hess (2007) found that anger expressions posed by Gabonese Canadians were largely similar to anger expressions posed by Quebecois Canadians save that the former group tended to widen their eyes while the latter group tended to narrow their eyes. According to Elfenbein's theory, such cultural variability in emotional expression may develop over time as the result of processes similar to those that create linguistic dialects (i.e., random drift and social stratification).

How Do Cultures Differ in Their Emotion-Related Beliefs and Values?

Many cultural psychologists have turned their attention to studying systematic relationships between cultural beliefs and values and culture members' emotional experience, expression, and behaviors. Because of their complexity, characterizing cultural beliefs and values is challenging. One well-regarded framework for doing so is Hofstede's **cultural dimensions theory** (Hofstede, 2001, 2011). Originally based on surveys of IBM employee values in a wide range of cultures, Hofstede's model includes six dimensions of cultural orientation: *individualism/collectivism, uncertainty avoidance, power distance* (i.e., importance of hierarchical relationships), advancement-oriented/ relationship-oriented (unfortunately called "*masculine/feminine*"), *long-term/ short-term focus,* and *indulgence/self-restraint.* While acknowledging that concentrating on only one dimension is an oversimplification, many cultural psychologists have primarily analyzed the first dimension: **individualism/ collectivism**. Individualism/collectivism is a dimension that represents one's relative valuing of the individual versus the group. Cultures high on individualism encourage personal autonomy, personal expression, and achieving personal goals. Cultures high on collectivism encourage allegiance to their group, maintaining group harmony, and subordinating personal to group goals. However, collectivistic cultures do differ among themselves in terms of how they define their groups, for example, in terms of family, country, and/or place of employment. To illustrate, allegiance to one's employment organization has historically been very strong in Japan but notably weaker in the United States. Corresponding to the individualism/collectivism dimension at the level of the group, the personal orientation of culture members is often described as **independent/interdependent** (Kitayama, Markus, Matsumoto, & Norasakkunkit, 1997). For example, an independence-oriented person might readily leave his or her current employment if a better job is offered, whereas an interdependence-oriented person might be more reluctant due to company loyalty.

Culture and Appraisal

Because appraisals are a key determinant of emotion elicitation, understanding relationships between cultural values and emotion requires consideration of differences in appraisal. Cultures may differ in terms of whether or how they apply the appraisal features that have been associated with a particular emotion in Western studies. For example, control of (i.e., responsibility for) an event is considered to be an important factor involved in the appraisal underlying anger. However, members of different cultures may differ in terms of who they consider to be responsible or in control. For example, Boiger, Uchida, Norasakkunkit, and Mesquita (2016) found that U.S. and Japanese college students both tended to blame the other person more than themselves for creating an anger-inducing situation. However, Japanese college students were more likely than U.S. students to also blame themselves for an anger episode that involved a person with whom they had a close relationship. Thus the collectivist values of Japanese students influenced their anger-related appraisals.

Emotion in Individualistic versus Collectivistic Cultures

To explore the emotional ramifications of individualism/collectivism, Kitayama, Mesquita, and Karasawa (2006) examined experiences of college students from Japan (an interdependence-oriented culture) and the United States (an independence-oriented culture). For a 2-week period, students were asked to record the most emotional episode of their day and rate how strongly they had felt each of 27 emotions. Students from both cultures reported experiencing both positive and negative emotions. However, the specific positive emotions they experienced were different. Japanese students reported experiencing socially engaging positive emotions (e.g., respect, sympathy, closeness, friendliness) more than socially disengaging positive emotions (e.g., pride, superiority, self-esteem). In contrast, U.S. students reported more socially disengaging than socially engaging positive emotions. With respect to negative emotions, both Japanese and U.S. students reported experiencing socially disengaging emotions (e.g., anger, frustration, sulkiness) more than socially engaging emotions (e.g., guilt, shame, indebtedness), but the tendency toward disengaging negative emotions was greater for the U.S. students.

To explore the influence of individualism/collectivism on emotional expressivity, Matsumoto, Yoo, Fontaine, et al. (2008) conducted an impressive questionnaire study involving more than 5,000 college students from 32 countries. Results showed that members of more individualistic cultures reported themselves to be more expressive overall than those from more collectivistic cultures. However, this finding was primarily driven by differences in the expression of positive emotions (i.e., happiness and surprise). In fact, members of individualist cultures were *less* expressive of negative emotions than members of collectivist cultures when interacting with outgroup individuals (i.e., persons with whom they did not have a close relationship). These findings are consistent with a view of individualistic cultures as both valuing the freer expression of emotion and distinguishing less between ingroup and outgroup individuals than do collectivistic cultures in their expression of negative affect.

Discussions of individualism/collectivism often appear to assume a categorical distinction between the two orientations and homogeneity among cultures that fall into the same category. Challenging these assumptions, a few researchers have empirically demonstrated differences between different collectivist cultures. For example, Ruby, Falk, Heine, Villa, and Silberstein (2012) compared college students from several collectivist cultures (Hong Kong, Japan, Mexico) in terms of the intensity of positive affect they prefer to experience. Consistent with research by Jeanne Tsai and her colleagues (Tsai, Knutson, & Fung, 2006), Ruby and colleagues (2012) found that Chinese participants reported a preference for experiencing low-intensity positive affect over high-intensity positive affect. Japanese participants also exhibited a preference for low-intensity positive emotions, but Mexican participants preferred high-intensity rather than low-intensity positive affect. According to Tsai's **affect valuation theory** (AVT; Tsai, 2007; Tsai et al., 2006), Asians' preference for low-intensity affect reflects a collectivistic disposition to adjust to their circumstances in contrast to an individualistic disposition to actively exert personal control over events. Because exerting control requires energy and high arousal while adjusting to circumstances does not, members of individualistic cultures (e.g., the United States) should prefer high-arousal emotions, whereas members of collectivist cultures (e.g., Asians) will prefer the opposite. Indeed, this has been consistently found in studies that compare Chinese and Western participants. However, as demonstrated by Ruby and colleagues (2012), members of some collectivist cultures may still value high-intensity positive affect, viewing it as a complement to interdependence rather than as in impediment to collective harmony. Thus differences in values and/or cultural dimensions other than individualism/collectivism may importantly influence emotional preferences.

Emotion Regulation across Cultures

Emotion regulation strategies may also differ across cultures in relation to different cultural dimensions. To investigate this possibility, Matsumoto, Yoo, Nakagawa, and the Multinational Study of Cultural Display Rules (2008) studied the self-reported use of reappraisal and expressive suppression by college students in 23 countries (e.g., Australia, Bangladesh, Brazil, Russia, Poland, United States, Zimbabwe). Participants completed the Emotion Regulation Questionnaire (ERQ; Gross & John, 2003), a measure with subscales for both regulation strategies. Drawing upon several available databases, each country was assigned a score representing its level of individualism/collectivism, power distance (hierarchy), long-term/short-term orientation, uncertainty avoidance, and affective autonomy (a dimension representing the individual's ability to seek out positive experiences). In addition, several databases were used to assign scores representing the overall level of well-being and maladjustment of each country's population. Results of their analyses showed that participants' greater use of expressive suppression was associated with country-level scores indicating higher levels of collectivism, long-term orientation, and greater importance of hierarchy. In contrast, participants from countries with greater affective autonomy and less emphasis on hierarchy reported lower levels of expressive suppression. Participants from countries with greater tolerance for uncertainty engaged in more reappraisal. With respect to emotion regulation and adjustment, participants' greater use of expressive suppression was related to lower country-level happiness scores. Lastly, and in contrast to the researchers' hypothesis, participants' greater use of expressive suppression was also associated with lower country-level scores on several indices of maladjustment (e.g., depression, anxiety, criminal activity, and drug use). To interpret this counterintuitive finding, the researchers suggested that countries that value social stability (and thus encourage expressive suppression) may provide fewer opportunities for crime and greater support for those who are emotionally vulnerable while simultaneously impeding individuals' pursuit of happiness.

Is Expressive Suppression Always Undesirable?

In discussing their findings, Matsumoto, Yoo, Nakagawa, and colleagues (2008) also acknowledged the limitations of using country-level measures of cultural values, happiness, and maladjustment in that associations at the level of the individual are not directly demonstrated. However, other studies have investigated within-individual associations in different cultures, particularly with respect to relations between expressive suppression and emotional outcomes. For example, Soto et al. (2011) asked European American and Hong Kong Chinese college students to complete measures of expressive suppression, life satisfaction, and depressed mood. Results showed that expressive suppression was related to lower life satisfaction and greater depression among European Americans but not Chinese students. Similar results were obtained in a study of European American and Asian American college students. In this study, Butler, Lee, and Gross (2007) administered measures of adherence to Western versus Asian values, use of suppression as a regulation strategy, and experience of negative emotions to women college students of varying cultural and ethnic backgrounds (but primarily European American and Asian American). Their data analyses confirmed that European American participants reported greater adherence to Western values than Asian American participants. For those who adhered more strongly to Western values, more expressive suppression was related to experiencing more negative affect. In contrast, for those who subscribed more strongly to Asian values, more expressive suppression was related to experiencing less negative affect. Both these studies suggest that expressive suppression has a negative impact on European Americans' emotional experience. However, their findings also must be viewed in light of a dissimilar conclusion reached in Webb et al.'s (2012) meta-analytic investigation of 190 studies primarily involving Europeans or European Americans. Somewhat surprisingly, these investigators found that expressive suppression was accompanied by a significant (albeit very small) decrease in negative affect. Given these conflicting findings, the question of how expressive suppression and emotional experience are related both within and across cultures requires further investigation.

Cultural Differences in Other Values

The relationship between values and emotional preferences was also demonstrated by Tamir et al. (2016) in a study of college students from eight cultures (Brazil, United States, Singapore, Germany, Poland, Ghana, China, and Israel). Participants completed a questionnaire measure of their personal values with subscales for self-transcendence (e.g., valuing benevolence), self-enhancement (e.g., valuing achievement, recognition, or power), openness to change (e.g., valuing self-directed action), and conservativeness (e.g., valuing conformity and tradition). Participants also rated how much they wanted to experience each of 26 emotions that were categorized as self-transcending (e.g., love, affection), self-enhancing (e.g., pride, anger), opening (e.g., interest, excitement), conserving (e.g., calmness, contentment), nonopening (e.g., sadness, depression), or nonconserving (e.g., fear, anxiety). Although the investigators were unable to make direct cross-cultural comparisons for statistical reasons (i.e., lack of scalar invariance), hierarchical linear modeling demonstrated significant associations between categories of values and related categories of desired emotions in all eight cultures. Perhaps surprisingly, informal inspection of the data suggested that participants in all cultures rated self-transcending values (presumably related to interdependence/collectivism) higher than self-enhancing values (presumably related to independence/individualism). In addition, openness was rated higher than conservativeness in all cultures save Ghana. Such data suggest that traditional assumptions about the characterization of some cultures may need to be reconsidered in light of increasing globalization of values—at least among college students.

GENDER AND EMOTION

Personality, Expressivity, and Emotional Experience

As indicated above, temperament in adulthood is often represented in terms of personality factors, most notably the Big Five. In their meta-analysis of gender differences in adults' personality across cultures, Costa, Terracciano, and McCrae (2001) reported significant but small differences for several emotion-related facets subsumed under the five factors as measured by the NEO Personality Inventory. In particular, women scored higher for positive emotions, anxiety, and depression within the United States and in a range of other countries. No significant gender difference in angry hostility was found for U.S. adults, although (surprisingly) women in other countries reported higher levels than did men.

Regarding emotional expressivity, in one large-scale survey, Simon and Nath (2004) found that women generally rate themselves as being more expressive than men for both positive and negative emotions (with the exception of anger). Regarding emotional experience, women reported experiencing more sadness than did men, and no gender differences in self-reported anger were obtained. Men reported experiencing positive emotions more than women did, a result that appears inconsistent with the findings for positive emotions in Costa et al.'s (2001) personality study. One possible explanation is that different positive emotions were considered by participants in the two studies, arguing for the value of querying participants about distinct emotions rather than broad affective categories.

Focusing on self-conscious emotions, Else-Quest, Higgins, Allison, and Morton (2012) conducted a meta-analysis that evaluated gender differences in the self-reported experience of embarrassment, shame, guilt, hubristic pride, and authentic pride. Data from studies of both children and adults were analyzed in their investigation, and age was included as a potential moderator. However, the great majority of studies involved adult participants. Results showed small gender differences, with females reporting that they experienced more authentic pride (i.e., pride in one's accomplishments), guilt, shame, and embarrassment than males. Males reported experiencing more hubristic pride (i.e., global pride in oneself). Moderator analyses showed that the gender differences for guilt were found in adults but not in children. Importantly, the researchers also examined the effects of different study methodologies. These methodologies included procedures in which participants reported on recent specific events during which they experienced the emotion, those in which they reported their self-perceived general tendencies to experience the emotion, and those in which they reported specific events that may have occurred in the more distant past. Gender scholars (e.g., Brody, Hall, & Stokes, 2016; Shields, MacArthur, & McCormick, 2018) have argued that the first type of study is least likely to be contaminated by self-stereotyping (i.e., beliefs about oneself that reflect cultural stereotypes more than one's actual experiences). Evidence of self-stereotyping was found for guilt, shame, and authentic pride. That is, studies that analyzed reports of participants' recent specific experiences generated significantly smaller gender differences than studies that utilized the other methodologies. Although inconsistencies across some studies remained, gender scholars have increasingly moved toward focusing on social and contextual determinants of gender-related behaviors rather than trying to pinpoint context-invariant differences between women and men. This point is illustrated below.

Socialization and Stereotyping

Contemporary scholars emphasize the socialization origins, as well as the context dependency, of gender differences in emotion seen in adulthood (Brody et al., 2016; Shields et al., 2018). For example, men may be encouraged to be less expressive than women in most situations—but it may be acceptable for them to show heightened emotion in the context of athletic competitions or when they express morally justified anger and distress (Gallegos, Vescio, & Shields, 2019; Shields et al., 2018). Broadly conceived, context also can include aspects of one's identity other than gender, for example, ethnicity, professional status, or religion (Brody et al., 2016). These may interact with gender to affect how one appraises a situational context and thus one's emotional reaction.

The emotion of anger provides a good example of the effects of both gender and context on emotional expression. Anger is considered by many laypersons to be both more common and more appropriate for men than for women (Shields et al., 2018). However, many studies find no gender difference in self-reports of anger experience (as noted above and in reviews by Averill, 1983, and Brody et al., 2016). At the same time, research has shown that, depending on the context, anger expressed by women may be associated with a variety of negative evaluations. For example, Brescoll and Uhlmann (2008) presented participants with scenarios in which a male or female business professional lost an important account and obtained judgments of the professional's status, competence, and merited salary. Results showed that female professionals portrayed as showing anger received lower ratings than female professionals portrayed as showing sadness or no emotion. In contrast, male professionals were not so penalized. However, if a reasonable justification for anger was provided in the scenario (e.g., a coworker's negligence), then justified angry females were rated higher than unjustified angry females. Thus anger in females was more acceptable if it appeared justified by the situational context. Such context-related differences in the acceptability of female anger may well underlie differences found in women's expression—but not their experience—of this emotion.

The Female Advantage in Adults' Emotion Understanding

A female advantage in adults' emotion recognition is consistently seen across studies. In two early meta-analytic investigations that included primarily adults, Hall (1978, 1984) found an advantage that was moderate in size for studies that involved recognizing visual and visual-plus-auditory expressions, although not for auditory expressions presented alone. As noted in Chapter 4, gender differences in emotional intelligence (EI) emerge during early adolescence. Throughout adulthood, the EI advantage for women has been found to persist and to be small to moderate in size (Cabello, Sorrel, Fernández-Pinto, Extremera, & Fernández-Berrocal, 2016; Joseph & Newman, 2010). In Cabello et al.'s study, significant gender differences were obtained for all four branches of ability EI and were moderate in size for total EI and for the understanding branch. Given their developmental history, presumably women's better scores on EI measures reflect their socialization experiences beginning in childhood and extending into adulthood.

NEUROBIOLOGICAL UNDERPINNINGS

Brain Functioning: Are There Emotion Programs in the Brain?

In 2015, Walt Disney Pictures released *Inside Out*, a movie about emotions inspired in part by a screenwriter's experiences with his teenage daughter. In that movie, five basic emotions are represented by personified figures who operate a console that controls a young girl's emotional responses. In doing so, the filmmakers (probably unwittingly) aligned themselves with those basic emotion theories that arose at the end of the previous century and that propose the existence of discrete emotion programs in the brain (Ekman, 1971; Izard, 1977; see Chapter 1). Such theories clearly have intuitive appeal, but how has the idea of emotion programs in the brain held up in light of recent research?

The development of new neuroimaging tools has allowed neuroscientists to empirically investigate this question, primarily by means of functional magnetic resonance imaging (fMRI) studies. Although this effort is ongoing, a picture is emerging that suggests a more complicated story than was first envisioned. Originally, emotion programs were conceived as residing in different and nonoverlapping locations in the brain. This **locationist view** has been investigated in numerous studies that involve inducing emotions in participants as they lie in an MRI scanner, for example, by showing them emotional pictures or asking them to recall personal emotional events. Brain scans taken during these procedures allow investigators to identify (with good—though imperfect—precision) those areas of the brain that are activated during the experience of different emotions. Recent meta-analysis of these studies has demonstrated that the locationist view is not accurate. In particular, Lindquist, Wager, Kober, Bliss-Moreau, and Barrett (2012) analyzed data from 91 studies and found that virtually all areas of the brain that responded to emotion actually responded to more than one of them. For example, several early studies had tied the amygdala to fear (Davis, 1992). However, when a wider range of investigations were considered, the amygdala was found to respond at a significant level to disgust as well.

Because Lindquist et al.'s (2012) findings had been foreshadowed by some of the individual studies included in their meta-analysis, many scholars have abandoned a strictly locationist position in favor of a network approach to emotion and brain functioning (e.g., Adolphs, 2017; Hamann, 2012; Pessoa, 2019). One possible proposal within this framework is that emotions are characterized by discrete networks rather than discrete locations—that is, each emotion should be distinguished by a discrete pattern of synchronized activation in a particular set of brain areas. One novel way used to investigate this proposal has been through the use of multivoxel pattern analysis (MVPA). For example, Saarimäki and colleagues (2016) evoked six basic emotions in participants undergoing fMRI by either presenting them with brief movies or asking them to mentally recreate the target emotion. Using MVPA, they were able to successfully identify neural signatures for each emotion that were consistent across both methods of emotion induction. Consistency across emotion induction methods is an important criterion that must be met in order to infer that the neural patterning characterizes the emotion itself rather than some feature of the induction method.

Although Saarimäki et al. (2016) found consistency across induction methods within their own investigation, differences have been observed in other studies. To integrate the range of findings across studies, Wager et al. (2015) conducted meta-analyses that included data from 148 studies involving five emotions (happiness, sadness, fear, anger, and disgust). Using Bayesian modeling, the researchers analyzed patterns of brain activity accompanying each emotion in each study and identified a best-fitting overarching pattern for each emotion. Importantly, the investigations included in the meta-analysis involved a variety of different means for evoking each emotion, and these differences were statistically controlled in the data analyses. Results of the analyses showed that the best-fitting overarching patterns could be used to correctly classify approximately 67% of individual emotion episodes, ranging from 86% of fear episodes to 43% of anger episodes. In all cases, classification accuracy was greater than chance (i.e., 20%, given that the choice was among five emotions); however, it was far from perfect. Each of the identified patterns included activity in multiple brain regions, including the cortex, amygdala, and thalamus. Furthermore, components of each pattern also participate in other brain networks (e.g., networks that support perception). Thus, as with Lindquist and colleagues (2012), this study's findings are inconsistent with a locationist view of the emotional brain. However, they are also inconsistent with a network view that posits a discrete, dedicated network whose components are uniquely associated with a single emotion.

In part to accommodate this complex picture of emotion-related brain activity, a radical alternative has been proposed by Lisa Barrett. Consistent with Barrett's (2017a, 2017b) theory of constructed emotions (see Chapter 1), she proposes that emotions themselves do not exist in nature as discrete entities, that is, as **natural kinds,** each having a well-defined set of necessary and sufficient features that include a dedicated neural network. Instead, emotions are psychological categories that may have a conceptual (and statistical) prototype—but in actuality this prototype is derived from a set of differing individual episodes that we have come to identify as exemplars of the emotion. Therefore, substantial variability must be expected and built into emotion modeling. This proposal forms an important pillar of Barrett's theory of constructed emotion. Barrett's controversial theory has generated a great deal of vigorous discussion among emotion psychologists and correspondingly stands to energize a great deal of future research.

Autonomic Nervous System (ANS): Do Response Patterns Differ across Emotions?

Even before the advent of fMRI, many researchers investigated presumed downstream effects of presumed emotion programs on the ANS. Interest in emotion-related ANS functioning has a long history, inspired by William James's early theory that proposed emotion to be the perception of situationally evoked body responses (see Chapter 1). Investigation of this topic is ongoing, and controversies continue to this day.

Although no one disputes that episodes of emotion may typically include ANS responses, the emotion-specific patterning (often termed **coherence**) of these responses is subject to debate. Strong claims regarding ANS response coherence parallel strong claims regarding the existence of emotion-specific programs or brain networks. Some studies have indeed produced results consistent with such claims. For example, Ekman, Levenson, and their colleagues (Levenson, Ekman, Heider, & Friesen, 1992) measured ANS responding in participants from both the United States and Sumatra who were instructed to produce facial muscle movements corresponding to prototypic expressions for several emotions (i.e., happiness, sadness, disgust, fear, anger). Their theoretically based assumption was that producing these expressions generates the corresponding emotion via feedback to the brain from the face (known as the **facial feedback hypothesis**). The investigators reported distinct ANS patterning for each emotion. For example, heart rate acceleration was greater when posing fear than disgust for participants from both cultural groups. In a more recent study, McGinley and Friedman (2017) used three other methods for generating emotion that are currently more common in the emotion literature: viewing film clips, imagining events portrayed in a story, and recalling personal experiences. Four emotions (amusement, contentment, sadness, fear) plus a neutral (control) state were investigated and a number of ANS responses were measured (e.g., heart rate, systolic and diastolic blood pressure, respiration rate). Using discriminant function analysis, the researchers found that ANS patterns could be identified for three emotions (amusement, contentment, fear) that allowed for a significant number of emotion episodes to be correctly classified. However, classification hit rates (i.e., number of correct identifications of an emotion/ number of correct identifications + number of missed identifications) were not high: 36.4% for fear, 34.1% for contentment, 29.8% for amusement, and 18.4% for sadness versus 20% for chance. Success in identifying reliable ANS patterning also differed for the three induction methods. Within each of two methods (film clip viewing and imagining emotion events), ANS patterns for amusement, contentment, and fear were identified that allowed a significant number of episodes to be correctly classified. However, no reliable pattern could be identified for sadness using either the film-viewing or imagining-events method, and no reliable pattern could be identified for any emotion using the personal-recall method. Furthermore, no consistent set of necessary and sufficient (i.e., core) features were identified for any emotion. Still, the investigators interpreted their findings as yielding "further support for autonomic specificity of emotion" (p. 48)—while at the same time emphasizing that induction method also influences ANS responding (McGinley & Friedman, 2017).

Siegel et al. (2018) reached a radically different conclusion in their subsequent meta-analytic investigation of ANS responding in over 200 studies. They conducted six separate meta-analyses using multivariate pattern classification analysis, one analysis each for happiness, anger, fear, disgust, sadness, and neutral emotion. They also ran several moderator analyses to investigate effects of sample characteristics (gender distribution, student vs. community samples), study characteristics (e.g., induction method), and quality (e.g., use of emotion manipulation checks). Results showed that the ANS pattern identified for anger had the highest hit rate (19.1%). Hit rates for the other emotions were substantially lower: 2.1% for happiness and disgust, 1.7% for fear, and 5.8% for sadness. Youden's J statistic for anger (representing both the hit rate and the true negative rate) was 0.3 on a scale of 0–1, indicating it was closer to being a "useless" classifier than a "perfect" classifier. Further analyses demonstrated significant heterogeneity among studies in the results for happiness, anger, and fear. There were also a few differences between mixed-gender studies and studies involving all women and between studies involving student versus community samples. Because hit rates were low and heterogeneity was high, the researchers concluded that their results supported Barrett's (2017a, 2017b) constructivist theory rather than ANS specificity.

Hypothalamic–Pituitary–Adrenal (HPA) System

Adults show a typical diurnal cortisol rhythm involving a gradual increase overnight followed by a further spike after awakening that lasts for approximately 30–45 minutes (known as the cortisol awakening response [CAR]). The CAR is followed by a gradual decline of cortisol secretion during the day (Gaffey, Bergeman, Clark, & Wirth, 2016; Wilhelm, Born, Kudielka, Schlotz, & Wüst, 2007). However, substantial individual differences in cortisol rhythms also have been noted. For example, in a study of healthy adults (mean age = 36 years) by Smyth and colleagues (1997), 51% of the sample showed the typical trajectory of decline that was consistent across 2 consecutive days, 17% showed a flattened trajectory on both days, and 34% were inconsistent, showing a decline on one day and a flattened trajectory on the other. Flattened trajectories can represent either a failure to show the normative decline across the day, and thus a higher overall cortisol level, or, alternatively, a failure to show the normal increase overnight or in the morning and thus a consistently low cortisol level.

To shed light on the implications of such individual differences, some researchers have investigated associations between stress-related or emotion-related variables and HPA functioning in adulthood. For example, in a study of men, Franz et al. (2013) found that participants' experience of childhood adversity (i.e., low paternal socioeconomic status, low maternal education, separation from parents, and/or large family size) was associated with higher levels of daily cortisol in middle adulthood. In a study of both men and women, Stawski, Cichy, Piazza, and Almeida (2013) found that cortisol levels were higher on days when participants reported experiencing stress in comparison with stress-free days.

With respect to emotion, several researchers have hypothesized that persons who experience more negative affect should also exhibit atypical HPA functioning. This hypothesis has sometimes—but not always—been confirmed. For example, in a study of adults' self-reported affect, Polk, Cohen, Doyle, Skoner, and Kirschbaum (2005) found that more negative experiences were associated with higher cortisol levels for men but not for women. In a study of adults ranging from 33 to 84 years of age, Piazza, Charles, Stawski, and Almeida (2013) found that more negative affect was related to higher levels of cortisol for older participants but not for younger adults.

Poorer emotion regulation skills might contribute to nonnormative cortisol levels. Consistent with this possibility, Otto, Sin, Almeida and Sloan (2018) found that higher scores on the suppression subscale of the ERQ were associated with a stronger CAR and flatter diurnal cortisol trajectory. In an investigation of both stress and emotion regulation, Roos, Levens, and Bennett (2018) found that adults who scored higher on both expressive suppression and relationship stress exhibited a stronger cortisol response to a public speaking task.

Considering cultural differences in values related to emotions (as described earlier), corresponding differences in the relationship between emotion and HPA functioning might also be expected. In addition to valuing expressive restraint, persons from Asian cultures are often considered to be more accepting of the experience of negative emotion in comparison with persons from Western cultures (De Vaus, Hornsey, Kuppens, & Bastian, 2018). If so, negative emotions should be experienced as less stressful by Asians. Consistent with this portrayal of meta-emotional differences across cultures, Park, Kitayama, Miyamoto, and Coe (2020) found that self-reported negative affect by American adults was associated with a flattened diurnal cortisol trajectory, but no significant association between negative affect and daily cortisol measures was found for Japanese adults. A similar pattern of findings across the two cultures was reported for several other health-risk biomarkers.

EMOTIONAL INTELLIGENCE (EI)

As noted in Chapter 4, most contemporary research on adults' emotion understanding conceptualizes it within the framework of EI. In their large-scale developmental study, Cabello and colleagues (2016) found that ability EI was higher in middle adulthood (32–42 years) than young adulthood (17–31 years). Older adults scored lower than both of the other age groups.

Interest in adults' EI by both professionals and laypersons has increased exponentially since the late 1990s, due in part to claims made in Daniel Goleman's (1995) popular trade book that portrayed emotional intelligence as the key to success in a variety of domains, including careers and socioemotional relationships. Correspondingly, researchers have continued to conduct systematic research in these areas. Based on this research, several meta-analyses have evaluated the influence of EI on various aspects of employee functioning and SWB in the workplace.

Does EI Affect Employee Satisfaction and Performance?

Interestingly, ability EI (as described in Chapter 4) often appears to make less of a contribution to adaptive occupational functioning than trait EI (emotion-related dispositions such as optimism and social responsibility) and mixed models of EI (those incorporating both ability and trait components). In one meta-analytic study, Miao, Humphrey and Qian (2017b) found that all three forms of EI were significantly related to job satisfaction but that the contribution of ability EI was considerably weaker than the contribution of both other types. For all three types of EI, both job performance and on-the-job self-reported affect mediated the relationship between EI and job satisfaction. In addition, the relationship between trait EI and job satisfaction was moderated by the amount of emotional labor required by the job. The relationship was strongest for workers in jobs requiring more interpersonal skills, such as in the health care and service industries. In a second meta-analytic study, Miao, Humphrey, and Qian (2017a) focused on good organizational citizenship (behavior that promotes the functioning of the organization but is not explicitly rewarded) and counterproductive workplace behavior (behavior intended to hurt the organization or members of the organization). Similar to their previous findings, results showed that all three forms of EI were significantly related to positive citizenship and counterproductive behavior (in the predicted directions), but the strength of the relationship for ability EI was considerably weaker than for both other types. In a third meta-analytic investigation, Sánchez-Álvarez, Extremera, and Fernández-Berrocal (2016) found that SWB also was significantly associated with all three types of EI. However, again, the relationship of ability EI to SWB was not as strong as the relationship between SWB and the other two EI measures. When the components of SWB (i.e., life satisfaction, positive affect, and negative affect) were examined separately, all three types of EI measures were related to life satisfaction more strongly than to the affect measures.

Does EI Influence Social Behavior and Relationships?

Why do trait and mixed EI measures predict some desirable outcomes better than ability EI measures? This pattern of findings may reflect the fact that trait and mixed measures also tap other dispositions and abilities that significantly influence how persons act upon their emotion knowledge (e.g., their motivation to act in a socially desirable manner; Lopes et al., 2012; Mayer et al., 2016). Still, one recent meta-analysis (Miao, Humphrey, Qian, & Pollack, 2019) did find that trait EI and ability EI were both equally (and negatively) associated with two members of the Dark Triad of personality traits related to undesirable social behaviors (i.e., Machiavellianism and psychopathy/ antisocial behavior), although not to the third member (i.e., narcissism).

Although meta-analyses are not currently available, several studies have found positive associations between ability EI and social interactions and relationships. For example, Lopes, Salovey, and Straus (2003) asked college students to complete a measure of ability EI (the MSCEIT), as well as two measures of their interpersonal relationships, one reflecting general relationships with others and the second reflecting their specific relationships with their closest parent and their closest nonromantic friend. In analyses that controlled for verbal intelligence and personality variables, the researchers found that students who scored higher on the managing emotions branch of the MSCEIT reported more positive relationships with others, more perceived social support from parents, and fewer negative interactions with friends. Higher MSCEIT scores on the understanding emotions branch and the using emotions branch were also related to fewer negative interactions with friends. In a study that focused on romantic relationships, Brackett, Warner, and Bosco (2005) recruited college-age couples who had been together for at least 3 months and asked each member to complete the MSCEIT and three measures of relationship quality and satisfaction. Data analyses showed that couples in which both partners scored low on EI tended to be least satisfied and have the lowest relationship quality.

SUMMARY AND FINAL THOUGHTS

Global surveys of life satisfaction and affect indicate that most adults are relatively happy and satisfied with their lives as long as their basic needs are being met. Still, analyses of the Gallup Organization's surveys suggest that people residing in Anglo regions report themselves to be happier and more satisfied than average.

Participants from Western cultures are able to match facial configurations considered prototypic expressions for the Big Six basic emotions to stories and verbal labels representing these emotions with significant "accuracy"—that is, they make choices that conform to predictions based on basic emotion theories. However, rates of recognition are considerably lower when participants are asked to provide their own labels or when they come from non-Western cultures. Furthermore, when members of different cultures are asked to pose their own versions of emotional expressions, variable degrees of overlap have been found among cultures and between each culture's poses and the prototype expressions. Lastly, recent studies have raised questions about the ecological validity of these expressions. Together, these findings suggest that emotional expression includes both universal and variable components, that emotion is only one factor determining facial behavior, that multimodal cues to emotion should be considered, and that future research should focus on how emotion is expressed in the natural environment.

Temperament in adulthood is often represented in terms of personality factors, most notably the Big Five factors. Normative trends in personality change across adulthood have been described that include declines in Neuroticism (roughly corresponding to the temperamental factor of negative emotionality) and increases in Conscientiousness (related to EC) and

Agreeableness (related to affiliativeness). The emotion-related personality factor of Neuroticism has been associated with greater negative affect experienced in daily life and greater use of maladaptive emotion regulation strategies.

Adult attachment status is associated with more effective parenting, although the mechanisms underlying this association have not been fully explicated. Other studies have shown that one's parenting quality is influenced by additional aspects of one's experiences (e.g., harsh treatment by one's own parents that includes their expression of hostile and angry emotion). However, many adults successfully adopt a more desirable parenting style than the one they experienced. In the future, more emotion-relevant parenting behaviors need to be studied, and particular attention should be paid to moderating factors that might enable breaking the transmission chain of negative attachment and parenting.

James Gross's process models of emotion and emotion regulation designate a number of strategies that may be implemented at different steps of the emotion process. Circumventing issues regarding the conceptualization of emotion regulation, research findings appear to show the desirability of having a variety of strategies at one's disposal that can be flexibly employed when appropriate to the encountered situation. This principle applies even to cognitive reappraisal and expressive suppression, strategies that are generally considered desirable and undesirable, respectively. One's personality can influence strategy selection for better or worse. Adults may regulate their expressive behavior when interacting with acquaintances more than with close friends. Expressing negative emotion toward one's partner (particularly contempt) or expressing no emotion at all (stonewalling) is associated with unsuccessful marriages. In workplace settings, regulation of one's emotional expression may be required and can engender dissatisfaction and stress. In contrast, successful regulation of one's emotional experience (i.e., deep acting) engenders fewer costs. However, these studies generally take place in Western individualist cultures, and findings may not generalize to collectivist cultures in which the prioritization of group values is normative.

Recent research has raised questions about the universality of emotional facial expressions considered prototypic based on earlier cross-cultural studies. Current evidence suggests both universality and cultural variability in expressions for a range of emotions going beyond the Big Six. Cultural values influence both the experience and expression of emotion. Members of collectivist cultures may experience more socially engaging emotions than members of individualistic cultures, that is, more emotions that reflect their focus on the group. Members of individualistic cultures may be more expressive of their emotions overall. Although individualism/collectivism is the dimension most widely studied, other cultural values also play an important role. The use of emotion regulation strategies also differs across cultures. Some strategies (particularly expressive suppression) may be related to negative affect and poorer well-being in individualistic cultures but not in cultures that prioritize group harmony over self-expression. However, this question has not yet been resolved.

Small gender differences in emotional expressivity continue to be seen in adulthood and are likely due to socialization influences. Stereotypes also influence how the expressions of particular emotions by men versus women are evaluated, but such evaluations are also context dependent. For example, anger may be acceptable for women only in some circumstances. The same is true for displays of sympathetic distress by men. A small to moderate female advantage in ability EI is seen in adulthood.

Traditional discrete emotion theories proposed that basic emotions each have a dedicated program in the brain in the form of a specific anatomical location or network of neural connections. For several decades, scientists have struggled without much success to obtain convincing evidence for this hypothesis. For an even longer period of time, psychologists have sought evidence for a dedicated set of ANS responses associated with each emotion. Similarly, strong evidence for this position has been elusive. Consequently, many contemporary researchers are abandoning the search and instead are seeking alternative ways of conceptualizing how the nervous system functions during emotional experiences. One emerging conceptualization views emotion episodes as constructions involving highly variable appraisals, feelings, and responses that are each supported by situationally adaptive neural activity. Adversity and negative affect have been related to disrupted HPA functioning in Western cultures. However, these relationships may not exist in Asian cultures that have a more accepting attitude regarding negative emotion.

Ability measures of EI (i.e., the MSCEIT) assess emotion recognition and understanding, while trait and mixed measures also assess one's disposition to engage in positive social interactions. All three types of EI are significantly related to job satisfaction, organizational citizenship, and life satisfaction. Ability EI also has been related to more satisfactory interpersonal and romantic relationships.

CHAPTER 6

Later Adulthood

65+ Years

Life expectancies both in the United States and worldwide have changed substantially in the past 50 years (Worldometer, 2020). In 1970, life expectancy in the United States was 71 years and, worldwide, 58 years. In 2020, U.S. life expectancy was 79 years, and worldwide life expectancy was 73 years. Thus adults who retire at 65 years in the United States must prepare for a substantially longer postwork life than ever before. Fortunately, corresponding to this increase in life expectancy, our views about emotional well-being in later adulthood have also experienced an upswing.

EMOTIONAL EXPERIENCE AND EXPRESSION

Emotional Well-Being

During much of the last century, portrayals of aging were uniformly bleak, focusing on declines in cognitive functioning, health problems, and loss of social contacts with the death of friends and family. Although all of these challenges indeed exist, most older persons who are in reasonably good health actually report an increasingly favorable balance between their positive and negative emotional experiences. For example, Carstensen et al. (2011) conducted an experience sampling study in which participants ranging in age from 18 to 94 years were paged 5 times per day and asked to rate their current experiencing of 8 positive emotions (e.g., happiness, excitement, contentment) and 11 negative emotions (e.g., anger, sadness, fear).

Affect balance scores were computed by subtracting the average rating of the 11 negative emotions from the average rating of the 8 positive emotions. Results showed that these affect balance scores increased until the age of 64 and then somewhat declined—but they never receded to the level of those of participants in their 20s. This showed that older persons experienced a greater proportion of positive relative to negative affect during the course of their days. Not surprisingly, physical health (assessed at the beginning of the study) also predicted positive affect balance scores, suggesting that it too is important for emotional well-being in later adulthood (Sliwinski & Scott, 2014). Older persons who suffer debilitating health problems may not necessarily experience an affect upswing.

Other studies have investigated positive and negative emotions separately and produced a more nuanced picture of emotional experience in later adulthood. For example, Charles, Reynolds, and Gatz (2001) found that negative affect decreased linearly from about 15 to 60 years of age but then remained fairly level up to about 85 years. Positive emotion was fairly stable up to about age 55 but then gradually declined until about age 85. Still, positive affect was higher than negative affect even at the oldest age. Data on people older than 85 years are scarce, and study participant numbers are very small. One study found that life satisfaction ratings were below the neutral midpoint for participants at 97 years or above (Gerstorf et al., 2008). Still, another study (Jopp & Rott, 2006) found that centenarians who were in reasonably good physical and mental health reported themselves to be just as happy as a middle-aged control group.

Among older adults, high levels of positive emotion are associated with better cardiac health and markers of immune system functioning, and the relationship is likely bidirectional (Steptoe, Deaton, & Stone, 2015). According to one study (Freedman, Cornman, Carr, & Lucas, 2019), effects of poor physical functioning on emotional well-being can sometimes be buffered by economic resources such that more severe physical impairments are not always accompanied by lower well-being. But, somewhat surprisingly, this buffering effect was seen only for participants in the two middle-income quartiles and not for those in either the bottom or the top quartile in Freedman et al.'s study. In attempting to interpret their unexpected findings for upper-income participants, the researchers suggested that "persons who have experienced very low levels of stress and adversity over the life course may not have developed skills to adapt to such adversity, whereas their counterparts who experienced modest stress develop efficacious coping skills" (Freedman et al., 2019, p. 486). Although speculative, this interpretation is consistent with the proposal that the emotional effects of one's experiences are dependent on how one appraises and responds to the circumstances that are encountered.

Focusing on negative affect, one important finding is that different negative emotions have different developmental trajectories. In particular, anger tends to decrease from middle adulthood through later adulthood, whereas sadness remains relatively stable until it begins to increase slightly starting at around age 75 (Kunzmann, Richter, & Schmukle, 2013; Kunzmann, Rohr, Wieck, Kappes, & Wrosch, 2017; Stone, Schwartz, Broderick, & Deaton, 2010). High levels of self-reported anger—but not sadness—have been associated with more chronic illness and higher levels of interleukin-6 (a biomarker of chronic low-grade inflammation) in a study of adults ranging in age from 59 to 93 years (Barlow, Wrosch, Gouin, & Kunzmann, 2019).

Theories of Positive Affect in Later Adulthood

Several theories have been advanced to account for consistent findings that a positive affect balance is maintained in later adulthood (Sands, Ngo, & Isaacowitz, 2016). Of these, three have received the most attention: (1) **selection, optimization, and compensation (SOC**; Baltes & Baltes, 1990); (2) **socioemotional selectivity theory (SST**; Carstensen, Isaacowitz, & Charles, 1999); and (3) **strength and vulnerability integration (SVI**; Charles, 2010; Charles & Luong, 2013). All three theories propose that older individuals are more motivated (i.e., biased) toward experiencing positive emotion than are younger individuals. However, this positivity bias in motivation is embedded in a larger set of age-appropriate goals and mechanisms for reaching those goals that differ somewhat among the three theoretical perspectives.

According to the SOC model, an individual's adaptive goals shift from focusing on growth (i.e., developing and achieving new skills and resources) to focusing on maintenance of one's skills and resources as well as prevention of losses as one ages (Ebner, Freund, & Baltes, 2006). The term *selection* refers to the choice of age-appropriate goals, *optimization* refers to choosing the best means for achieving these goals, and *compensation* refers to the process of using one's available resources to maintain functioning as high as possible and to prevent or minimize losses. In order to more explicitly incorporate emotion, Urry and Gross's (2010) **SOC-emotion regulation model (SOC-ER)** proposes that older individuals seek to maintain positive emotion as one of many goals related to adaptive functioning and they do so by optimally selecting and utilizing emotion regulation strategies (see further discussion of emotion regulation later in the chapter).

SST focuses more exclusively on emotion-related goals. According to SST, an individual will shift from focusing on future-oriented knowledge-related goals (e.g., cognitive achievements) to more present-oriented positive emotion goals as they age (Carstensen et al., 1999). An important tenet of this theory is that the shift in goals is motivated by a shift in the older person's time perspective, that is, the realization of a time-limited future now that they have reached later adulthood. Similar to SOC, SST also predicts that the individual will engage in emotion-related regulation behaviors that will enhance his or her experience of positive emotion.

Building upon SST, SVI seeks to specify circumstances and factors that may impede as well as facilitate older adults' maintenance of positive affect. Older adults' strengths include their ability to avoid negative emotional experiences or to modify them so as to reduce their impact (i.e., to use emotion regulation strategies involving situation selection or modification). However, cognitive and physical declines that accompany old age constitute vulnerabilities. That is, when older individuals are exposed to high levels of stress and/or experience high levels of negative affect, they may be less able to employ cognitively demanding emotion regulation strategies as effectively as younger individuals. In addition, they may produce stronger stress-related cardiovascular and neuroendocrine responses (e.g., increased blood pressure, greater cortisol reactivity) and be unable to return to baseline levels as quickly as younger individuals.

Because all three theories emphasize older adults' maintenance of positive affect, many findings in the relevant emotion literature can be interpreted as being consistent (or at least not inconsistent) with all three (Sands et al., 2016). However, Carstensen, Shavit, and Barnes (2020) interpreted findings in their study of 18- to 76-year-old adults' affective responses to the COVID-19 pandemic as more consistent with SST than SVI. Older adults reported greater emotional well-being than younger adults despite perceiving that they were at greater risk. Still, older retired adults may have found it easier to cope with pandemic restrictions and thus experienced less stress than younger individuals. Thus it remains for future research to further adjudicate or integrate these models.

Retirement and Emotional Experience: Are These the Golden Years?

Retirement is a life event that comes with both benefits and costs (Luhmann, Hofmann, Eid, & Lucas, 2012). Among the benefits are termination of work-related stress and increase in time available for leisure activities and social engagements. Among the costs can be diminished income, loss of opportunities to interact with coworkers on a daily basis, and lack of a dependable structure to one's day. In addition, retirees will eventually encounter health problems due to their increasing age.

In recent decades, older workers have been given more choice about when they retire, and the factors associated with this decision have been studied. In a systematic review of retirement-related decision making, Browne, Carr, Fleischmann, Xue, and Stansfeld (2019) reported that later retirement was associated with higher job satisfaction and job control (e.g., decision authority, predictability of work, influence at work, flexibility of work hours/place). Job demands (e.g., fast work pace, conflicting demands) were not consistently related to retirement decisions. However, in a meta-analytic investigation of early retirement, Topa, Depolo, and Alcover (2018) found that an unpleasant work environment (e.g., age discrimination), an attractive financial incentive, and poor health were all associated with workers' decisions to leave their employment before a mandatory retirement age. Still, effect sizes were small.

The emotional impact of retirement has also been investigated, although the literature is sparse. In one meta-analytic investigation, Luhmann et al. (2012) reported that the retirement event itself was accompanied by a decrease in life satisfaction, but affective well-being (i.e., reports of positive and negative affect) did not change. During the course of the first postretirement year, life satisfaction and affective well-being both increased, with life satisfaction returning to its preretirement baseline level. Thus, when older adults first confront their postretirement lives, they may be dissatisfied although not less happy. Shortly thereafter, they appear to adapt and even experience an increase in positive affect balance.

Factors contributing to greater satisfaction and affective well-being in retirement have also been studied. For example, Bye and Pushkar (2009) found that positive affect was related to better health, greater perceived control over one's life, greater use of problem-focused coping strategies, greater motivation to engage in cognitive activities, more actual engagement in cognitive activities, and the personality traits of Conscientiousness and Openness. Poorer health, less perceived control, and the personality trait of Neuroticism were related to greater negative affect.

Largely consistent with these findings, Pushkar et al. (2010) also reported that higher levels of activity were related to greater positive and less negative affect. Regarding types of activity associated with better adjustment, Choi, Stewart, and Dewey (2013) found that formal volunteering and providing informal help to others were associated with lower levels of depressive symptoms, but caring for a sick or disabled adult was associated with higher levels of depression. Caring for grandchildren was unrelated to depressive symptoms. With respect to marital relations, Kupperbusch, Levenson, and Ebling (2003) reported that positive affect expressed by retired husbands during conversations with their wives predicted their higher ratings of satisfaction with retirement. However, no significant association between affect expressed by retired wives and their retirement satisfaction was found. All these studies involved retirees from Western cultures, but Zhang, Zhang, Zhao, and Yang (2019) examined Chinese retirees' subjective well-being (SWB). Findings showed that Chinese retirees with larger social networks maintained higher levels of SWB. This relationship was partially mediated by a form of future time perspective that involved focusing on the opportunities remaining in one's life for gratifying experiences. Together, the findings in these studies are consistent with an earlier review by Melton, Hersen, Van Sickle, and Van Hasselt (1995), who concluded that retirement is generally a positive experience for those who are in good health, have an adequate income, marital compatibility, purposeful activity, and a social network. Thus retirement can enhance one's emotional well-being under many (but not all) circumstances.

Are Older Persons' Emotions Reflected in Their Expressive Behavior?

An interesting discrepancy exists between results obtained in two types of studies that investigate facial expressivity in later adulthood. In the first type of study, trained coders measure older and younger persons' facial behavior using anatomically based systems (e.g., Facial Action Coding System [FACS]; Ekman et al., 2002). These studies have most often found either no age differences or even greater expressivity by older individuals (see Fölster, Hess, & Werheid, 2014, for a review). For example, Levenson, Carstensen, Friesen, and Ekman (1991) found no differences between younger and older adults who were asked to mentally relive and then describe experiences of happiness, anger, sadness, fear, and disgust. Providing another example, Lwi, Haase, Shiota, Newton, and Levenson (2019) found that older adults produced more sadness expressions than younger adults while watching a sad film clip, even after controlling for participants' self-reported experience of sadness.

In the second type of study, untrained observers are asked to identify the emotion in older and younger persons' facial expressions. These studies most often find that older persons' expressions are identified more poorly (again, see Fölster et al., 2014, for review). For example, Ebner, He, and Johnson (2011) asked both younger and older participants to identify standardized facial configurations (i.e., prototypic expressions) for happiness, sadness, anger, fear, and disgust that were posed by both younger and older models. Observers chose the intended emotion for expressions posed by younger models significantly more often than they did for expressions posed by older models. Similarly, Craig and Lipp (2018) found that college-age participants chose the intended emotion more often and more quickly when shown pictures of prototypic angry and happy expressions posed by younger rather than older models. According to Fölster et al. (2014), differences in observers' ability to decode older versus younger faces are likely due to both differences in facial morphology (e.g., increased sags and wrinkles) and age-related stereotypes that influence observers' attributions (e.g., more readiness to attribute sadness to older individuals). Interestingly, differences in observers' ability to decode older versus younger persons' emotion faces seem to occur irrespective of the observers' own age (e.g., Ebner et al., 2011); that is, an older person's smiles and frowns might be misinterpreted by both younger persons and the older person's own peers.

PERSONALITY

Can Personality Change in Later Adulthood?

Although comparatively few studies have been conducted on normative personality development during later adulthood, both continuity and change have been reported. As summarized in Costa et al. (2019; see Chapter 5), both Extraversion and Openness continue to decline in later adulthood, as they do throughout early and middle adulthood. However, the trajectories of Neuroticism, Agreeableness, and Conscientiousness appear to change direction. That is, after an earlier period of decline, Neuroticism now increases. After an earlier period of increase, both Agreeableness and Conscientiousness now decrease.

Individual Differences in Personality and Adaptive Functioning

Irrespective of normative trends, a considerable body of research has found associations between older adults' personality characteristics and their physical, cognitive, social, and emotional functioning. Much of this research has examined two of the Big Five personality factors that most intrinsically involve emotion, that is, Neuroticism and Extraversion. For example, Luchetti, Terracciano, Stephan, and Sutin (2016) conducted a meta-analysis of prospective studies involving older adults (50–107 years) in which personality was measured at Time 1 and cognitive functioning was measured at two or more later time points. Results showed that Neuroticism was associated with greater declines in memory over time, whereas Conscientiousness and Openness were associated with smaller declines. Perhaps surprisingly, Extraversion was also associated with greater cognitive declines over time. In interpreting this finding, the investigators suggested that persons who are high in Extraversion may become more easily distracted from cognitive tasks as they age. Interestingly, extraverts also have been found to overestimate their own cognitive performance. Although effect sizes for the personality variables were small, Luchetti and colleagues (2016) noted that they were comparable to or greater than effect sizes that have been reported in the literature for a variety of other risk factors related to cognitive decline (e.g., smoking, obesity, hypertension, diabetes).

Other investigations have examined relations between personality and various measures of social and emotional well-being. For example, in a study of adults in their early 70s, Potter et al. (2020) found that lower Extraversion and higher Neuroticism were associated with lower SWB. In a study of adults ranging in age from 24 to 74 years, Stokes (2019) found higher Neuroticism to be related to lower self-esteem. In addition, Neuroticism exacerbated the relationship between lower self-esteem and lower levels of perceived social integration (i.e., feelings of connectedness to members of one's community). This effect was strongest for the oldest participants.

Several other studies have investigated relations between Neuroticism and daily emotional experience. For example, Mroczek and Almeida (2004) conducted evening telephone interviews with participants from 25 to 74 years of age who rated the extent to which they had encountered stressful experiences during the day and also rated their experience of several forms of negative affect (e.g., depression, sadness, nervousness, restlessness). Participants also completed a one-time short measure of Neuroticism. Data analyses showed that the relationship between daily stress and negative affect was stronger for older than for younger participants and was particularly strong for those older adults who scored higher in Neuroticism. In a later study, Ready, Åkerstedt, and Mroczek (2012) examined the relationship between Neuroticism and measures of affective complexity and well-being. Participants ranging in age from 34 to 84 years completed a short measure of Neuroticism and rated themselves on their experience of both positive and negative emotions during the preceding month (e.g., depression, sadness, nervousness, cheerfulness, good spirits, enthusiasm). Affective complexity was assessed by correlating participants' scores for the positive and negative emotions; a higher negative correlation was considered to represent a lesser degree of emotional complexity. Affective well-being was assessed by determining the participant's ratio of positive to negative affect. Data analyses showed that Neuroticism predicted both lesser well-being and lesser affective complexity, and these relations were particularly strong for the older individuals. In a study of older persons' adjustment to retirement, Ryan, Newton, Chauhan, and Chopik (2017) found that higher levels of positive affect were related to higher levels of Extraversion, Conscientiousness, and Openness, whereas higher levels of negative affect were related to greater Neuroticism and lower levels of Conscientiousness. Thus, although the relevant literature is small, research appears to consistently show that emotion-related personality traits, especially Neuroticism, are manifested in the individual's daily emotional experiences.

Influences on Personality Development

Most studies implicitly adopt the position that personality is the cause rather than the consequence of the other measures with which it is associated (e.g., Wettstein, Wahl, & Siebert, 2020). In contrast, Mueller, Wagner, Smith, Voelkle, and Gerstorf (2018) considered both directions of influence in their study of Neuroticism, Extraversion, and their relation to functional health in adults participating in a longitudinal study of aging. Using criteria that are often employed in aging research, participants were categorized as young-old (i.e., 70 to 84 years) or oldest-old (85+ years). Over subsequent years, they periodically completed measures of personality, hand grip strength, and visual acuity. Data analyses showed that increases in Neuroticism preceded and predicted declines in grip strength and vision for young-old participants. In contrast, declines in grip strength and vision preceded and predicted increased Neuroticism for the oldest-old group. Decreases in Extraversion and decreases in the functional health measure (i.e., grip strength) were reciprocally related in both age groups.

A few studies have explicitly explored experiential factors that might contribute to the development of higher levels of some personality variables. In particular, childhood adversity has been related to higher levels of Neuroticism. For example, Wilson et al. (2006) conducted a retrospective study in which older individuals (M_{age} = 80 years) rated themselves on a number of **adverse childhood experiences** (e.g., "made you feel afraid," "not enough to eat," "punished you with a belt"), rated themselves on six facets of Neuroticism (i.e., anxiety, angry hostility, depression, self-consciousness, impulsiveness, vulnerability), and also indicated the number of children, family, and friends with whom they interacted, how often they participated in six types of social activities (e.g., visit with a friend, attending religious services), and their feelings of emotional isolation. Data analyses showed that childhood adversity (particularly, emotional neglect and parent intimidation) was strongly related to all facets of Neuroticism and also to having a smaller social network and feeling more socially isolated in later years. Together, these studies highlight the potential malleability of personality in response to one's circumstances.

ATTACHMENT

As noted in Chapters 4 and 5, researchers studying attachment in adulthood have developed a variety of measures designed to capture distinctions similar to those introduced by Ainsworth and her colleagues in their seminal work with infants (see Chapter 2). However, as also noted, adult studies evaluate the individual's general state of mind regarding attachment relations rather than the quality of their attachment to particular people (e.g., their mothers). Unfortunately, prospective studies of attachment starting in infancy and reaching into later adulthood are nonexistent. However, a few longitudinal investigations have followed participants from adolescence into later adulthood or across later adulthood itself. These studies have not produced entirely consistent results.

Are There Normative Trends in Older Adults' Attachment Development?

In one longitudinal investigation, Zhang and Labouvie-Vief (2004) studied 15- to 87-year-old middle-class European Americans using a measure in which participants rated themselves on statements describing **secure, dismissing/avoidant, anxious/preoccupied,** and **fearful attachment** (e.g., "It is relatively easy for me to become emotionally close to others"; "I am comfortable without close relationships"; "I find that others are reluctant to get as close as I would like"; "I find it difficult to trust others"; Bartholomew & Horowitz, 1991). These categories are presumed to roughly correspond to the four attachment categories developed in infant attachment studies (see Chapter 2). Averaging across participants, data analyses showed that scores for both secure and dismissing/avoidant attachment increased in later adulthood, whereas anxious/preoccupied attachment scores decreased. While acknowledging that the increases in both secure and dismissing/avoidant attachment appear somewhat paradoxical, the authors suggest that older adults may cope with the loss of some attachment figures by simultaneously

investing more in those who remain (thus scoring high on secure attachment) while at the same time defensively placing greater emphasis on independence (thus scoring high on dismissive avoidance).

In a second study, Consedine and Magai (2006, as reported in Magai,
Frias, & Shaver, 2016) studied an ethnically mixed sample of less affluent
and less educated 72-year-old adults (60% African American, 40% European American) using a different self-rating measure of attachment. Results
showed that scores for both secure and dismissing attachment declined over
the 6-year duration of the study. In interpreting the findings from both their
own study and that of Zhang and Labouvie-Vief (2004), Magai et al. (2016)
suggested that older participants from different ethnic and SES backgrounds
may differ in experiences that lead to disparate attachment outcomes. In
particular, older adults from poorer backgrounds may suffer more personal
losses, as well as losses of material resources, than middle-class individuals.
Consequently, they may cope with their losses in a different way. That is,
these older adults may experience a decline (rather than an increase) in feelings of overall attachment security. At the same time, their greater dependence on the personal and emotional relationships that remain may lead to
a decline in dismissive/avoidant feelings.

More recently, data from several landmark longitudinal studies
of human development have been creatively mined to produce a picture
that could shed further light on normative changes in attachment from
adolescence into old age. To do so, Chopik, Edelstein, and Grimm (2019)
extracted data from the Block and Block (2006) longitudinal study, the
Intergenerational Studies (Eichorn, Clausen, Haan, Honzik, & Mussen,
1981), and the Radcliffe College Class of 1964 Sample (Stewart & Vandewater, 1993). Within each of these three studies, the California Q-sort had
been administered at a number of time points. This measure consists of
100 descriptive items (e.g., "is talkative," "has conservative values," "keeps
people at a distance," "is basically anxious") that are sorted into nine groups
that reflect how characteristic they are of the target person (Block & Block,
2006). Chopik et al. (2019) identified a subset of Q-sort items that were
judged to reflect anxious or dismissive/avoidant attachment and generated
scores for each of these two insecure attachment categories. Of note, security was assumed to correspond to low scores for both categories but was not
directly measured or interpreted. Using a variant of multilevel growth curve
modeling that enables researchers to combine data from studies with overlapping but nonidentical age-related measurement time points, the investigators found moderate stability from 13 to 72 years of age in the rank ordering
of individuals' scores in both attachment anxiety and avoidance. Regarding

normative development, mean scores for anxious attachment remained at the same level up to 40 years of age but then declined, whereas mean scores for dismissive/avoidant attachment declined over the age range studied. Men were higher than women in dismissive/avoidant attachment at each time point. Being in a relationship was related to lower levels of both categories of attachment insecurity. These results are generally consistent with an interpretation of age-related decreases in dismissive/avoidance for high-risk populations offered by Magai et al. (2016). That is, declines in insecure attachment scores are consistent with the increase in emotional investments that characterizes later adulthood as portrayed in SST (Carstensen et al., 1999). At the same time, Chopik et al.'s (2019) results conflict with those of Zhang and Labouvie-Vief (2004), who found an increase in dismissing attachment for older adults from presumably comparable middle-class backgrounds. Of course, this inconsistency may reflect other methodological differences between the two studies—but it also indicates that further work is needed to understand how insecure attachment should be conceptualized in later adulthood and how its development should be characterized.

Attachment and Well-Being

Secure attachment status in later adulthood has been related to greater well-being in several investigations. For example, Bodner and Cohen-Fridel (2010) found that secure older adults (64–85 years) rated themselves higher than anxious/preoccupied and fearful adults on seven quality-of-life measures focusing mainly on physical health—physical functioning, bodily pain, vitality, and general health—but also mental health, social functioning, and emotional functioning. As in Zhang and Labouvie-Vief's (2004) study, findings for dismissive adults challenged the interpretation of this category as necessarily representing a form of maladjustment. Dismissive adults rated themselves as high as secure adults on the quality-of-life measures, again suggesting that a high degree of self-reliance may characterize dismissive older individuals and help them to adapt to their circumstances in later adulthood. Consistent with this notion, LeRoy et al. (2020) found that higher scores on attachment avoidance were associated with better self-reported mental and physical health and fewer grief symptoms in older adults who had lost their spouses. Thus, as noted above, further research is necessary to understand the meaning of dismissive attachment for older individuals living in different ecological circumstances. Qualitative interview studies that directly probe their appraisal of these circumstances might provide a useful database from which quantitative measures could eventually be developed.

Whereas parents and peers are the primary attachment figures for younger individuals, older persons identify their own adult children, as well as religious figures (e.g., God), caregivers, deceased loved ones, and pets, as important objects of attachment (Van Assche et al., 2013). Even favorite television characters can serve as sources of companionship and are often named by those with anxious attachments who are asked to list people to whom they feel close. However, these **parasocial attachment figures** cannot provide older individuals with the same sense of security that is derived from real-life secure attachment relations. Among older individuals who score high on anxious attachment and have poor relationships with their children, greater attachment to television characters is associated with higher—rather than lower—levels of depression (Bernhold & Metzger, 2020).

Attachment and Discrete Emotions

Attachment security has been found to be associated with greater expressions of both positive and negative discrete emotions. For example, Consedine and Magai (2003) asked 65- to 85-year-old low-income adults to complete a questionnaire measure of attachment and also to indicate the frequency with which they experienced each of 10 emotions in their daily lives (i.e., the Big Six, along with interest, contempt, shame, and guilt). Results showed that higher scores on attachment security were associated with higher levels of joy, sadness, interest, fear, and anger and with lower levels of guilt, contempt, and shame. Higher dismissive attachment scores were associated with higher scores on interest and lower scores for joy, shame, and fear. Greater fearful/preoccupied attachment was associated with higher scores for joy, disgust, shame, and anxiety/fear. Interpretation of these data was hampered by the absence of information about the situational contexts in which the various emotions were experienced. However, Consedine and Magai (2003) identified several theoretically plausible relationships between attachment and emotion. For example, they argued that attachment security should be associated with a wider range of emotional experiences, as was indeed found in their study. In the attachment literature, dismissive attachment has been interpreted as reflecting an attempt to minimize the negative emotional consequences of early rejection (Cassidy, 1994), and this might result in the low levels of shame and fear found in their study for those who scored high in dismissiveness. Fearful/preoccupied attachment (as conceptualized within their study) has been interpreted as reflecting a strong investment in the attachment relationship along with anxiety about the dependability of the attachment figure. Thus one might plausibly expect high levels of both joy and negative emotions such as shame and fear. These findings point the way to future studies that might incorporate measures of the situational contexts in which participants' emotions are experienced.

EMOTION-RELATED INFORMATION PROCESSING

The Positivity Effect

Supporting older adults' increased motivation to experience positive emotions is an information-processing bias known as the **positivity effect** (Carstensen, 2019). The term refers to older persons' propensity to attend to and remember information related to positive affect more than negative affect. For example, Charles, Mather, and Carstensen (2003) asked young, middle-aged, and older adults to simply view a set of pictures designed to evoke positive, neutral, and negative affect (e.g., a beautiful landscape, a filthy toilet). Afterward, they were asked to write down a brief description of as many pictures as they remembered. Whereas younger adults recalled an equal number of positive and negative images, both the older and middle-aged adults recalled more positive than negative pictures. In addition, when shown both the previously viewed pictures and an equal number of never-viewed distractor images, younger adults recognized an equal number of positive and negative pictures, whereas middle-aged and older adults recognized more positive than negative images.

In a meta-analysis that included 100 studies, Reed, Chan, and Mikels (2014) found a robust positivity effect that also was moderated by an important methodological factor. In particular, the effect was substantially larger in studies that imposed fewer controls on participants' information processing, such as the study by Charles et al. (2003) described above. In contrast, when participants' responses were constrained by experimental instructions or tasks that overwhelmed their resources, the effect was smaller or did not occur. For example, Grühn, Smith, and Baltes (2005) failed to find a positivity effect in a study in which they explicitly instructed participants to remember as many words as possible from lists of emotion-related words. Similarly, Bucher, Voss, Spaniol, Hische, and Sauer (2020) failed to find a positivity effect when they explicitly instructed participants to determine whether a group of pictures included a greater number of happy or a greater number of angry facial expressions. According to SST, the positivity effect ultimately reflects age-related differences in individuals' motivation to experience positive emotions (i.e., a positivity bias) and thus may not emerge when experimental demands overwhelm this motivational preference.

Appraisal Biases

Another factor that may contribute to the experience of positive affect in later adulthood is an age-related shift in appraisal tendencies. As previously noted (see Chapter 1), most contemporary emotion theories consider appraisals to mediate between the situation encountered by a person and the person's emotional reaction. Young, Minton, and Mikels (2021) have proposed that older and younger adults may appraise some situations differently and consequently differ in their emotional responses. As previously noted, extant appraisal theories differ among themselves in their characterization of the appraisal process. However, virtually all include assessing control (i.e., who or what controls the initiation or outcome of the emotion situation) as one important feature. To explore possible age differences in appraisals of control, Young and Mikels (2020) presented older (mean age = 63 years) and younger adults (mean age = 23 years) with scenarios that were emotionally ambiguous (e.g., not hearing from your friends on your birthday about halfway through the day). Participants rated how much the eventual outcome of the situation would be controlled by themselves, by another person, and by circumstances beyond either's control. Additionally, participants rated how strongly they would feel each of several emotions (e.g., hope, joy, sadness, nervousness). Demonstrating a positivity effect, affect balance scores were greater for older than for younger adults. Similarly, difference scores representing self-minus-other control ratings were greater for older than younger adults, indicating that older adults reported themselves more in control of the situation than did the younger participants. Further analyses showed that the relationship between age group and positive affect balance was partially mediated by appraisals of relative control by oneself.

EMOTION AND DECISION MAKING

Does Affect Impair Decision Making in Older Adults?

Concerns about the cognitive declines that accompany aging have led to a growing body of research on decision making in older adults, including studies that investigate the role of positive and negative affect. Taken together, this research suggests that whether affect impairs their decision making depends on both the type of affect and the type of decision being made. One important distinction has been made between integral and incidental affect. **Integral affect** refers to feelings relevant to the decision to be made (i.e., one's affective responses to the various choices), whereas **incidental**

affect refers to affect one may be experiencing while making the choice but that is unrelated to the choice itself (e.g., how one is feeling when encountering the decision-making event). To illustrate, your choice of whether to watch a comedy or dramatic movie might depend both on both integral affect (e.g., which movie has your favorite actor) and incidental affect (e.g., whether you are in a good or bad mood when you make your movie choice).

Models and Frameworks

Most models that have been proposed for emotion-related decision making focus on integral affect. For example, **dual systems models** (e.g., Kahneman, 2003) posit that decision making relies on both an intuitive system and a deliberative system. The deliberative system is slow, deliberate, and analytical, while the intuitive system is fast, automatic, and spontaneous. Some (but not all) dual system models include affective responding as a component of the intuitive system. In addition, other decision-making models have been proposed that include different types of mechanisms involving integral affect (e.g., framing effects, affect heuristics; see Mikels, Shuster, & Thai, 2015, for a detailed review).

Although incidental affect has received less attention, the appraisal tendency framework (Lerner, Gonzalez, Small, & Fischoff, 2003; Lerner & Keltner, 2000) addresses the role it may play in the decision-making process. According to this model, a person's dispositional emotions (e.g., temperamental fearfulness or anger proneness), as well as his or her momentary (i.e., incidental) affect, can influence how he or she appraises a decision-making event and can thereby bias his or her choices. For example, a fearful person would tend to estimate the probability of an unfortunate event (e.g., a natural disaster) as being greater than would an anger-prone person and would be more likely to take precautionary measures. Affective arousal can also influence one's decisions. That is, high incidental arousal (e.g., positive arousal not caused by the decision event) may incline a person toward taking risks, whereas low arousal may have the opposite effect. Lastly, irrespective of one's emotional dispositions, incidental affect experienced for whatever reason (e.g., physical discomfort) can also bias one's appraisals of a decision-making event and thus one's final choices.

Positivity Bias and Positivity Effect

Research has shown that older adults' greater motivation to experience positive affect (i.e., their positivity bias) and their greater tendency to attend to and remember positive information (i.e., the positivity effect in information processing) both may play a role in their decision making. For example, Kim, Healey, Goldstein, Hasher, and Wiprzycka (2008) asked younger and older adults to list the positive and negative attributes of four products (i.e., pen, flashlight, mug, clipboard) and then choose the one they preferred to receive. The researchers found that older adults listed relatively more positive features than did younger adults and also tended to be more satisfied with their final choices. However, as suggested by Mikels et al. (2015), the positivity bias and/or effect may be disadvantageous if an older individual fails to think of a critically important disadvantage of a particularly important choice and thus is led astray. Consistent with this concern, older individuals more often than younger adults have been found to terminate exploration of decision choices prematurely when experiencing incidental positive affect (von Helversen & Mata, 2012). Providing another example, Chou, Lee, and Ho (2007) found that older adults were more likely than younger adults to choose a risky decision option after watching a positive film clip that was unrelated to the decision choice.

Health-Related Decision Making

Because health-related decision making is of particular importance to older individuals, a growing number of studies have explored their responsiveness to affective components of health care messages. To illustrate, Mikels et al. (2010) conducted a health care decision-making study in which younger adults (18–30 years) and older adults (65–85 years) were asked to choose between two options (e.g., between two health care plans) after being presented with a number of positive and negative features of each option. The number of features presented increased across trials, thus placing a progressively greater load on participants' working memory. Participants also were instructed to focus on the details of the features presented for each option (information-focus condition) or on their overall positive or negative affective response to each option (affect-focus condition) or were given no special instructions at all (control condition). No significant age differences were found for participants in the affect-focus or control conditions. However, older adults performed more poorly than younger adults in the information-focus condition, that is, they more often failed to choose the option with the best ratio of positive to negative features. For both older and younger adults, performance in the information-focus condition was related to a separate measure of their speed of information processing. Given these findings, it is not surprising that older adults prefer to engage in less deliberate and complex decision making than younger adults and prefer to decide among fewer options (Reed, Mikels, & Simon, 2014). For example, although a younger adult might like to shop in a grocery store that offers 26 different types of coffee, an older adult might be happier choosing among a smaller number of options.

In another investigation, Shamaskin, Mikels, and Reed (2010) asked younger and older adults to read pamphlets with positive or negative health care messages regarding the benefits of engaging in healthy behaviors or the risks associated with failing to do so. Participants rated each pamphlet for informativeness, seriousness of the health risk described, their own level of risk, and their likelihood of engaging in preventative or detection practices. They were then given a task that assessed their recognition of the specific messages that appeared in each pamphlet. Relative to younger adults, older adults gave higher ratings to the pamphlets for informativeness and seriousness and their own likelihood of engaging in preventative practices. In addition, older adults rated the positive pamphlets as more informative than the negative pamphlets, whereas no significant difference was found for the younger participants. Lastly, positive messages constituted a greater proportion of the total number of messages remembered by older adults in comparison with younger adults. These findings indicate that older persons may be more responsive to health care messages than are younger persons and may exhibit a positivity bias in their preference for such messages and a positivity effect in their memory for such messages.

Complementing these findings were the results of an investigation by Isaacowitz and Choi (2012) that focused on negative health care messaging. In their study, younger and older adults viewed videotapes with unpleasant images (e.g., pictures of skin damage due to sun exposure) along with risk-reduction information about skin cancer. Results showed that older individuals spent less time than younger individuals attending to the videotape and learned fewer facts about skin cancer. Nonetheless, the older adults responded more often than younger adults by changing their skin care practices (at least temporarily) after receiving the negative message. Together, these studies suggest that the positivity effect in information processing (as typically measured in the form of attention and memory) does not always dominate decision making in older adults. One possibility is that negative messages may sometimes be appraised as being particularly relevant and important. Thus, including an affective component in health care messaging may indeed improve its effectiveness. However, further research is necessary to better understand how younger and older adults respond to both positive and negative health care information.

EMOTION REGULATION

Is Emotion Regulation Impaired in Later Adulthood?

Much of the research on emotion regulation in later adulthood has been conducted within the framework of James Gross's (2015a, 2015b) process model of emotion regulation. As previously described (see Chapter 5), Gross's model outlines five categories (or families) of emotion regulation strategies: (1) situation selection, (2) situation modification, (3) attentional deployment, (4) cognitive change (e.g., reappraisal), and (5) response modulation. Research on older adults' use of these strategies has included laboratory investigations, questionnaire studies, and studies using experience sampling methods (ESMs). These have not always produced consistent results. However, overall, the research suggests that older adults can regulate their emotions as well as (and sometimes better than) younger adults, but they may sometimes use different strategies in order to do so.

Studies Using Experience Sampling Methods (ESMs)

Recent ESM studies have found that older adults use the various categories of emotion strategies as often as younger adults in daily life. To illustrate, Livingstone and Isaacowitz (2021) examined younger adults' (20–39 years), middle-aged adults' (40–59 years), and older adults' (60–79 years) daily experiences of emotion regulation in an experience sampling study. Participants were signaled by smartphone five times a day and rated their affect on a 7-point bipolar hedonic scale (–3 to +3). They also indicated whether they had "done anything to try to influence [their] emotions" since they were last prompted. If so, they indicated in which of the five regulation categories they had engaged: whether they had chosen to enter or avoid a situation, acted to change the situation, shifted their attention, changed their thinking, and/or changed their expression of emotion. They were also asked whether they had tried to increase or decrease their positive or negative affect. Results showed that there were no age differences in how often participants attempted to regulate their emotions, nor were there age differences in their relative preference for some strategies over others; instead, all age groups used situation selection and situation modification more than attentional change, which itself was used more than cognitive change, followed by response modification. Older individuals tried to increase their positive emotion more than younger individuals. Only one age difference was found for strategy effectiveness (indexed by the difference in affect scores before vs. after the regulation attempt). Specifically, situation selection was more effective for younger than older individuals.

Eldesouky and English (2018) asked both younger and older adult participants to complete daily diary reports on their use of six regulation strategies, including two from the cognitive change category: detachment and positive reappraisal. No age differences were found in participants' use of these two strategies or any of the other four that were measured, that is, one strategy each from the categories of situation selection, situation modification, attention deployment, and expressive suppression. However, in a daily diary study examining a wider range of responses, Puente-Martínez, Prizmic-Larsen, Larsen, Ubillos-Landa, and Páez-Rovira (2021) found that older adults used more of the regulation strategies considered to be more adaptive by the authors (e.g., reappraisal, humor) than did younger and middle-aged adults when they experienced particularly high levels of negative affect. Similarly, Burr, Castrellon, Zald, and Samanez-Larkin (2021) found that the older adults reported being able to control their desires (i.e., resist temptations) more than younger adults.

Questionnaire Studies

Eldesouky and English (2018) also collected questionnaire data by having participants complete a one-time measure of their habitual use of reappraisal and expressive suppression. Participants rated themselves on items taken from the ERQ (Gross & John, 2003), a measure with subscales for both regulation strategies. In contrast to results from analyses of the same participants' daily diaries, older adults reported more use of suppression than did younger adults. Although this inconsistency across measures may be difficult to explain, future research that examines strategy use in specific situational contexts may shed light on the discrepancy. For example, when participants complete the ERQ, perhaps older adults are thinking about more intense emotional situations than are commonly encountered in their daily lives.

In another type of questionnaire study, Fung, Carstensen, and Lang (2001) examined associations between older and younger adults' happiness ratings and both the size and composition of their social networks. Older persons reported having fewer social partners than younger individuals but tended to retain those with whom they had a close relationship. These close relationships appeared sufficient to bring them happiness. The investigators interpreted their findings within the framework of SST. They suggested that older adults may use avoidance (a situation selection regulation strategy) more often than younger individuals so as to selectively prune their social networks in a way that maximizes their positive experiences.

Laboratory Studies

Other examples of age differences in emotion regulation have been found in laboratory studies. In an investigation that illustrated the category of situation modification (Livingstone & Isaacowitz, 2015), older and younger individuals participated in a laboratory procedure during which they were presented with video episodes containing positive, neutral, or negative affect content. When given the opportunity, older individuals skipped over the negative episodes more often than did younger individuals. With respect to attention deployment, Isaacowitz, Wadlinger, Goren, and Wilson (2006) presented older and younger individuals with pairs of faces, one having a neutral expression and one having an emotional expression of happiness, sadness, anger, or fear. Consistent with the positivity bias, older participants looked more at the happy face than the neutral face and less at the angry face than the neutral face. Consistent with research showing an attentional bias toward threat stimuli at earlier ages (see Chapter 7), young adults' only preference was to look at the fearful face more than the neutral face.

For cognitive change, most investigators have focused on reappraisal, that is, thinking differently about an emotion stimulus. However, cognitive change can take several forms, and there may be age differences in their frequency of use or their effectiveness. To investigate the relative effectiveness of two forms of cognitive change, Shiota and Levenson (2009) presented older, middle-aged, and younger individuals with brief film clips having either sad or disgust content and instructed them to engage in either detachment (i.e., viewing the negative clips objectively) or positive reappraisal (i.e., thinking about the positive aspects of what they were seeing). In an additional condition (involving the fifth regulation category, response modification), participants were instructed to suppress their emotional behavior so that another person would not know what they were feeling. After each trial, all participants rated their experiencing of sadness and disgust, as well as other emotions. Comparisons of emotion ratings were made between these regulation trials and control trials in which participants were instructed to simply watch the film clips. Results showed that older individuals were successful in regulating their emotions in the positive reappraisal condition but not in the detachment condition, whereas the opposite pattern was seen in younger and middle-aged participants. Thus different variants within the same regulation category may be differentially effective when used by older versus younger individuals. Finally, with respect to suppression (a type of response modulation strategy), Shiota and Levenson (2009) found no differences in its effectiveness for younger versus older individuals in their laboratory study.

Looking across two different categories of regulation strategies, Scheibe, Sheppes, and Staudinger (2015) found age differences in older and younger adults' preferences for distraction (an attentional deployment strategy) and reappraisal (a cognitive change strategy). In their study, younger adults (19–28 years) and older adults (65–75 years) briefly viewed high- and low-intensity negative emotion pictures and were asked whether they thought distraction or reappraisal would most effectively help them feel less negatively about the picture. Subsequently, the picture was viewed again, and participants were instructed to enact their chosen strategy. After viewing the picture for the second time, participants rated their negative affect. Results showed that older adults chose distraction more often than younger adults and that this strategy was more effective than reappraisal in mitigating their negative affect. Younger adults showed no preference, and both strategies were equally effective. Irrespective of age, poorer performance on a measure of executive functioning was related to a greater preference for distraction, the less cognitively demanding regulation strategy.

CULTURE AND EMOTION

Is Socioemotional Selectivity Theory (SST) Universal?

SST, the most emotion-focused contemporary theory of aging, proposes that adults shift from focusing on achievement-oriented goals to focusing more on emotionally meaningful goals as they grow older (Carstensen et al., 1999). Correspondingly, they seek to regulate their emotions so as to maximize emotional well-being. Within the existing research, emotional well-being has been operationalized almost exclusively in terms of maximizing positive affect relative to negative affect (i.e., affect balance). However, because positive affect may be more highly valued in independence-oriented Western societies than it is elsewhere (Kitayama, Berg, & Chopik, 2020), several culturally oriented researchers have sought to empirically determine the extent to which SST can be generalized across cultures, particularly Asian cultures with different emotion-related values.

Only a very few studies have directly compared positive and negative affect in younger and older adults in non-Western cultures. However, in one such study, Pethtel and Chen (2010) asked younger and older adults from both mainland China and the United States to complete the **Positive and Negative Affect Scales (PANAS**; Watson, Clark, & Tellegen, 1988). This widely used self-report measure assesses a set of both positive and negative affective states (e.g., interest, excitement, distress, fear—although not happiness or contentment!?). Results showed that older participants in both cultural groups reported less negative affect than younger participants, whereas positive affect did not significantly differ across age for either group. Thus findings for affect balance in both U.S. and mainland Chinese participants were interpreted as being consistent with SST. At the same time, U.S. individuals in both age groups reported higher levels of positive affect than did Chinese individuals.

Using a different methodology to investigate a different Asian culture, Grossman, Karasawa, Kan, and Kitayama (2014) asked younger and older U.S. and Japanese adults to recall personal instances of pleasant and unpleasant situations involving social relations, work, study, or daily hassles (e.g., being caught in a traffic jam). Participants then rated the intensity of both their positive and negative affective responses to their personal exemplars. Consistent with results reported by Pethtel and Chen (2010), older U.S. participants reported lower negative affect scores than younger U.S. participants, whereas positive affect scores did not change with age. In contrast, no age differences in either positive or negative affect were found for Japanese participants, a pattern of results not consistent with SST. In interpreting their findings, the authors propose that well-being for older Japanese individuals may not involve the same factors as it does for older U.S. individuals. In particular, Japanese individuals may be more accepting of both negative and positive affect and thus have less desire to maximize positive and minimize negative emotion as they grow older. Furthermore, they suggested that older Japanese individuals may be more accepting of age-related physical and cognitive declines than are older individuals in Western cultures.

The Positivity Effect in Information Processing

Several studies have investigated potential differences in information processing between older individuals from different cultures. For example, Fung, Gong, Ngo, and Isaacowitz (2019) examined the relationship between visual attention and mood in younger and older European American and Hong Kong Chinese adults. Participants' mood was first manipulated by showing them either a negative or neutral film clip (e.g., the death of Mufasa scene from *The Lion King* or nature scenery). Subsequently, participants viewed a series of pictures that included positive, negative, and neutral images and rated their mood after viewing each picture. Eye-tracking technology was used to measure their visual attention (i.e., duration of gaze) at the most affectively relevant part of each image. Results indicated a positivity effect for European Americans, with older participants looking longer at positive images than did younger participants. No similar effect was found for Hong Kong participants. At the same time, analyses of the mood ratings showed that looking longer at positive pictures was associated with better mood for older Hong Kong participants but not for European Americans. In interpreting their findings, the researchers suggested that "an age-related positivity effect exists at the preference level for Americans but at the effectiveness level for Chinese" (Fung et al., 2019, p. 1414).

Affective Arousal

An additional consideration in evaluating older Asians' emotional well-being is their preference for experiencing high-arousal positive affect less than do European Americans (Tsai & Sims, 2016). Cultural preferences for high- and low-arousal emotions have been investigated principally within the context of **affect valuation theory (AVT**; Tsai, 2007; Tsai et al., 2006; see also Chapter 5). According to this theory, **ideal affect** (i.e., one's preferred level of affect intensity) is at least partially shaped by cultural factors that include values regarding personal behaviors, social relationships, and emotional responding. Of importance, AVT distinguishes between ideal affect and the actual affect one may experience in daily life. In a study that investigated AVT across adulthood, Tsai et al. (2018) asked European American, Chinese American, and Hong Kong Chinese younger, middle-aged, and older adults to rate how much they like to feel emotion-related states that were high in arousal and positive (HAP; i.e., enthusiastic, excited, elated), low in arousal and positive (LAP; i.e., calm, relaxed, serene), high in arousal and negative (HAN; i.e., fearful, hostile, nervous), and low in arousal and negative (LAN; i.e., dull, sleepy, sluggish). Participants were also asked to describe what experiences they looked forward to and what they dreaded about being 75 years of age or older. Positive outlook scores were computed by subtracting the number of negative experiences they described from the number of positive experiences. Data analyses showed that both middle-aged and older European Americans valued HAP states more than their Asian peers but also had lower positive outlook scores, thus indicating they had a less optimistic view of old age. These findings suggest that continuing to value HAP states (e.g., excitement) into later adulthood might lead to lower levels of life satisfaction, possibly because engaging in some types of exciting activities (e.g., skydiving) becomes less feasible with age. In addition, nonsignificant trends in the data showed that European Americans also valued LAP states more than did the Asian participants, whereas HAN and LAN states were valued more by Asian participants than by European Americans. Albeit nonsignificant, these trends are consistent with both Kitayama et al.'s (2020) and Grossman et al.'s (2014) proposal that older Asians are less focused on experiencing positive affect and more accepting of negative affect than are older adults from Western cultures.

GENDER AND EMOTION

Do Older Men and Women Differ in Emotional Experience and Regulation?

Gender effects have not been a key focus in research on aging and emotion. However, comparisons have been made in some studies, yielding results that are only partially consistent across investigations. In studies of participant-reported emotional experience that include adults spanning a wide range of ages (e.g., from 18 to 94 years; Carstensen et al., 2011), women sometimes have been reported to experience some or all emotions more strongly than men (e.g., Carstensen et al., 2011; Kunzmann et al., 2013; Shiota & Levenson, 2009). However, no gender differences have been found in other investigations (e.g., Charles et al., 2001). Furthermore, results specific to the older men and women in these studies are rarely reported. Still, in one study of positive and negative affect, Mroczek and Kolarz (1998) did find that age-related trajectories differed depending on gender. In particular, positive affect increased linearly for men but exponentially for women, whereas negative affect decreased across age only for married men. Thus both genders experienced an increase in positive affect balance, but this resulted from different trajectories of affect change.

In studies of emotion regulation with participants spanning a wide age range, gender effects are again rarely investigated. However, in a study that involved participants' reports about their daily use of various regulation strategies (Eldesouky & English, 2018), results showed that older women used suppression more than younger women, whereas older men used situation selection more than younger men. In a similar self-report study that included only older participants (i.e., 60–89 years), Brady, Kneebone, and Bailey (2019) found that men used suppression more than women, whereas women used reappraisal more than men. Reappraisal was associated with higher levels of positive affect for both genders and was related to lower levels of negative affect for women. Suppression was associated with higher levels of negative affect for men but unrelated to positive affect. Thus a few potentially interesting gender effects have been found in some investigations. However, effect sizes for these differences have not been reported and are likely to be small. Further research is needed to evaluate the robustness of these relationships and to understand their contextual determinants.

Emotion Understanding: Does the Female Advantage Persist in Later Adulthood?

Overall, the female advantage in emotional intelligence (EI) appears to persist into later adulthood (Cabello et al., 2016). In fact, Cabello and colleagues found that the female advantage for perceiving emotion, the first of the four EI branches, is greater in older adults than in younger adults. Several studies using non-EI measures of emotion recognition also have found a female advantage in older adults (Campbell, Ruffman, Murray, & Glue, 2014; Ruffman, Murray, Halberstadt, & Taumoepeau, 2010; Sullivan, Campbell, Hutton, & Ruffman, 2017).

NEUROBIOLOGICAL UNDERPINNINGS

Brain Functioning

Although brain mass (including both gray and white matter) decreases with age, two areas importantly related to emotional functioning are relatively well preserved—the amygdala and the ventromedial prefrontal cortex (vmPFC; Mather, 2016). At the same time, different forms of emotion functioning include a variety of cognitive processes (e.g., attention, memory, speed of processing) and thus may be affected by age-related changes in brain structures and neural functioning related to these processes. For example, age-related breakdowns in white matter might affect overall speed of information processing. Decreases in hippocampal volume and activity might affect memory for emotion material. Production of some emotion-related neurotransmitters (e.g., dopamine, norepinephrine) also declines with age. In addition, older individuals show less specificity in their neural responses to various cognitive tasks in comparison with younger individuals, and this may translate into more errors in their behavioral responding (see Gutchess,

2019). At the same time, observed increases in overall prefrontal cortex (PFC) activity (Park & Reuter-Lorenz, 2009) may partially compensate for some of these declines. Consequently, a complex picture of brain functioning in later adulthood is beginning to emerge based on findings of both similarities and differences in the neural correlates of emotion functioning in younger and older individuals.

In an attempt to integrate the findings from functional magnetic resonance imaging (fMRI) studies comparing younger and older adults, Mac-Cormack et al. (2020) conducted a meta-analysis of investigations that presented participants with positive and/or negative affective stimuli and measured either their perception or experience of affect or emotion along with their brain activity. Data analyses were conducted to identify areas of the brain that were reliably (i.e., most often) activated in conjunction with positive or negative affect and affect at high versus low levels of arousal. Further analyses examined temporal co-occurrence among these areas within individual studies to identify "nodes" of coactivation and characterize nodes in terms of their centrality (e.g., number of connections to other nodes) and efficiency (i.e., distance from other nodes). Results were interpreted in terms of two proposals regarding age-related differences in brain functioning that have received attention in the literature. According to the theory of maturational dualism (Mendes, 2010), age-related structural changes in the peripheral nervous system (e.g., decreased myelination) may lead to lesser communication with the brain and correspondingly less activation of brain regions involved in autonomic regulation and interoception (i.e., the brain's representation of the activity of internal organs, tissue, hormones, and immune system). According to SST, older adults' positivity bias may be supported by greater activity in brain areas involved in mentalizing, autobiographical memory, and self-referential (i.e., introspective) processing (Mather & Carstensen, 2005; Martins & Mather, 2016). These two theories are considered complementary rather than mutually exclusive, and findings provided partial support for both theories. For example, younger adults showed more reliable activation than older adults in brain areas involved in autonomic regulation (e.g., amygdala, thalamus, posterior insula). Older adults showed more reliable activation in some of the brain areas considered to support the type of emotion processing described within SST (e.g., dorsal medial PFC). Although promising, the authors acknowledge that findings from this study are provisional due in part to the relatively small number of available studies. This may have precluded their ability to separate studies that focused on different specific emotions or to contrast emotion perception versus emotion elicitation.

Neural Correlates of Emotion Regulation

The neural correlates of emotion regulation in older and younger adults is an area of particular interest to neuroscientists. Using Gross's model of emotion regulation (Gross, 2015a, 2015b), strategies that are introduced at earlier steps of the emotion process (e.g., situation selection, attention deployment) have been proposed to be favored by older persons over strategies that are employed later (e.g., during the cognitive response step). Early regulation of emotion is considered advantageous because the strategies that are used at later stages are presumed to require more cognitive resources (Urry & Gross, 2010). Indeed, a preference by older adults for distraction (an attentional deployment strategy) over reappraisal (a cognitive change strategy) has been observed in some often-cited laboratory investigations (e.g., Scheibe et al., 2015, described earlier in this chapter). Therefore, the neural correlates of attentional strategies (e.g., distraction) and cognitive change strategies (e.g., reappraisal) are two forms of regulation that have often been investigated.

In a meta-analysis of fMRI studies on cognitive reappraisal, Buhle et al. (2014) found that younger adults tend to activate the parietal lobe and the cognitive control areas of the PFC (i.e., dorsal medial, dorsal lateral, and ventrolateral portions). These areas of the PFC decline over age in structure and function, and several studies have shown that older adults activate them less than younger adults during reappraisal (Mather, 2016). For example, Allard and Kensinger (2014) used fMRI to scan the brains of older (M_{age} = 69 years) and younger (M_{age} = 23 years) individuals as they viewed brief film clips depicting sadness, fear, and disgust scenarios. Participants were given different viewing instructions in different within-subject experimental conditions. In the passive viewing condition, participants were instructed to watch the film as they naturally would if they were at home. In the selective attention condition, they were instructed to attend to areas of the screen that would help them increase positive and decrease negative emotions. In the cognitive change condition, they were instructed to alter how they thought about the film (e.g., by using detachment and/or positive reappraisal). Both age groups showed greater activation of the PFC during cognitive change trials than during passive viewing or selective attention trials. However, differences between the age groups also were seen in terms of the areas within the PFC that were engaged. In particular, dorsal and lateral portions of the PFC showed increased activation in younger individuals, whereas more well-preserved ventromedial portions of the PFC showed increased activation in older individuals. Other studies have also found less lateral PFC activity accompanying use of cognitive change strategies by older individuals in contrast to younger individuals (Opitz, Rauch, Terry, & Urry, 2012; Winecoff, LaBar, Madden, Cabeza, & Huettel, 2011).

As noted above, some research also has suggested that older persons generate a less differentiated (i.e., less selective) set of neural responses during reappraisal than do younger persons. For example, Martins, Ponzio, Velasco, Kaplan, and Mather (2015) found that younger participants produced significantly lower levels of activity in the posterior medial cortex (PMC) during reappraisal than during distraction. In contrast, older participants showed similar levels of PMC activity during both types of regulation. Thus older persons demonstrated **dedifferentiation**, that is, activation of the PMC was less specialized. Such dedifferentiation might be expected to impair the effectiveness of some forms of emotion regulation (Gutchess, 2019). However, Martins et al. (2015) found no age differences in participant-reported affect ratings that followed their efforts at emotion regulation. Still, under circumstances in which cognitive load is very high, cognitive-oriented regulation processes such as reappraisal may be less successful in older individuals.

Focusing on distraction, this attention-oriented regulation process also is supported by activity of the parietal cortex, an area that plays a role in the voluntary control of attention. The parietal cortex is well maintained into later adulthood, and thus an age-related decline in the use of distraction would not necessarily be expected (Mather, 2016). Indeed, neither Scheibe et al. (2015) nor Livingstone and Isaacowitz (2021) found such a decline in their previously described studies of emotion regulation in younger and older adults.

Powerful Emotion Episodes

One striking characteristic of emotion is that some powerful episodes are characterized by acute onset, high arousal, and a narrowing of perceptual and cognitive focus. For example, when learning that your spouse has been killed in a car accident involving a drunk driver, you might be suddenly overwhelmed with intense grief and anger to the exclusion of everything else. Acute onset and high arousal may be readily explained by the acute nature of the stimulus. But why does this produce the attentional narrowing that may sometimes enhance but sometimes impede appropriate emotion responding? One potential explanation may come from an extension of the **GANE (glutamate amplifies noradrenergic effects) model** proposed by Mather, Clewett, Sakaki, and Harley (2016). According to this model, high arousal leads to increased release of norepinephrine from the locus coeruleus (LC), a small structure in the brainstem with long axons that project throughout much of the brain. Norepinephrine interacts with glutamate that has been released in areas of the brain that have been activated, in this case in relation to the emotion stimulus. This interaction further increases the activity of these areas while, at the same time, norepinephrine released in less active brain areas serves to further quiet their activity. Thus attention may be focused on the emotional event to the relative exclusion of other considerations. Whether the LC deteriorates with normal aging is as yet unclear (Mather, 2016). However, its deterioration does appear to accompany two diseases that tend to target older individuals: Parkinson's and Alzheimer's diseases. Thus these older individuals might be expected to differ from others in their experience of powerful emotion episodes.

Autonomic Nervous System (ANS)

Aging brings multiple changes in ANS activity and the functioning of body organs it controls (Shiota & Neufeld, 2014). Heart rate reactivity during physical exertion decreases, along with skin conductance. At the same time—as is well known—blood pressure tends to be higher in older adults.

Corresponding to age-related decreases in response to physical challenges, heart rate reactivity in response to emotion stimuli also appears lower in older adults. In a meta-analytic review of laboratory studies that involved emotion- or stress-related procedures, Uchino, Birmingham, and Berg (2010) found an association between older age and lower heart rate reactivity, as well as increased systolic blood pressure. Exemplifying such studies, Burriss, Powell, and White (2007) presented participants with pictures that had been previously rated for valence and arousal and found that younger adults (mean age = 22 years) responded to the emotion stimuli with greater changes in heart rate than did both older (mean age = 72 years) and middle-aged (mean age = 48 years) adults. At the same time, both the older and middle-aged groups rated the pictures higher in terms of valence and arousal than did the younger participants. Thus the lesser heart rate reactivity of the older two age groups was not attributable to their being less affected by the stimuli.

Other studies have examined the possibility that different emotions of the same valence (e.g., anger vs. fear vs. sadness) may differ in age-related physiological changes. For example, Seider, Shiota, Whalen, and Levenson (2011) presented older, middle-aged, and younger adults with sad, disgust, and neutral film clips and found that older participants reported greater sadness in response to the sad film than did the younger age groups and correspondingly were more physiologically reactive (i.e., showed increases in ANS-related measures, including heart rate, respiration, and skin conductance). No age differences were found in either subjective or physiological responses to the disgust films. Parallel findings for both subjective and physiological responses suggested that physiology tracked the subjective emotional impact of the stimuli for both age groups. Also of importance, older adults were no less physiologically reactive than younger adults. These findings thus suggest that age differences in emotion-related physiological reactivity may differ depending on stimulus characteristics. That is, film clips (such as those used by Seider et al.) may be more powerful elicitors than still photographs (such as those used by Burriss et al.) and thus produce fewer age differences in emotion responding.

Hypothalamic–Pituitary–Adrenal (HPA) System

As noted in Chapter 5, adults show a typical diurnal cortisol pattern involving a spike after awakening (i.e., the CAR), followed by a gradual decline of cortisol secretion during the day. Although findings across studies are somewhat inconsistent, Gaffey and colleagues (2016) concluded, in their review of the literature, that this broad pattern continues in later adulthood, although overall levels of cortisol may increase. In addition, substantial individual differences have been noted, and three general patterns of daily activity have been identified that may differ in their distributions within different age groups. As described in Chapter 5, Smyth et al. (1997) found that 51% of their younger adult sample showed a consistent decline over the course of the day, 17% consistently showed a flattened trajectory, and 31% were inconsistent, showing a decline on one day and a flattened trajectory on the next. In comparison, in a study of older adults (mean age = 76 years), Ice, Katz-Stein, Himes, and Kane (2004) found an equivalent proportion of the typical pattern (50%) but a higher proportion of inconsistent trajectories (48%) and a lower proportion of flattened trajectories (2%) than were found in Smyth et al.'s (1997) study. In both investigations, no significant differences were found among the three cortisol patterns in terms of participants' demographics (e.g., socioeconomic status, marital status) or psychosocial variables (e.g., self-reported affect, stress, life events).

Other studies, however, have found significant relationships between demographic and/or psychosocial variables and atypical patterns of cortisol secretion in later adulthood. For example, in a large-scale study of almost 4,000 middle-aged and older adults (mean age = 61 years), Kumari et al.

(2010) found flatter daily cortisol trajectories in men who reported poorer quality diets, more stress, lower occupational status, and/or less financial security. For participants of both genders, flatter trajectories were associated with smoking, early rising, and/or getting less than 5 hours of sleep. Smoking, shorter sleep duration, and financial insecurity partly mediated the relationship between occupational status and cortisol functioning for men. In another study of over 1,000 middle-aged and older individuals (50–70 years), Samuel, Roth, Schwartz, Thorpe, and Glass (2018) found that higher education was associated with more typical diurnal cortisol patterning than intermediate (but not lower) levels of education. In their study, differences in household income and assets were unrelated to cortisol functioning. However, they did find that more African Americans had atypical patterns in comparison with participants from other racial groups, suggesting that race-related stress accumulated over a lifetime might have a significant impact on HPA functioning in older African American adults.

With respect to emotion, Adam, Hawkley, Kudielka, and Cacioppo (2006) asked middle-aged and older adults (50–68 years) to provide three saliva samples per day for cortisol assay and to rate their daily experience of 22 emotion-related variables (e.g., sadness, loneliness, tenseness, energy, anger). Higher levels of sadness, loneliness, threat, and lack of control predicted higher levels of the CAR on the following day. Additionally, higher reports of tension and anger were associated with a flatter cortisol trajectory on the day of the report. Piazza and colleagues (2013) also found an association between higher levels of negative affect and higher cortisol output during the course of the day for older (but not younger) individuals. Together, these findings suggest that affect may mediate associations between stress and atypical patterns of cortisol functioning that contribute to poorer health in later adulthood.

EMOTION UNDERSTANDING

One of the most robust findings in the aging literature is that younger adults are better able to identify emotional facial expressions than are older adults. In a recent set of meta-analyses, Hayes et al. (2020) confirmed this overall finding for studies that utilized both still photographs and dynamic video presentations of facial expressions for happiness, sadness, anger, fear, and surprise. Only disgust was identified equivalently by both older and younger participants. Aligned with the notion of a positivity effect in later adulthood, the age difference in recognition of happiness expressions was smaller than the age difference for all emotions other than disgust. Results consistent with a positivity effect were also obtained in a related study that involved affect intensity rating. In that study, Shuster, Mikels, and Camras (2017) found that older adults rated the affectively ambiguous expression of surprise as reflecting more positive affect than did younger adults.

Several theoretical proposals have been advanced that may account for these age-related differences. For example, all three theories of aging described earlier (i.e., SST, SOC, and SVI) acknowledge that aging is accompanied by cognitive declines but might also argue that older persons' motivation to maintain well-being and to focus on positive information would lead to relative preservation of happiness recognition and a bias toward interpreting surprise expressions as being positive in valence. However, these models cannot account for older and younger adults' equivalent recognition of disgust expressions. Neurobiological explanations have also been proposed that posit selective maintenance or decline in the functioning of brain regions associated with different emotions (Cacioppo, Berntson, Bechara, Tranel, & Hawkley, 2011). However, recent empirical research has not supported these hypotheses (see Mather, 2016, and Mather & Ponzio, 2016, for detailed reviews). Additionally, some studies have failed to find any age-related differences in brain activity accompanying the identification of different emotional facial expressions (e.g., Ebner, Johnson, & Fischer, 2012).

An alternative proposal posits that age differences in the recognition of emotional facial expressions is due to differences between older and younger individuals in their visual scanning of faces (Mather, 2016). More specifically, older individuals have been found to look more at the lower part of the face (i.e., the nose and mouth areas) and less at the upper part of the face (i.e., the eyes and brows) than do younger individuals (e.g., Wong, Cronin-Golomb, & Neargarder, 2005). Some researchers have proposed that the most distinctive facial movements for happy and disgust expressions occur on the lower face, whereas the most distinctive movements for anger, fear, and sadness expressions occur in the brows (Calder, Young, Keane, & Dean, 2000). Thus relative preservation of older persons' recognition of happiness and disgust and their greater decline in recognition of fear, anger, and sadness may be due to their differential attention to the upper and lower areas of the face rather than an overall decline in expression processing. However, this intriguing proposal requires further study. Several variants of the prototypic facial expressions have been described for some emotions (e.g., anger), and these may differ considerably in the distinctiveness of their constituent brow or mouth configurations. Thus further research is necessary in which the distinctiveness of different expression variants is more systematically measured.

Beyond the recognition of facial expressions, the importance of other emotion cues is becoming more widely acknowledged. Therefore, studies that examine age-related differences in emotion recognition based on multimodal cues (e.g., posture, gesture, vocal prosody, verbalizations) are of particular interest. Unfortunately, such studies are relatively few, and findings are mixed. Several studies have found that younger and older persons are equally able to identify expressive stimuli that include both facial and vocal cues (e.g., Chaby, Luherne-du Boullay, Chetouani, & Plaza, 2015; Hunter, Phillips, & MacPherson, 2010; Wieck & Kunzmann, 2017). Regarding expressions that involve body movement, Noh and Isaacowitz (2013) found no difference between older and younger adults in their identification of anger and disgust expressions that included both facial expressions and gestures. In contrast, Foul, Eiten, and Aviezer (2018) reported that younger adults were better able than older adults to identify expressions that included both facial and postural cues for happiness, sadness, anger, and fear.

Surprisingly, there are even fewer studies that include information about situational context, although situational cues may be critically important for accurate inference of emotion. To illustrate, one's interpretation of a mother's crying will differ dramatically depending on whether it occurs at her child's wedding or her child's funeral. Measures of ability EI include consideration of situational cues in the branch that covers understanding of emotion, as well as facial cues in the branch that covers perceiving emotion (see Chapter 4). In their study of ability EI across adulthood, Cabello et al. (2016) found that scores on all four branches declined between 57 and 76 years of age.

SUMMARY AND FINAL THOUGHTS

Emotional well-being remains high in later adulthood. Positive affect may decline slightly across this time period but is still higher than in early adulthood. Anger declines more precipitously. Sadness remains fairly stable but may increase slightly after age 75.

Several theories of development in later adulthood have been proposed that either include or focus exclusively on emotion. In the latter category, SST proposes that individuals become increasingly invested in emotion-related goals as they become increasingly aware of their time-limited future. Seeking to experience more positive affect, they engage in regulatory behaviors that enhance their positive experiences. Many older adults do so in the context of retirement.

Emotional expressivity does not appear to decrease in later adulthood. However, emotional facial expressions may be more difficult for observers to accurately perceive due to age-related changes in facial morphology.

The few studies of normative personality development in later adulthood suggest that Extraversion, Openness, Agreeableness, and Conscientiousness all decline, whereas Neuroticism appears to increase. Both high levels of Neuroticism and high levels of Extraversion have been associated with less effective cognitive functioning. Neuroticism appears to exacerbate the relationship between stress and the experience of negative affect. At the same time, greater experience of negative affect in later adulthood (e.g., due to declines in health or childhood **maltreatment**) may lead to higher levels of Neuroticism.

Attachment status may change in later adulthood. However, results are inconsistent across studies. For example, both increases and decreases in dismissive attachment have been reported. Although plausible explanations for these inconsistencies have been offered, they have not yet been systematically evaluated. Differences in the specific emotions experienced by secure versus insecure older individuals also have been reported and merit further investigation to understand the eliciting circumstances and appraisal processes underlying these differences.

Supporting the positivity goals of older individuals is an information-processing bias, that is, the positivity effect. When given the opportunity, older individuals attend to and remember more positive information relative to negative information. Older individuals may also appraise emotion-eliciting circumstances in ways that support the experience of more positive and/or less negative affect.

Decision making is influenced by both incidental affect (i.e., the affect one brings to the decision-making event) and integral affect (i.e., one's affective responses to the decision choices). Although affect influences the decisions of persons at any age, older adults more than younger adults may prefer to rely on their affective responses to the available choices when a cognitively complex decision must be made. Whether this is adaptive or maladaptive depends on the nature of the particular decision (e.g., whether it has implications for the individual's physical health or choice of leisure activities).

In their daily lives, older adults appear to use the several categories (or families) of emotion regulation strategies as often as do younger adults. However, they may use different strategies within each category more or less frequently and use them in the service of different goals. Although reappraisal has been widely acclaimed as a regulation strategy (see Chapter 5), distraction may be more effective for older individuals. At the same time, reappraisal may be more effective for older adults than detachment, another cognitive change strategy.

Results consistent with SST have been found in studies of Chinese but not Japanese younger and older adults. Different variants of the positivity effect in information processing have been shown in studies of older Chinese versus European American individuals. European American adults value high-arousal positive emotions more than either Chinese American or Hong Kong Chinese adults. This may lead them to have a less optimistic view of old age when opportunities to experience high-arousal positive emotions might be expected to decline.

Gender differences in older adults' emotional experiences and expression have not been consistently demonstrated. Older men may use suppression as a regulation strategy more than women, whereas older women may use reappraisal more than men. The female advantage in emotion understanding continues to be seen in later adulthood.

Although the amygdala and vmPFC are relatively preserved in later adulthood, deterioration in other brain areas, as well as deterioration in several types of neural processing (e.g., speed of synaptic transmission), might have an impact on emotion functioning. Simultaneously, compensatory mechanisms or processes might offset some age-related declines. Therefore, empirical study is necessary to understand the neurobiological underpinnings of emotion functioning in older adults. In response to emotion stimuli, older adults activate areas of the brain that support autonomic arousal less than younger adults but activate areas related to introspection and autobiographical memory more. Older and younger adults appear to activate different areas within the PFC when engaging in cognitive reappraisal. In addition, some studies have found greater dedifferentiation (i.e., overlap) in areas of the PMC activated during reappraisal and distraction by older adults in comparison with younger adults. Consistent with the parietal cortex's relative preservation in later adulthood, older adults prefer distraction over reappraisal to a greater degree than do younger adults. The GANE model offers a potential explanation for the attentional narrowing that accompanies high-arousal emotions.

Older adults show less heart rate reactivity to some emotional stimuli (e.g., pictures) than do younger adults—even to stimuli that are rated equivalently by both age groups in terms of valence and arousal. However, they appear to respond similarly to stronger emotional elicitors (e.g., video clips of emotional events).

Equivalent numbers of older and younger individuals show the typical pattern of daily cortisol levels (about 50% in each age group). However, the atypical inconsistent pattern is shown more often and the atypical flattened pattern is shown less often by older individuals. Atypical patterns also are found more often among those subject to greater stress and/or those who have other health risk factors. Older adults reporting high levels of negative affect also show atypical patterns or higher overall cortisol levels more often.

Older adults are less able than younger adults to identify emotional facial expressions. One current hypothesis suggests that older adults' less efficient scanning of faces results in their failure to perceive important facial emotion cues. Further research is required to evaluate this proposal. Older adults may be better able to recognize multimodal emotional expressions that include nonfacial cues. However, few studies have investigated this possibility, and findings have been somewhat mixed.

CHAPTER 7

Some Specific Emotions

One noticeable feature of many early emotion studies was their emphasis on negative more than positive emotions. Indeed, four of the Big Six basic emotions originally studied by Ekman and Friesen (1971) were negative (i.e., anger, fear, sadness, and disgust), whereas only one positive emotion (happiness) and one arguably neutral valence emotion (surprise) were included. According to several contemporary emotion scholars, this emphasis on negative emotions was no mistake. Experiencing, attending to, and learning from negative emotions is considered to have particular evolutionary survival value in that doing so enables one to better anticipate and respond to undesirable events and circumstances (Vaish, Grossmann, & Woodward, 2008). For example, a person who is afraid of bears would be more likely to carry bear-repellent spray on a hike and thus may not need to run when she sees a bear in the woods. Of course, this argument favoring negative emotions can be readily countered by pointing out the equal importance of experiencing, expressing, and responding to positive emotions in order to cement personal relationships that also enhance survival (Fredrickson, 1998). For example, a person who is generally cheerful might tend to hike with a chatty group and thus minimize the probability of even seeing a bear. Additionally, as described in Chapter 6, positive emotions appear to assume special importance in later adulthood. Without necessarily arguing for the dominance of one or the other end of the valence dimension, a number of researchers have delved more deeply into specific emotions or families of negative or positive emotions to better understand their development and role in our emotional lives. This chapter presents some of their work.

SELF-CONSCIOUS EMOTIONS

Michael Lewis's Model

After the first year of life, a new set of emotions are thought to develop that are presumed to require a sense of the objective self (i.e., awareness of the self as a potential object of others' attention). These include embarrassment, guilt, shame, pride, and hubris. The most well-developed and well-recognized model for the development of these emotions is that of Michael Lewis (Lewis, 2014, 2016b, 2019). Lewis's model is closely tied to his interest in the development of human consciousness, a topic that has challenged scholars from many disciplines for many centuries (e.g., Hilgard, 1980).

According to Lewis, an objective sense of self emerges during the middle of the second year as an accompaniment to the development of consciousness. Previous to this, the infant may engage in purposeful actions (e.g., reaching for and picking up a colorful ball), but these do not qualify as conscious behaviors. In addition, the infant is not aware that others may be watching her and cannot experience embarrassment if she accidentally drops her ball. To investigate the development of the objective self, Lewis has used a **mirror-recognition task** (e.g., Lewis, Sullivan, Stanger, & Weiss, 1989). During this procedure, the experimenter surreptitiously applies a spot of red rouge on the nose of an infant or toddler and places the child in front of a mirror. Before about 15 months of age, most toddlers will treat their mirrored image as if it were an independent entity. However, upon seeing the red mark, older toddlers will touch their own noses, thus demonstrating objective self-awareness. Lewis considers objective self-awareness to also be evidenced by toddlers' use of personal pronouns and forms of pretend play that emerge at around the same age.

Lewis makes an additional distinction between self-conscious emotions that do or do not involve an evaluative component, that is, evaluation of the self against a standard, rule, or goal (SRG). Among the emotions that Lewis considers not to involve such self-evaluation are exposure embarrassment, envy/jealousy, and empathy. The best (and least controversial) example of these is exposure embarrassment. Exposure embarrassment is elicited simply by paying attention to the child (e.g., staring or pointing). It can even be evoked by lavishing praise. In these situations, the child will often behave in a way that suggests ambivalence between approach and avoidance (e.g., smiling while alternately glancing to and away from the other person). This constellation of gaze and facial behavior is considered an expression of embarrassment by Lewis, as well as other researchers (e.g., Tracy, Robins, & Schriber, 2009).

Whereas nonevaluative self-conscious emotions are thought to emerge between 18 and 24 months, the evaluative self-conscious emotions begin to emerge after the child reaches 2 years of age. These emotions include guilt/regret, shame, and pride. Preceding their emergence, the toddler must develop some understanding of "good–bad" or "right–wrong" and what types of events or actions are considered to fall into each category according to externally imposed social standards. Learning these externally imposed standards can take place through the same socialization processes that have been described for emotion socialization in general, that is, demonstrative modeling by others, contingent responding by others, explicit teaching, and/or niche selection (see Chapter 3).

Through such socialization processes, the child may also acquire achievement goals or behavioral goals and eventually evaluate him- or herself according to whether he or she succeeds or fails to achieve his or her goals. However, this evaluation involves more than just recognizing the objective outcome of one's endeavors (i.e., success or failure). An additional important factor is whether children attribute their success or failure to some unalterable global characteristic of the self (e.g., one's intrinsic adequacy or inadequacy) or to circumstantial features that made the outcome a reflection of the situation rather than one's own basic competence. More specifically, success or failure that is attributed to one's intrinsic self will evoke hubris or shame, whereas success or failure perceived as situation-specific will evoke pride or guilt. To illustrate, a 2-year-old child might feel either guilt or shame when he accidentally breaks a toy depending on whether he considers himself to have been momentarily careless or to be inherently clumsy. Notably, this analysis is similar to Carol Dweck's influential model of achievement orientation (Dweck & Leggett, 1998; Hong, Chiu, Dweck, Lin, & Wan, 1999).

To provide support for his model, Lewis and his colleagues have conducted a number of studies to examine relationships between children's evaluations of their success or failure and their emotional responses. For example, in one study (Lewis, 2019), preschool children participated in a puzzle task that appeared obviously easy (because there were few pieces) but that all children failed because they were given very little time to complete the puzzle. Afterward, children were asked whether they thought the task was hard or easy, and their nonverbal responses considered to reflect embarrassment, pride, and shame were coded. Children were classified as performance-oriented or task-oriented based on whether they said the puzzle task was easy or hard. They were classified as performance-oriented if they said the task was hard, presumably because they focused on their own fail-ure rather than the characteristics of the task. They were classified as task-oriented if they said the task was easy, presumably because they focused on the characteristics of the task rather than their own performance. Performance-oriented children showed more shame than pride or embar-rassment after failing the easy task, whereas task-oriented children showed more pride and embarrassment than shame. Although it is perhaps puzzling as to why any of the children would show pride after failure, these results were interpreted as supporting the general hypothesis that emotions depend upon attributions (or appraisals) regarding the causes of success or failure as much as the success or failure itself.

Distinguishing Shame from Guilt

Rather than coding children's expressive responses, some investigators have relied on their instrumental behaviors to identify shame and distinguish shame from guilt. Illustrating this approach, Karen Barrett and her col-leagues (Barrett, Zahn-Waxler, & Cole, 1993) observed 2-year-old children who were led to believe that they had broken a toy while the experimenter was out of the room. When the experimenter returned, some children (i.e., 46%) told her about the mishap and attempted to repair the damage, whereas other children (i.e., 38%) tried to avoid looking at or interacting with the experimenter. Barrett and colleagues (1993) proposed that those children who confessed and attempted repair might be considered to be showing guilt, whereas those who avoided the experimenter might be con-sidered to be showing shame. This interpretation has emerged as a point of consensus among many developmental researchers.

Nonetheless, other studies have questioned whether young children always feel guilty when they show reparative actions. In an interesting varia-tion of the broken-toy procedure, Vaish, Carpenter, and Tomasello (2016) designed an experiment in which the collapse of a toy tower appeared to be caused by either the child participant or an adult experimenter, and the mishap either upset or was shrugged off by a third person who had ostensi-bly built the tower. Two-year-old children made greater efforts to restore the broken tower when the builder appeared upset rather than neutral about the mishap, thus displaying a sympathetic response. However, 3-year-old children made an additional distinction between the conditions in which the mishap was caused by themselves or the adult, that is, they made greater restorative efforts when they themselves had (inadvertently) caused the mishap. The investigators interpreted these findings as indicating that only the 3-year-old children experienced feelings of guilt.

Temperament and Parenting Influences

Both temperament and parenting are considered sources of individual differences in self-conscious emotions (DiBiase & Lewis, 1997; Lewis, 2019). For example, in her long-term research program, Grazyna Kochanska and her colleagues (Kochanska, 1991, 1995; Kochanska & Aksan, 2006) found that the temperamental factors of fearfulness and effortful control (EC) interacted with parenting to influence the development of an internalized conscience (conceptualized as a moral orientation that includes feelings of guilt over transgressions). More specifically, in Kochanska's research, fearful toddlers were most responsive to parenting that minimized power assertion. For less fearful toddlers, secure attachment was more strongly associated with conscience development. Irrespective of fearfulness, higher levels of EC also were related to higher levels of internalized conscience.

Representing the other side of the coin, Lewis and his colleagues have investigated relations between the self-conscious emotions and maladaptive development. For example, Bennett, Sullivan, and Lewis (2010) examined relations between shame proneness, guilt proneness, and self-reported depressive symptoms in 7-year-old neglected and non-neglected children. Shame proneness and guilt proneness were measured using an age-appropriate version of the Test of Self-Conscious Affect for Children (TOSCA-C; Tangney, Wagner, Burggraf, Gramzow, & Fletcher, 1990). The TOSCA-C is an interview procedure developed by Tangney and her colleagues during which children are presented with scenarios describing situations that might be expected to evoke a variety of self-conscious emotions, including shame and guilt. In Bennett et al.'s (2010) study, the children were asked to rate their likelihood of feeling shame or guilt after each scenario. Results showed that the neglected children reported more shame and more depressive symptoms—but not more guilt—than the non-neglected children.

Maladaptive Outcomes

In another investigation, Bennett, Sullivan, and Lewis (2005) examined shame, anger, and sadness responses to task failure by maltreated 3- to

7-year-old children and the relationship of their responses to teachers' ratings of the children's problem behavior. In this study, results showed that a history of greater physical abuse (but not greater neglect) was related to more displays of shame following task failure. However, irrespective of the children's abuse or neglect history, associations between shame, anger, and teacher-rated behavior problems conformed to the investigators' proposed model in which anger mediates the relationship between shame and children's behavior problems.

Consistent with these findings is Lewis's further proposal that shame may often be converted to anger as a way of avoiding self-blame. To illustrate, Gold, Sullivan, and Lewis (2011) investigated abuse, shame, blame, and violent behavior in adolescents who were incarcerated in a juvenile detention facility. The adolescents reported on their experience of harsh parental discipline and their own violent behavior. Shame and blame measures were derived from the adolescents' responses to an age-appropriate version of the TOSCA. Data analyses showed that more adolescent-perceived harsh parenting was significantly related to a greater tendency to avoid shame and self-blame in response to scenarios in which shame would be considered appropriate. In addition, the avoidance of shame and self-blame was related to greater delinquency and was presumed to also involve greater anger.

Relations between self-conscious emotions and anger have also been studied in more representative participant samples. For example, Tangney, Wagner, Hill-Barlow, Marschall, and Gramzow (1996) investigated such relations in grade-school children, adolescents, college students, and adults using various versions of the TOSCA. Participants also completed questionnaires asking how they would respond in hypothetical situations likely to evoke anger. Across all ages, greater shame proneness was related to greater aggression, as well as self-directed hostility (e.g., berating oneself). In contrast, guilt proneness was related to corrective actions, nonhostile discussion with the target of anger, and cognitive reappraisal of the target's intentions (e.g., deciding that they had not meant any harm).

In light of these studies, it is somewhat surprising that Spruit, Schalkwijk, van Vugt, and Stams (2016) found higher levels of shame, as well as guilt, to be related to lower levels of delinquency and criminal behavior in their meta-analytic investigation. However, the effect size for shame was small, and the presence or absence of anger was not considered. Nonetheless, when discussing the implications of their findings for treating delinquency, the researchers recommended "staying away from shame promoting interventions . . . [that] can easily be felt as an attack on the self and trigger adverse defense mechanisms, such as aggression" (Spruit et al., 2016, p. 19).

Is Shame Equally Toxic across Cultures?

A different perspective on shame emerged in a provocative cross-cultural study of socialization. Fung (1999) conducted detailed observations in which she documented parents' frequent use of shame as a socialization tool for toddlers in nine Taiwanese families. Miller, Fung, Lin, Chen, and Boldt (2012) subsequently compared the Taiwanese families' practices to those of U.S. families and reported that U.S. families rarely used shame as a socialization technique. However, these investigators did not systematically distinguish shame-inducing from guilt-inducing socialization behaviors (e.g., criticizing the child as a person vs. criticizing the child's specific action), and thus it is possible that Taiwanese families utilized guilt-inducing practices as much as (or even more than) shame-inducing practices. Still, assuming that Taiwanese practices do indeed reflect shame rather than guilt, the implication of these differing socialization practices has been energetically debated. However, several studies have shown a relationship between parental shaming and depression for Chinese and Chinese American (as well as European American) adolescents (Camras et al., 2012; Camras, Sun, et al., 2017; Cheah, Yu, Liu, & Coplan, 2019). In a meta-analysis of 108 studies, Kim, Thibodeau, and Jorgensen (2011) concluded that both shame and maladaptive guilt (i.e., taking exaggerated responsibility, free-floating guilt not associated with specific contexts) were significantly related to depressive symptoms with moderate effect sizes. Ethnicity (i.e., Asians vs. Caucasians) did not significantly moderate these effects.

EMPATHY

Although there is a wide consensus that empathy is a desirable emotional response, scholars' conceptualizations of empathy often diverge from those of laypersons and sometimes from those of other scholars. Herein, I adopt a model that reflects increasing agreement among developmental scholars to define empathy as a process through which an emotion may be generated. Similar to emotion contagion, empathy occurs when one perceives another's emotion and matches that feeling. However, fully developed **empathy** differs from emotion contagion in that an empathic person retains awareness that the source of his own emotion is another being. For example, fear contagion occurs when one becomes afraid of a bear only after sensing that one's hiking partner is afraid. Empathic fear occurs when one experiences the emotion while listening to one's friend's account of confronting a bear.

From a theoretical perspective, one can experience empathic versions of any emotion—fear, anger, happiness, distress, and so forth. Still, most research on empathy focuses on empathic distress and its potential relation to prosocial behavior. Accordingly, this is the focus in this section.

Martin Hoffman's Model

Perhaps the most comprehensive and influential model of empathy development is that of Martin Hoffman (2000, 2008). With a focus on distress, Hoffman described four steps that lead to the development of empathic responding in infants and young children. The first stage (termed *global empathy*) is actually characterized by emotion contagion, a process that Hoffman considers to be automatic and natural. Emotion contagion is exemplified by newborn infants' automatic crying in response to the crying of other babies (e.g., Sagi & Hoffman, 1976). The second stage (*egocentric empathy*) occurs toward the end of the first year, when infants experience contagious distress but are still unable to clearly distinguish between their own distress and that of another person. Therefore, when confronted with another's distress, the infant seeks comfort only for herself and not for the other person. The third stage (*quasi-egocentric empathy*) occurs during the middle of the second year, when infants begin to develop an objective sense of self and thus can distinguish between their own and others' distress more clearly. At this point, they can begin to show empathic concern (i.e., sympathy). For example, they may seek to comfort the other person, although they will do so using behaviors more appropriate for comforting themselves (e.g., bringing a distressed peer to one's own mother rather than the peer's mother). In the fourth stage (*veridical empathic distress*), the young child can generate more appropriate responses to the distressed person. A subsequent important development (not tied by Hoffman to a specific age) involves the ability to empathize with the distress of others when it is portrayed more abstractly (e.g., by descriptions of another's expressions of distress or his distressing circumstances).

Hoffman's model has proved useful by describing a set of empathy-related behaviors that can be readily observed during early development. However, the interpretation of those behaviors has been challenged, and alternative models have been proposed (see Spinrad & Eisenberg, 2019, for a brief review). For example, Davidov, Zahn-Waxler, Roth-Hanania, and Knafo (2013) have argued that the emotion contagion observed during the infant's first year does not really reflect an inability to distinguish between self and others but rather an inability to regulate his or her own distress. Irrespective of this, it seems clear that the capacity for effective prosocial responding to others' distress increases across the early years of development.

When Does Empathy Lead to Prosocial Behavior?

Prosocial responding to others' distress can include behaviors such as help-ing, sharing, and cooperation. However, the experience of empathic distress does not always lead to a prosocial response. Building upon thinking and research in social psychology (see Batson, 1998), Eisenberg and her colleagues have proposed a model that distinguishes two possible forms of empathic responding when perceiving another's distress. First, one's empathic distress may be embedded in a more complex emotion-related response termed **sym-pathy,** that is, "feeling sorrow or concern for another (rather than feeling the same emotion)" (Spinrad & Eisenberg, 2019, p. 352). Sympathy also may be generated based on more abstract cues, for example, by memories or descriptions of others' distress or distressful circumstances. Sympathy is an emotion-related response that is likely to lead to prosocial behaviors. In contrast, a second possible form of empathic distress is **personal distress.** Personal distress occurs when a person is overwhelmed by his empathic dis-tress and is motivated to terminate his own feelings of overarousal and dis-comfort. In this case, the person is less likely to engage in prosocial behavior and more likely to try to escape the situation.

The experiences of sympathy and personal distress are influenced by both situational and personal factors. For example, the degree of distress displayed by the other person, as well as one's attribution of its cause, play an important role. To illustrate, Hepach, Vaish, and Tomasello (2013) observed that 3-year-old children displayed significantly more sympathy for an adult who showed extreme distress when she appeared to accidentally close a heavy box lid on her finger than for an adult who showed extreme distress when she closed the lid on the sleeve of her blouse.

Temperament and Parenting Influences

In addition to the factors discussed above, children's (and adults') tempera-mental characteristics are also important influences on empathy. More specifically, the temperament factor of negative emotionality increases the likelihood of experiencing personal distress when encountering the distress of another, but self-regulation abilities may have a countering influence. To illustrate, Guthrie et al. (1997) measured school-age children's sympathy and distress responses to a distress-portraying film and compared them with parents' and teachers' rating of the children's negative emotionality and self-regulatory abilities. Results showed that children who responded to the film with greater sympathy (as evidenced by facial expressions of sadness) were rated higher on their self-regulation abilities, whereas children who responded with greater personal distress (as evidenced by expressions of fear as well as sadness) were rated higher on negative emotionality.

Parenting styles and practices also would be expected to influence children's empathy and sympathetic responding. Indeed, in a meta-analysis, Boele et al. (2019) found a significant (albeit small) effect size for the association of better parent–child relations with children's empathy and empathic concern (i.e., sympathetic feelings). Interestingly, peer relationship quality was also related to children's empathy, with an effect size that was significantly greater than that found for parent–child relations.

Attachment security might be expected to influence children's empathy and sympathy in that a secure internal working model (IWM) of attachment includes the valuing of social and emotional relationships. Consistent with this expectation, Beier et al. (2019) found a significant relationship in 3- to 5-year-old children between attachment quality and comforting, a prosocial behavior considered to reflect empathic concern. However, somewhat surprisingly, Stern and Cassidy (2018) found only mixed evidence for a significant association between attachment security and empathic concern in their narrative review of the research involving infants and children. In contrast, they consistently found significant relations in studies involving adolescents. As suggested by the authors, inconsistent results across investigations of children may reflect the moderating effects of variables such as the identity and portrayal of the empathy target. In addition, measures of attachment security used with adolescents (e.g., the Adult Attachment Interview) typically consider the individual's broader views regarding the value of emotional relationships in general; these general attitudes may bear a stronger relationship to empathic concern than attachment as measured at earlier ages with its narrower focus on parent–child relations.

How Is Empathy Socialized?

Other studies of parenting influences on empathy have been conducted within the framework of Eisenberg's model of emotion socialization (Eisenberg, Cumberland, & Spinrad, 1998; Eisenberg, Spinrad, & Cumberland, 1998; see Chapter 3). For example, as part of a longitudinal investigation, Zhou et al. (2002) measured the emotional responses of school-age children and their parents as they viewed a set of positive, negative, and neutral slides at two time points—when the children were approximately 10 years old and again 4 years later. Children first viewed the slides with an experimenter and then with their mothers, who were allowed to talk with their children as they viewed the slides together. At both times, mothers and teachers also completed questionnaires to assess the children's externalizing behaviors (e.g., aggression) and social competence (e.g., socially appropriate behavior and peer relations). Children's positive expressivity while viewing the positive slides and negative expressivity while viewing the negative slides served as measures of their empathy. Parents' positive expressivity while viewing the slides was also measured. Lastly, parental warmth during interactions with their children between slide viewings was rated based on the parents' facial, vocal, verbal, and physical behaviors. Although results for the two time points were not entirely consistent, structural equation modeling (SEM) did yield evidence that parents' positive expressivity mediated a relationship between parental warmth and children's empathic responses to the positive slides (particularly at Time 1). In addition, children's empathic responses particularly toward the negative slides mediated the relation between parents' positive expressivity and lower levels of externalizing behaviors and higher levels of social competence (particularly at Time 2). Evidence was also found for children's effects on parenting, although the child-driven structural equation models (SEMs) did not fit the data as well as the parent-driven SEMs. In summary, the study suggested that parents' warmth and positive expressivity encourages the development of children's empathy and that children's empathy is associated with more desirable social functioning broadly defined. Of note, similar relations between maternal warmth and positive expressivity experienced during childhood and adolescence have been associated with empathic concern (i.e., sympathy) measured even in adulthood (Eisenberg, VanSchyndel, & Hofer, 2015).

An important component of Eisenberg's socialization model (Eisenberg, Cumberland, & Spinrad, 1998; Eisenberg, Spinrad, & Cumberland, 1998) is the nature of parents' responses to their children's emotions. In another longitudinal study, Taylor, Eisenberg, Spinrad, Eggum, and Sulik (2013) investigated the relation between mothers' supportive reactions to their children's negative emotions and the children's empathy and prosocial behavior. Mothers' supportive responding was measured using the CCNES (described in Chapter 3) when the children were 18 months of age. When the children were 24, 30, 42, 48, and 54 months old, mothers completed a questionnaire to assess the children's empathic responding. Teachers rated the children's prosocial behavior at 72 and 84 months. Children's ego resiliency (i.e., ability to cope adaptively in a somewhat stressful situation) was also rated by both mothers and nonparental caregivers at 18 months. Results showed that mothers' support of their children's emotions and the children's ego resiliency were both related to children's empathy at older ages. Children's empathy mediated the relation between maternal supportive responding and children's prosocial behavior, as well as the relation between children's ego resiliency and prosocial behavior.

Emotion discussion has rarely been studied in relation to children's empathy and prosocial behavior. However, Brownell, Svetlova, Anderson, Nichols, and Drummond (2013) investigated associations between parents' discussion of emotion in the context of a story-reading procedure and their preschool children's empathy-related helping. Helping responses were measured during a procedure that involved an adult who expressed a distressing state (i.e., sadness, cold, or frustration) that could be alleviated if the child interrupted her play activity in order to provide help or comfort. Results showed that parent–child engagement in emotion-related discussion while reading the story was indeed related to children's helping. Of particular interest, results were driven by the parent's elicitation of emotion-related comments by the child rather than the amount of emotion-related talk produced by the parent.

Neurobiological Underpinnings

The neural concomitants of emotion contagion, empathy, and empathic concern (sympathy) have been investigated in a comprehensive program of research by Jean Decety and his colleagues. Based on studies using both functional magnetic resonance imaging (fMRI) and electroencephalography (EEG), Decety has developed a model that depicts empathic responding as involving a set of distributed but connected neural areas and systems that underlie three overarching sets of functional components comprising the empathy process (Decety & Michalska, 2020). These are: (1) affect sharing via contagion, a bottom-up process proposed to involve the brainstem, amygdala, basal ganglia, and orbitofrontal cortex; (2) awareness of emotion in oneself versus others, a process proposed to involve the medial prefrontal cortex (mPFC), ventromedial PFC, and temporo-parietal junction; and (3) executive functioning skills (e.g., cognitive perspective taking, appraising the situational context, regulating emotion and behavior), processes also involving areas of the PFC. Developmental changes are seen in the functioning of these components reflecting an increasing ability to form more sophisticated cognitive representations of others' distress, to regulate one's own corresponding distress, and to integrate these with appropriate behavioral responses.

Perhaps because empathic responses to others' physical pain are readily observed and experienced in everyday life, many investigations have used pain as a model system for studying the neural underpinnings of empathy in adults. Two procedures are commonly used for this purpose, one involving the presentation of pictorial cues and the other involving presentation of more abstract cues for pain. In the picture-based paradigms, participants lying in the scanner see pictures of hands or feet appearing to receive a pain stimulus (e.g., an injection) or not receiving a pain stimulus. In the second procedure, participants are presented with abstract cues (e.g., a picture of a square or a circle) that are said to indicate whether another person present in the room is about to experience pain (e.g., an electric shock) or is not about to experience pain. Note that during both procedures, no facial, vocal, or bodily expressions of pain are presented. Importantly, both paradigms also include episodes in which the participant him- or herself does or does not receive a pain stimulus. Thus each paradigm involves a 2 (pain vs. no pain) × 2 (other vs. self) design and can be used to identify neural activity selectively involved in either self-experienced pain or empathic responses to another's pain. In a meta-analysis of nine such studies, Lamm, Decety, and Singer (2011) found evidence for shared neural components of experienced and empathic pain, as well as differences that correspond to participants' ability to distinguish between them. In addition, they found differences across the two paradigms reflecting the fact that they required different forms of cognitive processing to link the experimental stimuli (i.e., pictures of pain vs. abstract cues) to an understanding that pain was about to be experienced. Thus the findings from this study illustrate relations among the three sets of components constituting Decety's model, as described above. Interestingly, empathy-related responding in humans does not appear to involve several areas of the brain that have received considerable attention in the popular press, that is, areas analogous to those that include the mirror neurons identified in studies of primates (Decety, 2011).

Is Empathy More Common in Some Cultures Than Others?

Studies of empathy across cultures have not attempted to distinguish between empathy and sympathy. Instead, many studies of culture and empathy have focused on the laudable goal of encouraging effective communication between health care professionals (e.g., nurses, doctors, therapists) and those patients or clients who come from different cultural backgrounds (see Lorié, Reinero, Phillips, Zhang, & Riess, 2017, for a review). However, a few investigations have explored cultural differences in the circumstances that evoke empathy, as conceptualized in this chapter.

Illustrating these studies, Trommsdorff, Friedlmeier, and Mayer (2007) videotaped the empathy-related responses of preschool children from Germany, Israel, Malaysia, and Indonesia to an experimenter who displayed sadness when her toy balloon accidentally deflated during a play session. Importantly, this accident did not appear to be caused by either the experimenter or the child. Coders from the children's own cultural group viewed the videotapes and rated the children's sympathy (i.e., sad expressions directed toward the experimenter), other-focused distress (i.e., expressions of tension while focused on the experimenter), and self-focused distress (i.e., expressions of tension while turning away from the experimenter). Prosocial behaviors (e.g., attempts to comfort or help the experimenter find a new toy) also were coded. Results showed that sympathetic responses were positively related to prosocial behaviors and that self-focused distress was negatively related to prosocial behaviors. Also, children from the two Asian cultures showed less sympathy and less prosocial behavior than those from Germany and Israel. In interpreting these cultural differences, the investigators suggested that Asian children may have shown fewer sympathetic responses because of the value traditionally placed on emotional restraint in those cultures. In addition, the importance of face saving and respecting hierarchical relations in Asian cultures may have discouraged the children from initiating prosocial behaviors directed toward an unfamiliar adult. Thus, studying empathic responding in a wider range of situations (e.g., those involving parents or peers rather than unfamiliar adults) would be necessary to understand how empathy functions in children from different cultural groups.

Using a different methodology to study adults, Atkins, Uskul, and Cooper (2016) investigated East Asian (EA) and White British (WB) participants' empathic responses to physical or interpersonal distress. In their studies, participants viewed videotapes of physical pain (i.e., a WB woman's hand appearing to receive an injection) or interpersonal distress (i.e., a WB or EA female speaker describing a relationship breakup or being bullied). Participants provided ratings of their own affect and their perception of the target's affect using the Positive and Negative Affect Schedule (PANAS; Watson et al., 1988, as described in Chapter 6). Additionally, participants rated themselves on a set of empathy-related feelings (i.e., compassion, sympathy, being moved, tenderness, warmth, and softheartedness) that provided a measure of empathic concern for the distress target. Paralleling results of Trommsdorf et al.'s (2007) study, the researchers found that WB participants reported stronger affective responses and more empathic concern than did the EA participants irrespective of whether they viewed a WB or EA person in the videos. However, EA participants more accurately perceived the self-reported affect of both EA and WB speakers. In interpreting their results, the investigators emphasized that they saw no evidence of an **ingroup advantage** effect for either empathic concern or affect identification; that is, participants were not more accurate or concerned about members of their own culture as opposed to another culture. Instead, the authors suggested that empathy may take different forms in different cultures, with EAs emphasizing cognitive empathy (i.e., emotion recognition) and WBs emphasizing affective empathy (i.e., experienced affect and empathic concern). Still, although explicit and accurate emotion recognition may occur, it does not alone meet criteria for empathy according to the conceptual framework presented above. Thus, Atkins et al.'s (2016) study illustrates some of the divergent definitions of empathy extant in the literature. More consistent with Trommsdorf et al. (2007), an alternative interpretation of Atkin et al.'s (2016) results would be that EAs' lesser affective responding, as well as their lower scores on empathic concern, are both reflections of the value traditionally placed on emotional restraint in Asian cultures. An interesting question for future research would be whether the cultural differences found in their study would also translate into differences in adults' prosocial behavior.

POSITIVE EMOTIONS

Like many psychologists of his era, Martin Seligman spent the first decades of his academic career studying topics related to negative emotions, most notably making a name for himself by introducing and investigating the concept of learned helplessness (Seligman, 2019). Then he had a change of heart. In an epiphanic moment, Seligman recognized that the presence of optimism is just as relevant to healthy psychological functioning as is the absence of negative emotions. Thus the initial seed for the **positive psychology** movement was planted. Decades later, the positive psychology movement is still growing strong.

Barbara Fredrickson's Broaden-and-Build Theory

Although Seligman's own work was the early inspiration for this movement, others have also contributed to developing theoretical models of positive emotion and conducting empirical research to evaluate them. Of these, one influential current model is Barbara Fredrickson's **broaden-and-build theory (BBT;** Fredrickson 2013; Fredrickson & Cohn, 2008). According to this theory, positive emotions induce a broadening of attention, thinking, and action that allows for the building of social, cognitive, and physical resources. These increased resources naturally generate an increase in positive emotion that in turn leads to further resource development, creating an "upward spiral" that contributes to adaptive functioning. To illustrate, a person who is happy will be more open to making new friends and more willing to learn a new skill than a person who is depressed. That person may then be able to find employment opportunities that involve using his newly acquired skills by networking with his newly acquired friends.

From an evolutionary perspective, Fredrickson (1998) argues that negative emotions function to narrow the focus of attention, thinking, and behavior to facilitate immediate coping with specific undesirable events and circumstances. In contrast, positive emotions function to promote the development of resources that can be made available whenever needed (e.g., knowledge, cognitive skills, social networks, behavioral repertoires). At the same time, the BBT acknowledges boundary conditions for the benefits of positive emotions. For example, excessive positive emotion can sometimes degrade performance of a task that requires a narrow focus of attention. And, of course, it is negative emotions that are adaptive in threat situations.

A number of laboratory studies have provided support for the first component of BBT, that is, the hypothesis that positive emotions broaden attention, cognition, and action. To illustrate, Fredrickson and Branigan (2005) showed participants brief video clips designed to evoke amusement, contentment, or neutral affect and then presented them with a visual comparison task in which they chose one of two options as being most similar to a target (e.g., a pyramid made of squares). One option resembled the target only in its global configuration (e.g., a pyramid that was made of triangles rather than squares), whereas the second option resembled the target only in its detailed components (e.g., squares arranged in a nonpyramid configuration). Results showed that participants who had viewed either of the positive videos tended to choose the global match significantly more often than those who viewed the neutral video.

Extending the broadening hypothesis into the realm of social cognition, Nelson (2009) studied the influence of emotion on U.S. college students' responses to individuals showing culturally normative or nonnormative behaviors. In this study, participants first read a set of statements designed to evoke positive, negative, or neutral affect (e.g., "Most people like me"; "My classes are hard"; "It snows in Idaho"). Subsequently they read a story in which the protagonist showed culturally expected behavior (e.g., disappointment when their achievements were unrecognized) or culturally unexpected behavior (e.g., extreme embarrassment when they were singled out for recognition). Participants then responded to items assessing their empathic concern for the protagonist as well as their perspective taking (i.e., whether they thought the protagonists' behavior was understandable). Results showed that participants in the neutral and negative affect conditions reported less empathic concern and perspective taking for culturally dissimilar protagonists in comparison with culturally similar protagonists. However, these differences were not found for participants in the positive affect condition. Thus, positive affect appeared to broaden their thinking about persons exhibiting unfamiliar emotional responses and may serve to enhance relationships and interactions with persons from a different culture.

Other studies have provided support for the second component of BBT, that is, the building hypothesis that proposes positive emotions to engender better social, cognitive, and physical resources. For example, Fredrickson, Cohn, Coffey, Pek, and Finkel (2008) increased participants' experiences of 10 positive emotions by means of a loving-kindness meditation workshop and additionally obtained baseline and postworkshop measures of their psychological, social, and physical resources (e.g., self-acceptance, social support, positive relations with others, minor illness symptoms). Results showed increases in all 10 positive emotions. In turn, these increases in positive emotion were related to increases in many (although not all) of the psychological, social, and physical resources that were themselves related to increases in measures of adaptive functioning (i.e., increased life satisfaction and decreases in depressive symptoms).

One interesting effect of positive emotions is that they can aid in the recovery from some of the physiological effects of strong negative affect. In one of Fredrickson's first studies, she and Levenson (1998) showed participants a fear-inducing video clip followed by a video that induced amusement, contentment, or a neutral response. Measures of cardiovascular activity (e.g., heart rate) were taken throughout the procedure and increased significantly in response to the fear video. For participants who then viewed one of the positive videos, cardiovascular activity returned to baseline levels significantly faster than it did for participants who viewed the neutral video. This demonstrated what Fredrickson called the "undo effect."

Does Positive Affect Influence Health?

A considerable amount of research has investigated the relationship between positive affect and various physical health outcomes. For example, Wilson et al. (2017) conducted a three-wave study of positive affect and the effectiveness of antiretroviral therapy in almost 1,000 women with HIV. At the first two time points (spaced 6 months apart), participants rated their experience of both positive affect and negative affect during the previous week. Based on these ratings, participants were categorized as high in positive affect if they reported experiencing it on all or most days at both time points (36% of participants). Each participant's HIV viral load was also assessed at all three time points and scored as suppressed or not suppressed using Centers for Disease Control (CDC) criteria. Data analyses showed that participants with high positive affect at the first two time points were significantly more likely to show viral suppression 6 months later at the third time point, and this was especially true for participants who also had scored low for negative affect.

In a thoughtful narrative review, Pressman, Jenkins, and Moskowitz (2019) raised a number of issues that should be considered when evaluating the research in this area but concluded that "there is now impressive evidence that [positive affect] short-term states and long-lasting traits have extensive correlations with an array of health and health-relevant outcomes" (p. 628). These outcomes include mortality (i.e., lifespan), morbidity (i.e., disease onset and duration), cardiovascular health, and outcomes for cancer and HIV treatments. For example, Scherer and Herrmann-Lingen (2009) found that hospital inpatients' ratings of their ability to "enjoy things as much as before" significantly predicted their survival after 1 year. Importantly, this relationship held even when the data analysis adjusted for their physicians' prediction of 1-year survival based on their medical conditions. Several models have been proposed to account for such findings. These include a stress-buffering model that posits positive affect to mitigate stress and thereby increase the likelihood of a person engaging in healthy behaviors that influence their immune and cardiovascular systems and thus decrease the likelihood of disease progression.

Given the associations found between positive affect and health outcomes, it is not surprising that a substantial number of intervention programs have been developed to increase positive affect in persons living with chronic illness. These programs may seek to boost positive affect by encouraging participants to engage in acts of kindness, gratitude, optimistic thinking, and/or some form of meditation. Most programs include more than one of these strategies, making it difficult to compare their relative effectiveness. Still, overall, they do appear to increase positive affect and other indices of well-being with small to medium effect sizes (Bolier et al., 2013). However, in their review, Pressman et al. (2019) concluded that there are too few studies to permit conclusions regarding the effectiveness of intervention programs on objective measures of health and disease.

THREATS AND FEAR

An interesting and provocative body of research has emerged on the question of whether humans develop a **negativity bias** (i.e., "propensity to attend to, learn from, and use negative information . . . more than positive information"; Vaish et al., 2008, p. 383). For example, consistent with this proposal is the observation that news media typically report more crimes and disasters than celebrations and charity. But if a bias toward negative information indeed exists, how might its development proceed? One proposal asserts that an attentional bias toward threatening stimuli emerges early in life and that such a bias will subsequently facilitate adaptive fear-learning (Burris et al., 2019; LoBue, 2013; LoBue, Rakison, & DeLoache, 2010; Öhman & Mineka, 2001).

Do Infants Preferentially Attend to Threat-Related Facial Expressions?

Studies of infants' attentional responses to facial expressions appear to substantiate at least part of this proposal. In particular, starting between 5 and 7 months of age, a number of studies have found that infants look longer at prototypic fear expressions than happy expressions and take longer to disengage from them (e.g., Peltola, Hietanen, Forssman, & Leppänen, 2013; Peltola, Leppänen, Mäki, & Hietanen, 2009). To illustrate, Nakagawa and Sukigara (2012) studied infants at 12, 18, 24, and 36 months of age in an **overlap procedure** during which they were presented with a neutral, happy, or fear facial expression in the center of a display screen, after which an attractive object (i.e., a distractor) appeared on one side of the face. At each age, mothers also completed measures of their infants' temperament. Results showed that infants of all ages disengaged from the fear expression in order to look at the distractor less quickly than they disengaged from happy or neutral expressions. In addition, 12-month-old infants who were judged higher in negative emotionality by their mothers were found to fixate longer on the fear expressions than those low in negative emotionality. Interestingly, this relationship between temperament and attention was not found in older infants, suggesting that other factors may intervene at later ages to influence the strength of this attention bias (Burris et al., 2019).

Several hypotheses have been advanced regarding the mechanisms underlying infants' attentional bias toward fear expressions (LoBue, Kim, & Delgado, 2019). One possibility is that recognition of these expressions as signs of fear is an innate ability that emerges in the middle of the first year. However, arguing against this hypothesis, researchers have also observed that infants of that age do not themselves show fear when they attend to fear expressions (LoBue & Rakison, 2013; see also discussion of expression recognition development in Chapter 2). An alternative hypothesis is that infants' attention is captured by the unfamiliarity and intensity of the pro-totypic fear expression. This fortuitous propensity would position infants to later learn the important functional meaning of fear expressions, as well as what types of environmental stimuli should be feared. A third (compromise) possibility is that infants' attention is indeed selectively captured by fear expressions (not just intense novel expressions in general) through some mechanism that does not require recognition of the expression's meaning. Still, this innately determined perceptual bias could prepare infants for later learning about fear. Further research would be helpful to scholars seeking to adjudicate among these possibilities.

One interesting observation about fear expressions is that they do not actually represent a threat by the expresser (although presumably they do represent the presence of something in the environment that the expresser deems deserving of fear). In contrast, anger expressions might be considered as threats in and of themselves. Therefore, several developmental research-ers have expanded their own focus of attention to include anger as well as fear expressions. For example, using a procedure similar to that used by Nakagawa and Sukigara (2012, as described above), Leppänen, Cataldo, Enlow, and Nelson (2018) found that 7- to 36-month-old infants showed an attention bias for fear expressions, but only the 36-month-olds showed a bias for anger expressions. In contrast, Morales et al. (2017) found evidence for an attention bias toward both anger and happy expressions in younger infants (i.e., 4- to 24-month-olds) using a similar procedure but not including fear expressions. No significant effect for infant age was obtained in their study. However, results did show that mothers' ratings of their own anxiety-related symptoms were associated with greater attention biases in their infants. Fur-thermore, in a study of older children and adolescents from the United States, Netherlands, Ireland, and China (Abend et al., 2018), an attentional bias toward angry faces was found to be associated with both social anxiety and school phobias.

Other studies have investigated early attention to angry faces using an infant-appropriate version of the **dot-probe paradigm**, a procedure fre-quently used in research with adults. Infants first are presented with an emo-tional expression (e.g., anger) and a neutral expression on a display screen, after which the two expressions are replaced by a probe (typically an asterisk) positioned where either the emotional face or the neutral face was previ-ously seen. Infants' latency to fixate on the probe when its position is either congruent or incongruent with the previously viewed emotion face is measured. Bias is indicated if the latency to fixate on the incongruently placed probe is significantly longer than the latency to fixate on the congruently placed probe (Burris, Barry-Anwar, & Rivera, 2017). In studies involving infants ranging in age from 4 to 24 months of age, a significant attention bias has been reported for both angry and happy expressions (e.g., Pérez-Edgar et al., 2017). However, as with fear expressions, no evidence indicates that anger expressions elicit fear in the infants. Furthermore, it is unclear when in the 4- to 23-month age range infants begin to recognize the emotion meaning of this expression (see Chapter 2 for a more general discussion of infant expression recognition).

Attention to Snakes and Spiders

Other studies of infants' responses to threat have involved objects rather than faces. In particular, snakes and spiders have been investigated, as they have often been proposed as natural elicitors of fear due to the danger they posed in our evolutionary past (Öhman & Mineka, 2001; Seligman, 1971). For example, in a series of experiments, Öhman and his colleagues found that adult participants could be conditioned to associate snakes or spiders with a mild (but unpleasant) electric shock more readily than they could be conditioned to associate flowers and mushrooms with the same level of electric shock (see Öhman & Mineka, 2001, for a review of these and other studies). Results of some developmental studies (not involving electric shocks) suggest that infants and children also preferentially attend to snakes and spiders. For example, DeLoache and Lobue (2009) found that 7- to 16-month-old infants will associate a video of a moving snake with the sound of a fearful voice but will not associate the fear voice with videos of other moving animals. Preschool children can detect a snake or spider embedded in an array of flowers more readily than they detect a flower (or a frog or caterpillar) embedded in an array of snakes (Lobue & DeLoache, 2008). However, similar to observations made in the facial expression studies described above, neither infants nor children show any signs of fear during the experiments but appear instead to show interest.

As for threat-related facial expressions, the mechanisms underlying infants' and children's attentional biases to snakes and spiders, as well as the role of these biases in fear learning, warrant further study. In any case, it seems important to emphasize that the presence of attentional biases supporting fear learning does not in any way preclude the idea that fear learning in both children and adults can occur for stimuli that do not originate in our evolutionary past. To illustrate, several studies (e.g., Subra, Muller, Fourgassie, Chauvin, & Alexopoulos, 2018; Zsido, Deak, & Bernath, 2019) have shown that adults respond to modern threats (e.g., guns) more readily than to ancient threats (e.g., snakes). Furthermore, like many things in life, one can have too much of a good thing when it comes to attentional biases toward threat. In a narrative review of the existing literature on adults, Van Bockstaele et al. (2014) concluded that causal relations between anxiety and attentional bias to threat are bidirectional. That is, stronger attentional biases can lead to greater anxiety, while at the same time high levels of anxiety can exacerbate threat-related attentional biases. In a meta-analysis of studies with children, Dudeney, Sharpe, and Hunt (2015) similarly found that more anxious children showed significantly stronger threat biases, a relationship that further strengthened with age.

Do Infants Fear Strangers and Heights?

As noted above, investigators of attentional biases have refrained from concluding that infants and younger children (or at least most of them) are actually afraid of snakes, spiders, or anger and fear faces. At the same time, other stimuli have been proposed as normative elicitors of fear during infancy (e.g., strangers, heights). In a recent review, LoBue and Adolph (2019) concluded that stranger fear is indeed normative toward the end of the first year but that fear of heights is not. Their argument raises provocative questions about how to identify fear (or any other emotion) in preverbal infants and toddlers and what we mean when we say "X is afraid of Y." LoBue and Adolph point out that there is no gold standard for identifying emotion and argue that at least two of the following three emotion indicators should be present: facial expression, behavior (e.g., avoidance for fear), and physiological changes that may be reasonably interpreted to reflect the emotion. This criterion appears to be met for stranger fears, but the researchers question whether it is met for fear of heights. They note that infants may avoid going over the edge when confronted with a drop-off, but they do not necessarily retreat from it. Instead, infants often explore the edge and may even smile while doing so (LoBue & Adolph, 2019). But does this mean that they do not fear heights? In a commentary on this issue, Walle and Dahl (2020) presented a functionalist approach to the question. Reflecting Campos and Barrett's (1985; Barrett & Campos, 1987) theoretical perspective (see Chapter 1), they argue that emotions are relational phenomena that may be manifested by any form of behavior that accomplishes the functional goal of the emotion (e.g., avoidance of harm for fear). Therefore, exploring the edge of a drop-off while refraining from going over it may be said to indicate a fear of heights, even if the infant is not currently experiencing fear. Viewed from another perspective, infants may be engaging in a type of emotion regulation described in James Gross's (2015a, 2015b) influential process model of emotion (see Chapter 5). That is, they may be engaging in situation selection or situation modification in the service of avoiding harm, while also satisfying a desire to explore. In reflecting on the perennial question of "What is an emotion?," Pollak, Camras, and Cole (2019) acknowledged that consensus in the field is lacking but urged investigators to clearly articulate their own views or assumptions in order to provide a context for understanding their measurement criteria and interpretation of their findings when studying preverbal infants or even older children and adults.

Fears in Older Children

Regarding the measurement of fear at older ages, a different set of issues arises (Gullone, 2000; Muris & Field, 2011). The vast majority of studies with children rely on verbal or written reports that may be collected by very different methods. These include face-to-face interviews with an experimenter, spontaneous listing of a child's fears by parents, teachers, or children themselves, or completion of a survey on which a predetermined set of common fears is listed, and each is rated by the respondent. One popular measure is the Revised Fear Survey Schedule for Children (FSSC-II; Gullone & King, 1992) that lists 75 fears that are each rated on a 3-point scale ("not scared" to "very scared"). This scale has been revised several times to incorporate common fears that emerged after the original version was created (e.g., AIDS).

Each method of fear measurement has its advantages and disadvantages and has generated somewhat different results. However, a number of general findings have emerged, as summarized by Gullone (2000). First and perhaps foremost, studies have shown that almost all children report some number of fears. However, estimates of the average number have varied rather widely, ranging from about three to about nine. A second finding is that most fears are temporary and appear to spontaneously diminish or disappear as children grow older. Third, some common categories of fears have been identified for children of different ages. In preschool children, common fears include animals, being alone, and darkness. During the elementary school years, new fears may emerge, including fear of supernatural beings (e.g., the "boogie man"), bodily injury, school failure, and criticism by others. In adolescence, fears also may relate to economic or political events about which the young person has now become aware. To summarize, as children become more cognitively sophisticated, they can imagine dangers that are not immediately present and that may involve psychological rather than physical harm.

Demographic differences are also seen. For example, girls typically report more fears than boys, perhaps reflecting gender differences in fear socialization. In addition, lower-SES children report more fears than higher-SES children, perhaps reflecting the realities of living in more dangerous environments. Cultural differences have also been found that reflect different sources of potential harm. For example, Dong, Yang, and Ollendick (1994) found that fear of school failure is rated higher in China than the United States, presumably reflecting the more intense pressure for school performance in China.

ANGER

Can Babies Get Angry?

Reflecting differences among researchers in their conceptualization of infant emotional development, determining when the emotion of anger first appears has proved problematic. According to Izard's differential emotions theory (DET), anger emerges between 2 and 3 months of age, when the infant version of the prototypic anger facial expression can first be seen (Izard & Malatesta, 1987). However, as noted earlier (see Chapter 2), this expression initially occurs in a wide range of eliciting circumstances, including many that would not be considered to evoke anger. Other theorists propose that anger cannot be said to be present until cognitive abilities that underlie the appraisal of anger (e.g., perceiving intentionality on the part of the offending agent) are present (Sroufe, 1996), until consciousness emerges (Lewis, 2014), or unless anger-related functional behaviors or thoughts are generated (e.g., resisting obstruction to one's goals or thinking about doing so; Barrett & Campos, 1987). Before those additional indices appear, the infant may be said to be experiencing more diffuse negative affect (e.g., distress; Camras, 2011), precursor emotions (e.g., frustration; Sroufe, 1996), or pre-emotional expression–action patterns (Lewis, 2014). Considering these criteria together, it appears that a consensus regarding the emergence of anger finally is reached when the infant is in the middle of his or her second year, although some researchers will identify anger at earlier ages.

To illustrate, Braungart-Rieker, Hill-Soderlund, and Karrass (2010) studied the development of emotional reactivity in infants at 4, 8, 12, and 16 months. At each age, mothers completed Rothbart's (1981) Infant Behavior

Questionnaire (IBQ), which includes two scales considered by Braungart-Rieker et al. (2010) to be measures of anger and fear—that is, **distress to limitations** and **distress to novelty**, respectively. During a laboratory visit, infants participated in a number of procedures. These included an episode of mother–infant toy play and two episodes based on Goldsmith and Rothbart's (1996) Laboratory Temperament Assessment Battery (Lab-TAB)—that is, stranger approach (for fear) and nonpainful arm restraint (for anger/frustration). Anger and fear were scored based on the infant's facial expressions, intensity of distress vocalizations, and intensity of body activity (i.e., struggle to escape). Interestingly, only the facial codes were distinct for the two emotions, and the final scores for anger and fear were based primarily on the intensity of vocal and bodily reactions that were similar in form across the two procedures. Thus whether the infants actually were experiencing anger and fear or simply distress at the younger ages depends upon one's theoretical point of view. Still, results showed an interesting age progression: both "anger" and "fear" reactivity as seen in the laboratory increased with age and were related to mothers' ratings on the temperament measures for these same variables. In addition, results showed that developmental trajectories were also influenced by other factors. In particular, maternal sensitivity measured during the toy play session was related to a slower age-related increase in fear reactivity during the stranger approach. Also, lower levels of negative affect were seen in infants who showed early signs of behavioral regulation (i.e., were able to distract themselves during the fear and anger episodes by attending to nonstressful objects in the laboratory room).

Temper Tantrums

The increases in anger-related reactivity observed by Braungart-Rieker et al. (2010) are consistent with the popular notion that the normative development of negative emotionality culminates toward the end of infancy in the "terrible twos." Also consistent with this notion is research on infants' and children's temper tantrums. As operationalized by Michael Potegal (2019), temper tantrums are brief episodes of behavior characterized by expressions and actions indicating both anger (e.g., hitting, screaming) and distress (e.g., crying, whining). Although results differ somewhat across investigations using different parent-report methodologies and participant samples, there is general agreement that temper tantrums are rarely seen before 15 months of age, are common in toddlers between 18 and 30 months, and decline in frequency thereafter (Potegal, 2019). For example, in a study of primarily middle-class European American children, Potegal and Davidson

(2003) found that 87% of their 18- to 24-month-old sample were reported by parents to have had at least one tantrum during the previous month. This prevalence rate increased to 91% for the 30- to 36-month-old children but was only 59% for the 42- to 48-month-old children. Thus tantrum frequency declined during the fourth year, although tantrums could still be seen at this older age and beyond. Extreme or frequent temper tantrums may be considered symptoms of behavioral disorders if combined with other symptoms (Belden, Thomson, & Luby, 2008). For example, according to the fifth edition of the *Diagnostic and Statistical Manual of Mental Disorders* (**DSM-5**; American Psychiatric Association, 2013), weekly tantrums are considered normative for preschoolers, but daily tantrums may be a symptom of **oppositional defiant disorder (ODD)**. In children older than 6 years of age, more than three tantrums a week may be considered a symptom of disruptive mood dysregulation disorder.

Laboratory studies have also shown that anger normally declines from late infancy to early childhood. To illustrate, Cole et al. (2011) studied children from 18 months to 4 years of age using a delay of gratification procedure during which children were given a boring broken toy to play with while waiting for their mothers to complete a lengthy set of questionnaires. An attractively wrapped gift was placed on a table in front of them, and the children were told they could open it after their mothers completed their task. After an 8-minute wait, the experimenter entered the room and gave the pair permission to open the package. During the 8-minute interval, the children's facial and vocal anger expressions were coded according to criteria developed by the investigators based on descriptions by previous researchers (particularly Ekman and Izard). The children's waiting-related activity was also coded, such as focusing on the gift, distracting themselves with the available toys, begging their mothers to finish, and/or opening the present. Results showed that anger expressions were relatively high at 18 and 24 months but then declined between 24 months and 4 years as children became better at distracting themselves during the waiting period.

Anger in Children and Adolescents

Normative anger levels remain relatively low across childhood. This may be due in part to the development of both behavioral and emotion regulation skills (Dollar & Calkins, 2019; Kopp, 1989). For example, children become more able to cope effectively if they encounter a blocked goal (e.g., by figuring out how to climb onto a chair to obtain an object placed out of their reach). Children also become more able to regulate their anger (e.g., to distract themselves in situations in which they are required to wait). In addition, they are more likely to perceive emotion regulation to be desirable (Saarni, 1979). Providing an example, Shipman, Zeman, Nesin, and Fitzgerald (2003) presented younger children (i.e., first and second graders) and older children (i.e., fourth and fifth graders) with stories in which the protagonist's anger or sadness was caused by either the child's mother, father, or best friend. In the story, the child protagonist responded in one of five ways (i.e., expressing the emotion verbally, expressing the emotion facially, crying, sulking, or being aggressive). For both anger and sadness, children in all grades indicated that verbally expressing the emotion would be most acceptable, whereas acting aggressively would be least acceptable—although aggression toward peers was more acceptable than aggression toward parents. Children also indicated their awareness of the negative consequences associated with aggressive responses (i.e., conflict with their social partners).

Despite the improvements in behavioral and emotion regulation abilities seen during childhood, anger may increase once again during adolescence. Two complementary explanations have been proposed. One ascribes this upsurge to increasing conflict between adolescents' goals for greater autonomy and the rules and regulations imposed by their parents (Dollar & Calkins, 2019). The second explanation proposes that adolescence (or more specifically puberty) is accompanied by increased sensitivity in the reward areas of the brain and that this increase is not yet offset by the full development of cortical areas involved in self-regulation (Casey & Caudle, 2013). This latter explanation has received considerable attention in the popular press, as well as the scholarly literature (see Chapter 4).

Temperament and Socialization Influences

Layered on top of the normative trajectory of anger development are important individual differences. These have been of particular interest to researchers because of their potential relationship to the development of anger-related behavioral problems and pathologies such as **conduct disorder (CD)**. Numerous studies have documented such relationships. For example, Brooker et al. (2014) studied infants at 6 and 12 months of age in laboratory procedures designed to elicit anger/frustration, that is, gentle arm restraint and restraint in a car seat. Infants' emotions were coded using the same system used by Braungart-Rieker et al. (2010), as earlier described. Two years later, parents completed a measure of their children's behavior problems using the Child Behavior Checklist (CBCL; Achenbach & Rescorla, 2000). At both 6 and 12 months, the researchers computed an average score for anger across the entire group of children. They then identified three profiles of anger development between 6 and 12 months: (1) consistently below-average anger, (2) consistently above-average anger, (3) increasing anger from somewhat below average at 6 months to somewhat above average at 12 months. This last profile was the most common and considered to represent the normative trajectory. Infants in this normative group were found to show significantly fewer behavior problems at 3 years of age than infants in the high-anger group, with infants in the low-anger group falling somewhere in between. In a study of older children, Nozadi, Spinrad, Eisenberg, and Eggum-Wilkens (2015) found that mothers' and teachers' ratings of children's temperamental anger at 4½ years (using Rothbart et al.'s [2001] Children's Behavior Questionnaire [CBQ]) was related to maternal ratings of conduct problems (primarily aggression) at 6 and 7 years of age.

Irrespective of any temperament-based differences in infant anger-related reactivity, socialization influences may come to have strong effects on both the elicitation and expression of anger in children. As described in Eisenberg's emotion socialization model (Eisenberg, Cumberland, & Spinrad, 1998; Eisenberg, Spinrad, & Cumberland, 1998), parents (and others) may influence children by means of demonstrative modeling, responding to, and discussing anger, as well as introducing or avoiding situations in which anger might be experienced. Through these means, children may learn that anger is expected, acceptable, and/or even appropriate under some circumstances and should be expressed in particular ways (see examples in work by Miller & Sperry, 1987, discussed in Chapter 3, and both Davies & Cummings, 1994, and Patterson, 1982, discussed in Chapter 8). At the same time, when parents (and others) fail to demonstrate or encourage the development of behavioral coping and emotion regulation strategies, then higher levels of anger also would be expected.

How Is Anger Related to Aggression?

The relationship between anger and aggression illustrates the complexity of relations between different components of the emotion process. Although aggression may serve the functional goal of anger (i.e., to remove an impediment to one's goals), not all anger episodes involve aggression, and not all aggression is motivated by anger. For example, a bully need not experience anger when attacking another child in order to steal his lunch; his victim may experience anger but complain to the teacher rather than counterattack. Researchers have partly captured the distinction between anger and aggression by differentiating between **proactive aggression** and **reactive aggression** (Dodge & Coie, 1987). Reactive aggression is defined as aggression produced in response to a perceived provocation, whereas proactive aggression is initiated by a child as a means to achieve a goal. Some research has suggested that reactive aggression is associated with more physiological arousal and anger-related behaviors than proactive aggression (Hubbard et al., 2002).

From an appraisal perspective, reactive aggression might indeed be expected to often involve anger. For example, according to Lazarus's (1991) appraisal theory of emotion (see Chapter 1), anger results when a provocation is perceived as intentional or due to inexcusable carelessness. One interesting line of research initiated by Kenneth Dodge and his colleagues suggests that children may differ in their propensity to perceive a provocation as intentional. For example, Dodge and Coie (1987) studied first- and third-grade boys who were categorized by their teachers as being proactive aggressive (i.e., tending to strategically use aggression to achieve their goals), reactive aggressive (i.e., tending to react aggressively when provoked), both proactive and reactive aggressive, or nonaggressive. The boys were presented with 12 video-recorded scenes, each portraying a provocation (e.g., one boy knocks down another boy's block tower as he walks by). By means of facial and verbal cues, the provocateur either signaled his intentions clearly or the provocateur provided ambiguous signals so that it was unclear as to whether the act was deliberate, accidental, or prosocial (i.e., the provocateur was actually trying to help). For each scene, the participating boys were asked to indicate how they perceived the action (i.e., as hostile, accidental, or prosocial) and how they themselves would behave in the depicted situation (i.e., do nothing, talk to the provocateur, tell the teacher, or get angry). Results showed that the groups did not differ significantly in their identification of the provocateur's intentions in scenes that included clearly portrayed signals of intention. However, when errors were made, those boys categorized as reactive aggressive or both reactive and proactive aggressive were more likely to attribute hostile intentions to the provocateur than were the proactively aggressive or nonaggressive boys. For scenes in which the provocation was ambiguous, those boys categorized as reactive aggressive or both reactive and proactive aggressive again attributed hostile intentions to the provocateur more often than the other two groups. Unfortunately, in analyzing the children's behavioral choices, anger responses were combined with "telling the teacher" to form a composite score for aggression. Thus the specific association between anger and reactive aggression was not directly examined. However, the study did demonstrate an association between reactive aggression and an anger-related **hostile attribution bias** in children (i.e., a tendency to interpret ambiguous cues as reflecting another's hostile intent). The relationship between aggressive behavior and a hostile attribution bias was confirmed in a more recent meta-analytic investigation (Verhoef, Alsem, Verhulp, & De Castro, 2019).

An Applicable Model of Socioemotional Information Processing

Dodge's early work heralded the subsequent development of general models of social information processing, that is, models that describe the psychological and behavioral processes through which children generate a response to a social encounter. For example, Crick and Dodge (1994) proposed a model that they initially applied to aggressive behavior. The model included five steps: (1) encoding and interpreting others' behaviors (e.g., observing someone knock over your block tower and deciding it was a deliberate act), (2) relating those behaviors to one's own personal and interpersonal goals (e.g., punishing the offender, maintaining his or her friendship), (3) considering various possible responses (e.g., asking for help in rebuilding, punching the offender), (4) deciding upon the most desirable option, and (5) enacting the chosen response.

Subsequently, this model was modified by Lemerise and Arsenio (2000) to more explicitly acknowledge the role that emotion plays in each step of the process. For example, the child may observe and recognize the provocateur's emotional expression (e.g., a sneer produced by the class bully), interpret the provocateur's action accordingly (e.g., as deliberate), respond with one or more particular emotions (e.g., anger and/or fear), decide upon the most desirable action (e.g., attack the offender), and proceed to enact the response—or fail to enact it due to competing considerations (e.g., fear of retribution by the bully). Although a considerable amount of research on children's social interactions is consistent with these models (e.g., studies of the hostile attribution bias), one potential objection is that both appear to portray social information processing as involving a deliberate and sequential decision-making process. However, researchers in this area hasten to emphasize that social information processing—like other forms of information processing—is often implicit, rapid, and automatic, particularly when it is based on past experience.

DISGUST

Among the negative emotions, disgust seems to be particularly popular among young children. A quick Google search for "disgusting candy" will yield a wide variety of options, including scorpion lollipops, oozing eyeballs, Snotz, and Original Bag of Poo. A search for "disgusting toys" yields such trendy hits as the Gross Body Lab, the Poopy Head game, and the Grossery Gang 10-pack of rotten groceries (presumably plastic). The enjoyment of emotions that are normally experienced as negative has been labeled *benign masochism* (Rozin, Guillot, Fincher, Rozin, & Tsukayama, 2013) and may reflect a feeling of mastery resulting from the successful practicing of emotion regulation when the emotion is experienced at a relatively low intensity and in a safe environment.

What Causes Disgust?

Several theories of disgust have been proposed based primarily on research with adults (see Rottman, DeJesus, & Greenebaum, 2019, for review). Currently, the most prominent theory holds that disgust evolved as a preventative mechanism to aid humans in the avoidance of pathogen contagion (Curtis, de Barra, & Aunger, 2011). However, because pathogens themselves (e.g., germs, viruses, plant toxins) cannot be seen with the naked eye, humans will use sensory cues that are often (but not always) associated with pathogens (e.g., rotten odors, slimy textures, bizarre abnormalities in appearance or behavior, such as foaming at the mouth). At the same time, considerable cultural differences in disgust responses are readily observed. For example, many Americans are disgusted by foods that are considered delicacies in another culture (e.g., sheep's head in Iceland). Some people also report feeling disgust in response to moral violations (e.g., exploiting the helpless). These phenomena suggest that social learning is key to the development of disgust responding in the individual, although it may overlay an evolutionary foundation.

Development of Disgust

Developmental research provides support for this proposal. Neonates and young infants respond to bitter tastes and sharp odors (e.g., from butyric acid) with facial expressions of disgust (i.e., nose wrinkling, upper lip raising; Soussignan, Schaal, Marlier, & Jiang, 1997), but no other disgust-related responding can be seen. For example, infants and toddlers do not show signs of disgust to feces, an elicitor that might be expected to be innate from a pathogen avoidance perspective (Rozin, Haidt, & McCauley, 2016).

Few studies have investigated the development of disgust responding in children. However, Stevenson, Oaten, Case, Repacholi, and Wagland (2010) examined responses to a range of potential disgust elicitors in parents and their children ranging in age from 2½ years to 14 years. The elicitors exemplified three empirically derived categories that were created based on statistical analysis of parents' reports of their children's disgust responses. These categories roughly conformed to three theoretically derived categories proposed on the basis of research with adults: (1) core elicitors, (2) animal elicitors, and (3) sociomoral elicitors. Core elicitors are those considered to reflect threats posed by oral consumption (e.g., rotting food), contact with body products (e.g., sniffing feces), violation of the body envelope (e.g., blood, dismembered body parts), or neglect of hygiene (e.g., touching a dirty sock). Animal elicitors are reminders of one's animal nature, including death (e.g., dead bird, cockroaches). Sociomoral elicitors are aberrant behaviors judged to be offensive within one's community (e.g., littering, stealing from a handicapped person). Ethically acceptable exemplars were created to be presented to children and their parents (e.g., a urine-smelling glob of fermented shrimp paste). Participants' ratings indicated how much they liked or disliked each elicitor. In addition, the investigators recorded whether participants were willing to approach or make contact with the elicitors and coded their disgust facial expressions. Results showed that a significant proportion of children at all ages responded to the core elicitors with avoidance, disgust expressions, and negative ratings. Responses to the animal elicitor emerged more gradually— avoidance at 2 years, 5 months; low ratings at 4 years, 5 months; and disgust facial expressions at 6 years, 8 months of age. Responses to the sociomoral elicitors emerged at 6 years, 8 months of age. Two other theoretically important findings were obtained. First, disgust responding was unrelated to children's cognitive understanding of contagion. Second, children's disgust responses to the elicitors were related to the parents' behavioral and expressive responses. Together, these findings suggest that disgust responses are largely socialized rather than being intrinsically innate or emerging spontaneously in conjunction with knowledge about contamination. Going beyond children's observation of others' avoidance behaviors and facial expressions, Rottman et al. (2019) has suggested that linguistic testimony (i.e., verbal labeling of an object or event as disgusting) may be an especially important means by which disgust responses are socialized in children (see Muris, Mayer, Borth, & Vos, 2013; Rottman, Young, & Kelemen, 2017). At the same time, some prominent theorists still maintain that true disgust can only be said to occur when disgust-related behavior (e.g., avoidance) is based on an understanding of contamination rather than just the testimony of others or observation of their behavioral responses to an object or event (e.g., Rozin et al., 2016).

Disgust as a Moral Emotion

Stevenson et al.'s (2010) findings regarding sociomoral elicitors also are relevant to larger debates about emotion and morality extant in the adult literature (see Rozin et al., 2016, for review). In brief, one prominent theory (i.e., the theory of **contempt–anger–disgust [CAD]**; Rozin, Lowery, Imada, & Haidt, 1999) proposed that disgust is related to offenses against divinity (i.e., spiritual purity, religious laws or beliefs), anger is related to threats against one's autonomy (i.e., ability to act freely), and contempt to violations of one's duty to uphold community standards or expectations. However, more recent research has called this simple trichotomy into question. In particular, anger has been observed as a common response to violations of divinity and community, as well as autonomy. Providing an example involving children, Stevenson et al. (2010) found that disgust was associated with sociomoral violations of community standards (i.e., littering). To explain these theoretical mismatches, Hutcherson and Gross (2011) have proposed that the emotion associated with a sociomoral violation (i.e., anger vs. disgust) will depend on its self-relevance. That is, the same offense (e.g., stealing a student's exam) will evoke anger if it is your own exam but disgust if some other student is the victim. Other research suggests disgust also may be recruited to establish and maintain social boundaries (e.g., avoidance of individuals or groups with lower social standing such as the homeless; see Rottman et al., 2019, for detailed review of this position).

CULTURE-SPECIFIC EMOTIONS

In recent years, several emotion terms not found in the English language have appeared in the popular press. Among these are *schadenfreude* (a German term for finding joy in another person's misfortune), *hygge* (a Danish and Norwegian term for coziness or feeling comfortable, warm, and relaxed), and *amae* (a Japanese term for feeling pleasurable dependence on another person). The existence of such culture-specific terms is important to highlight because they must be accounted for in any theoretical or empirical attempt to understand human emotion. As noted in Chapter 1, the existence of nonuniversal emotion terms has long been acknowledged by emotion theorists. For example, basic emotion theorists such as Izard and Ekman conceptualize them as referring to emotion states that consist of one (or more) basic emotions in combination with each other and/or occurring in particular culture-specified eliciting circumstances (e.g., another person's misfortune). *Schadenfreude* clearly fits within this conceptualization. However, some culture-specific emotion terms do not appear to refer to any specific basic emotion as a component (e.g., *amae*). Consistent with constructivist emotion theories, these terms may be more easily explained as referring to core affective states (i.e., combinations of valence and arousal) occurring in particular culture-specified contexts. Thus identifying and analyzing culture-specific emotions may be important for adjudicating among contemporary emotion theories. Perhaps even more important, identifying and understanding culture-specific emotions may make an important contribution to our efforts to improve intercultural understanding.

SUMMARY AND FINAL THOUGHTS

According to Michael Lewis's influential model, self-conscious emotions develop starting in the middle of the second year with the emergence of objective self-awareness. According to this model, the first self-conscious emotions to appear are exposure embarrassment, jealousy, and envy. These do not involve a self-evaluative component. Starting at around 2 years of age, new self-conscious emotions emerge that require an appraisal of one's success or failure in meeting some standard, rule, or goal (e.g., pride, shame, guilt).

Shame and guilt are two self-conscious emotions that have received considerable attention. Current views of these emotions consider shame to occur when one attributes failure to one's global inadequacy, whereas guilt occurs when one perceives oneself as having done something wrong. Shame is associated with an impulse to withdraw or hide, whereas guilt is associated with an impulse to remedy one's wrongdoing. However, reparative actions can also stem from other motivations. Both temperament and parenting can influence the development of children's propensities to experience guilt and/or shame. Historically, Chinese parents have used shaming as a socialization practice more than European American parents. At the same time, given recent social changes in China, shaming may now be used less often. Greater shaming is associated with higher levels of depression across cultures.

Empathy is an emotion process that involves experiencing the emotion one perceives in another person while still distinguishing between one's own emotional experience and that of the other. An empathic response to another's distress may lead to personal distress if one focuses primarily on one's own negative feelings. Alternatively, it may lead to sympathy (also called empathic concern) if one focuses primarily on the distress of the other person. Temperament and parental socialization both influence the development of empathic concern. Negative emotionality may bias the child toward personal distress, whereas better self-regulation may facilitate the development of sympathy. Attachment security measured during adolescence is more strongly related to empathy than attachment security measured at younger ages. Parental warmth, positive expressivity, supportive responding, and emotion-related discussions with their children are also related to empathy development, prosocial behavior, and social competence. According to Decety's model, the neural concomitants of empathy involve brain areas associated with affect sharing, self-awareness, and executive functioning. Cultural differences in empathic responding may be related to differences in values related to emotional expressivity and restraint.

Fredrickson's BBT proposes that positive emotions generate a broadening of attention, thinking, and action that allows one to build resources contributing to positive adaptation. Consistent with this theory, positive emotions (or positive affect) are associated with a variety of beneficial outcomes (e.g., self-acceptance, positive relations with others). Efforts to boost positive affect via intervention programs have been successful in their goal. However, the effect of these programs on physical health remains to be demonstrated.

Infants show a number of biases related to the perception of threat stimuli. Starting at 5 to 7 months of age, infants look longer at prototypic fear expressions than at expressions for most other emotions. There is also evidence that an attentional bias to anger expressions and other threat stimuli (e.g., snakes, spiders) emerge during infancy and early childhood. Interestingly, neither infants nor children show indications that they themselves are experiencing fear as they look at these stimuli. Still, these attentional biases may be adaptive if they prepare infants and children to more readily learn about environmental threats. At the same time, more powerful attention biases to threat stimuli have been associated with anxiety in children.

Whether infants are afraid of heights is currently being debated. This debate exemplifies the lack of a gold standard for identifying an emotion and thus the lack of a consensus about when it is appropriate to attribute emotion to infants. At the same time, it also raises interesting questions about our use of emotion language in everyday speech—for example, what exactly do we mean when we say that someone "is afraid" of something? If infants preemptively avoid going over the edge of a cliff, can we still say that they are afraid of heights but are regulating their emotion via situation selection or modification?

Interviews and questionnaire measures have been used to identify common fears in children. As they grow older, children's fears become increasingly related to threats that are abstract and psychological in nature. Specific threats also change over historical time as new environmental dangers emerge (e.g., COVID-19) and old ones disappear (e.g., smallpox). Children living in different types of environments may have different fears depending upon their perception of the dangers that exist (e.g., neighborhood violence, school failure).

When infants can be said to first experience anger is also subject to disagreement. Some investigators are willing to attribute anger to infants early in the first year, whereas others believe that young infants experience a more general negative affective state, that is, distress. However, investigators do concur that anger can be seen in infants by the middle of the second year.

Normative anger development appears to culminate toward the end of infancy, when temper tantrums become common (i.e., starting at around 18 months). Anger begins to decline during the third year and remains relatively low across childhood. However, children who continue to show high levels of anger (e.g., frequent temper tantrums) may be diagnosed with ODD or disruptive mood dysregulation disorder. Normally, children learn how and when they should regulate their anger and become better able to do so. However, anger may increase again during adolescence as parent–child conflicts become more common. Socialization processes that influence anger are the same processes that influence emotional development in general, as discussed in previous chapters.

Anger does not necessarily lead to aggression, and aggression does not always stem from anger. Yet the two are closely related. Reactive aggression may occur more often in children who have an anger-related hostile attribution bias. Social information-processing models specify a series of steps that lead from encountering a social event (e.g., a provocation by another child) to enacting a behavioral response to the event (e.g., an aggressive response). Although early models focused on cognitive processes, emotion has been incorporated more fully into recent social information-processing models.

Disgust may have evolved as a defense against pathogens, but it is heavily influenced by sociocultural factors. Disgust responses to core elicitors (i.e., those related to protecting body integrity and health) are the first to develop, followed by reminders of one's animal nature, followed by sociomoral violations. However, whether this sequence holds across all cultures has not yet been determined. The relationship between disgust and particular types of moral offense is currently a topic of active investigation.

Although some emotions may be universal, others are culture specific. Any comprehensive emotion theory must be able to adequately explain these emotions.

CHAPTER 8

Adversity, Adaptation, Problems, and Interventions

Both emotion researchers and clinical practitioners are often motivated by a desire to help others lead a better emotional life. But what does such a life entail? As noted earlier, cultures may differ in their emotional values and thus in their conceptualization of "healthy" emotional adjustment. Emotional proclivities that are optimal (i.e., adaptive) in one culture may be maladaptive elsewhere. Because most research on emotional adjustment has taken place in Western societies, our conceptualization of healthy adjustment largely reflects contemporary Western values. This must be kept in mind when considering the research on adversity, psychopathology, and emotion-oriented intervention programs presented in this chapter.

ADVERSITY

Adversity is in the mind of the beholder, and circumstances that are generally perceived as adverse (e.g., low income) can affect different people in different ways. Still, measures of circumstances typically experienced as adverse may sometimes be significant predictors of emotional adjustment. In recent decades, the construct of **adverse childhood experiences (ACEs)** has become popular in both the medical and clinical psychology literature (Portwood, Lawler, & Roberts, 2021). As originally conceptualized (Felitti et al., 1998), this construct initially included three categories of child **abuse**

251

(physical, psychological, sexual) and four categories of household dysfunction (substance abuse, mental illness, household violence, criminal behavior). Thereafter, three other categories were added as part of an ACEs measure that has been widely adopted (i.e., parents' divorce/separation, physical neglect, emotional neglect; California Surgeon General's Clinical Advisory Committee, 2020). An individual's adversity score is computed by adding the number of adversity categories he or she experienced (i.e., 0–10), and a score of 4 or more is considered to indicate significant risk for a variety of emotional and health problems. Although widely used, the adequacy of this measure has been questioned on a number of grounds. For example, several researchers have argued that merely adding up the number of categories experienced fails to capture the important influences of exposure duration (Hamby, Elm, Howell, & Merrick, 2021), the ages at which adversity is experienced (Hawes et al., 2021), and multiplicative effects of particular forms of adversity experienced together (Briggs, Amaya-Jackson, Putnam, & Putnam, 2021). In addition, race-related stressors are not included on the standard questionnaire (Hampton-Anderson et al., 2021). These critiques illustrate the challenge of capturing the complexity of adverse experiences in both research and clinical assessment (Smith & Pollak, 2021). Still, the importance of addressing adversity dictates that efforts toward this end should continue to be made.

ENVIRONMENTAL SENSITIVITY

As noted above, the same adverse circumstances do not affect all individuals in the same way. Similarly, not all individuals benefit from the same high-quality environments. In an attempt to understand these differences, several potential forms of responsiveness to one's environmental circumstances are currently being explored.

Three Models

In a thought-provoking paper, Pluess (2015) described three models of **environmental sensitivity** that have received increasing attention in recent decades. According to the **diathesis–stress model,** some individuals are seen as more vulnerable than others to the negative effects of adversity. For example, some maltreated children will develop anxiety and depression, but this does not occur in all cases. The diathesis–stress model has historically been highly influential in research focusing on the development of psychopathologies in both children and adults. The **vantage sensitivity model** offers an opposite perspective by proposing that some individuals may benefit more than others from a high-quality environment (Pluess & Belsky, 2013). For example, an impulsive child might benefit from a highly responsive mother, that is, might show fewer externalizing behaviors than impulsive children with unresponsive mothers. In contrast, less impulsive children might show similar levels of externalizing behavior irrespective of their mothers' responsiveness (Slagt, Dubas, & van Aken, 2016). Merging these two perspectives, the **differential susceptibility model** takes a better-or-worse approach, proposing that certain individuals may be particularly responsive to both positive and negative influences. That is, if placed in a positive environment, they will do better than others; however, if placed in a negative environment, they will do worse (Belsky & Pluess, 2009). For example, a 3-year-old child who displayed high negative emotionality in infancy may show less compliance (i.e., do worse) than one who displayed low negative emotionality in infancy if both have mothers who are relatively unresponsive (i.e., provide them with a relatively negative environment). However, if both children have highly responsive mothers, then the child who displayed more negative emotionality in infancy may actually show greater compliance (i.e., do better) at the later age (Kim & Kochanska, 2012).

Importantly, these three models are not considered mutually exclusive. Different models may apply to different individual characteristics, environmental factors, and outcomes. For example, Nofech-Mozes, Pereira, Gonzalez, and Atkinson (2019) studied the later development of externalizing problems and internalizing problems in infants who had been securely or insecurely attached to their mothers and who produced either high or low levels of cortisol during the Strange Situation procedure. Results supported a diathesis–stress (i.e., vulnerability) model for internalizing symptoms but a differential susceptibility model for externalizing symptoms; that is, infants with high levels of cortisol were later (i.e., at 5 years of age) found to show more internalizing problems than infants with low cortisol levels if they were insecurely attached to their mothers (who presumably provided a less favorable emotional environment). However, cortisol was unrelated to internalizing problems in more securely attached infants. For externalizing problems, infants with high cortisol levels also did worse (i.e., showed more symptoms) than infants with low cortisol levels if they were insecurely attached (i.e., exposed to a poorer environment), but they showed *fewer* externalizing problems (i.e., did better) than infants with low cortisol levels if they were securely attached. That is, with respect to externalizing problems, the infants with low cortisol responded more strongly to either the positive experience of attachment security or the negative experience of attachment insecurity.

Rabinowitz and Drabick (2017) conducted a set of meta-analyses that evaluated the three models across multiple studies of young children involving a variety of outcomes related to social and emotional adjustment. They reported evidence for the diathesis–stress model in 60% of the studies, whereas 32% of the studies provided evidence of differential susceptibility, and 8% provided evidence for vantage sensitivity. In a meta-analysis focusing on infant temperament as a presumed marker of differential susceptibility, Slagt, Dubas, Deković, and van Aken (2016) found that infants scoring high in negative emotionality were more sensitive to both positive and negative parenting relative to infants scoring low in negative emotionality. However, this support for the differential susceptibility model was found only when negative emotionality was assessed in infancy rather than later in development, possibly reflecting the influence of parenting on the later development of temperament itself, as described in previous chapters.

Integrating the Three Models

In an attempt to theoretically integrate the three models, Pluess (2015) presented an overarching theoretical framework. This meta-model proposes that the three strategies coexist to represent evolutionary "bet-hedging" and conditional adaptation as viewed from a group perspective. Simplifying this complex explanation, it starts by acknowledging that neither individuals nor groups can predict the environmental circumstances into which they will be born. Therefore, it is beneficial (from a group perspective) for a population to hedge its bets by including a number of individuals who can adapt to either particularly positive or negative environments and thus can carry the group forward if such extreme circumstances arise. Focusing on those exhibiting differential susceptibility, some of these individuals will carry *sensitivity genes* (e.g., the short allele form of *5-HTTLPR*) that lead to their having greater sensitivity to sensory input of any type (Slagt, Dubas, van Aken, Ellis, & Deković, 2018). This in turn makes them more responsive to whatever type of environment they encounter. Thus, if they are raised in a largely positive environment, they will exhibit vantage sensitivity, that is, greater responsiveness to the positive input they receive in comparison with other individuals. In a largely negative environment, they will exhibit vulnerability, that is, greater responsiveness to the negative input in comparison with their peers. From an individual's perspective, adaptive responding to adverse circumstances may be maladaptive (or pathological) if circumstances change. For example, aggressiveness may be adaptive (i.e., provide a degree of protection) for youth raised within the context of a high-violence neighborhood. However, if their families are able to move to a more peaceful neighborhood, then their aggressiveness may incur social costs with little or no accompanying advantages.

Note that Pluess (2015) posits a genetic foundation for environmental sensitivity, and, indeed, many studies have examined a number of gene variants that are hypothesized to serve as its basis (see Rabinowitz & Drabick, 2017, Table 1). However, as illustrated above, other studies have used nongenetic variables as presumed markers of sensitivity (e.g., negative emotionality, cortisol responsivity, respiratory sinus arrhythmia [RSA], behavioral inhibition [BI]). Because such measures may be imprecise markers of sensitivity, Lionetti, Aron, Aron, Klein, and Pluess (2019) recently developed an observational rating system designed to more directly measure this construct.

CHILDHOOD MALTREATMENT

Child abuse and **neglect** are forms of adversity that have been widely studied. **Abuse** is an active form of adverse caregiving (e.g., harsh physical punishment, verbal threats), and **neglect** is a passive form (e.g., failure to provide proper care). Because abuse and neglect tend to co-occur, they are often considered together under the heading of child **maltreatment**. Recent reviews and meta-analyses have confirmed that maltreatment is associated with a variety of unfortunate consequences, including disorganized attachment and lower self-esteem (Cicchetti, 2016), depression and anxiety (Gallo, Munhoz, de Mola, & Murray, 2018; Infurna et al., 2016), antisocial behavior (Braga, Cunha, & Maia, 2018), lower language skills (Sylvestre, Bussières, & Bouchard, 2016), cognitive impairments (Masson, Bussières, East-Richard, R-Mercier, & Cellard, 2015), and academic failure (McGuire & Jackson, 2018). Maltreated children also are more likely to have difficulties with peer relations due in part to social cognitive biases that may predispose them to aggressive behaviors (e.g., a hostile attribution bias as described in Chapter 7; see also Cicchetti, 2016). Some may be diagnosed with posttraumatic stress disorder (PTSD; Masten et al., 2008). Still, it is important to recognize that not all maltreated children manifest any or all of these difficulties (Collishaw et al., 2007).

Do Maltreated Children Show Atypical Emotion Responding?

In an investigation of children's emotional reactivity, Shackman and Pollak (2014) compared the responses of maltreated and nonmaltreated 7- to 10-year-old boys during a frustration task. Frustration was induced by informing the participating boy that his reward for taking part in the study hinged on the performance of his partner, another child who was supposedly playing a video game in the next room. The participating boy was told he could observe the performance of his (actually nonexistent) partner on a computer screen. In response to the partner's winning or losing moves, the boy was told to provide feedback by pressing a button that would produce either a positive or negative sound (i.e., cheering or aversive honking). Results showed that maltreated participants produced more aversive feedback to their partners than did nonmaltreated boys and also produced more negative facial expressions.

Maltreated children may also have problems with emotion regulation. To illustrate, Milojevich, Levine, Cathcart, and Quas (2018) asked 10- to 17-year-old maltreated and nonmaltreated adolescents to describe personal experiences of sadness and anger and then to describe what they did to "make their feelings go away." Narratives were coded in terms of the nature of the emotion elicitor, severity of any physical harm that may have occurred, the emotional intensity of the event, and the coping strategies that were described. Coping strategies included many responses often studied under the rubric of emotion regulation (e.g., reappraisal, suppression, distraction). Results showed that some maltreated adolescents described maltreatment-related events (29% for anger; 11% for sadness), but most did not. Irrespective of whether or not they described maltreatment-related episodes, maltreated adolescents reported using disengagement (e.g., avoidance, ignoring) in response to sadness more than did nonmaltreated participants. Those adolescents who described maltreatment episodes reported using antisocial strategies (e.g., violence, self-harm, drugs, suicide attempt) more than did the nonmaltreated controls. Both disengagement and antisocial responses are considered less adaptive in comparison with alternatives such as problem solving and support seeking. Interestingly, however, logistic regression analyses yielded no significant differences between maltreated and nonmaltreated participants in use of these more adaptive strategies. In addition, no significant group differences were found for reported strategy use in anger episodes.

Maladaptive emotion communication is thought to contribute importantly to many of the problems of maltreated children. Yet relatively little research has been conducted in which the emotional expressions of these children are directly observed. However, Camras and colleagues (1990) videotaped and coded facial expressions produced by both maltreated and nonmaltreated children and their mothers during a laboratory play session and several mealtime observation sessions that took place in their homes. Significant associations were found between mothers' and children's facial behavior, particularly in their frequency of smiling. Somewhat surprisingly, no differences were found in facial expressivity between maltreating and nonmaltreating mothers or between their children—possibly because the presence of observers constrained mothers' expressions of negative affect. Still, Camras et al.'s (1990) results suggest that demonstrative modeling—a component of Eisenberg's emotion socialization framework—takes place in both maltreating and nonmaltreating families.

Do Maltreated Children Show Atypical Neurobiological Activity?

A variety of paradigms have also been used to study the neurobiological concomitants of maltreatment. For example, De Bellis and Hooper (2012) examined maltreated and nonmaltreated adolescents' neural responses as they completed an *emotional oddball task* while in a functional magnetic resonance imaging (fMRI) scanner. Participants were presented with a series of pictures and were instructed to press a button when they saw a designated target image (e.g., an oval shape). Interspersed in the series were distractor images, including some portraying sadness (e.g., a crying woman). Maltreated participants differed from nonmaltreated participants in that they showed greater amygdala activation when viewing the sadness images and less activation in brain regions related to cognitive control when viewing the target images. Consistent with these findings, a meta-analysis of 20 studies (Hein & Monk, 2017) also found greater amygdala reactivity to emotion faces in maltreated compared with nonmaltreated individuals.

A number of studies have investigated brain activity of maltreated and nonmaltreated children and adolescents during efforts at emotion regulation. To illustrate, McLaughlin, Peverill, Gold, Alves, and Sheridan (2015) presented physically abused and nonabused adolescents with positive, negative, and neutral pictures, each accompanied by an instruction to either: (1) just look at the pictures and let their emotions unfold naturally, (2) use the cognitive change strategy of detachment (i.e., think about the pictures as being distant, unreal or irrelevant), or (3) use cognitive change to make the pictures feel closer, more real, or more relevant. After viewing each picture, participants rated the intensity of their emotion on a 5-point scale. No differences were found between the maltreated and nonmaltreated groups in their emotion ratings. In addition, no differences were found in their neural responses to the positive pictures in any condition. However, differences were found between the two groups in their neural activity when viewing the negative pictures. In the passive just-look condition, maltreated adolescents showed greater activation in brain areas involved in the salience network (a neural network that responds to salient stimuli and includes the amygdala, putamen, anterior insula, and thalamus). When attempting to down-regulate their emotional response using detachment, both groups showed less amygdala activation when viewing negative pictures compared with the just-look condition and greater activation in several regions of the prefrontal cortex (PFC). Although the resulting amygdala activation levels did not differ across groups, maltreated adolescents showed greater activation of PFC regions (presumably related to cognitive control) than did the nonmaltreated participants. The investigators interpreted their findings as suggesting that maltreatment increases the salience of negative emotion information as an adaptation in the service of detecting potential threats and that regulating their greater emotional response requires greater effort on the part of maltreated individuals.

Blunted autonomic nervous system (ANS) responding also has been found in maltreated children and adolescents. For example, Leitzke, Hilt, and Pollak (2015) found that nonmaltreated youth (9–14 years of age) responded to a stressful public speech task with an increase in both negative affect and blood pressure, but maltreated youth responded with only an increase in negative affect. Similarly, McLaughlin, Sheridan, Alves, and Mendes (2014) found lower levels of sympathetic nervous system (SNS) reactivity in maltreated adolescents during a task that required them to perform mental arithmetic in front of a panel of judges.

Disrupted functioning of the hypothalamic–pituitary–adrenal (HPA) system is also characteristic of maltreatment as manifested in lower cortisol levels. For example, Trickett, Gordis, Peckins, and Susman (2014) found that 9- to 12-year-old maltreated children showed less cortisol reactivity in response to a social stressor in comparison with nonmaltreated children. In a particularly interesting study, Romens, McDonald, Svaren, and Pollak (2015) found greater methylation (i.e., blocking) of the glucocorticoid receptor gene (a gene involved in regulation of the HPA system) in physically maltreated compared with nonmaltreated children. In a meta-analytic investigation, Bernard, Frost, Bennett, and Lindhiem (2017) found lower levels of cortisol at awakening in maltreated children. Children who have experienced extreme neglect in the context of institutional child rearing also have consistently been found to show signs of hypocortisolism (Koss & Gunnar, 2018). Overall, the findings for both HPA system functioning and ANS responding are consistent with proposals that chronic stress produces physiological dysregulation.

Problems in Emotion Understanding

Maltreated children show clear deficits in their identification of emotional facial expressions. For example, in an early study, Camras, Grow, and Ribordy (1983) presented maltreated and nonmaltreated preschool children with brief stories describing typical emotion-eliciting situations for the Big Six emotions (e.g., "Her mother died and she feels sad"). Children were shown three pictures of prototypic emotional facial expressions and asked to choose the expression that matched the story. Maltreated children scored lower than nonmaltreated children and were also rated as less socially competent by their teachers.

Subsequent research by Seth Pollak and his colleagues produced a more nuanced picture of maltreated children's responses to facial expressions. Using the same materials and procedure that were employed by Camras et al. (1983), Pollak, Cicchetti, Hornung, and Reed (2000) examined the two major subtypes of maltreatment separately (i.e., physical abuse vs. neglect). Results showed that children in both maltreatment categories performed more poorly than nonmaltreated participants but that the physically abused children performed significantly better than the neglected children. Data analyses also revealed a unique pattern of responding to anger and sadness expressions. Physically abused children recognized anger as well as did nonmaltreated children, whereas neglected children recognized this expression more poorly. In contrast, neglected children recognized sadness expressions as well as nonmaltreated children did, whereas physically abused children were less accurate. Additionally, signal detection analyses indicated that physically abused children showed a response bias for angry faces (i.e., a tendency to select angry faces when they made errors in their responses to nonanger stories). In contrast, neglected children showed a response bias for sad faces. In later studies, Pollak and his colleagues (Pollak, Messner, Kistler, & Cohn, 2009; Pollak & Sinha, 2002) also demonstrated that physically abused children could identify anger expressions more readily than nonmaltreated children when presented with perceptually degraded stimulus faces.

Perlman, Kalish, and Pollak (2008) extended the study of maltreated children's emotion understanding to include emotion situations. To do so, they presented 5-year-old physically abused children and nonabused children with positive or negative facial expressions paired with either a positive, negative, or ambiguous eliciting event (e.g., a smiling woman paired with either a child writing on a wall or a woman hugging a child). The children were asked to indicate whether they thought the expression and event could really go together. Results suggested that the abused children considered positive, negative, and ambiguous situations to be equally plausible antecedents of negative emotion, whereas nonmaltreated children selectively endorsed the negative situations as likely elicitors of the negative facial expressions. Taken together, these studies suggest that physically abused children's heightened exposure to anger and aggression engenders heightened sensitivity to anger cues, along with an expectation that such negative emotions may occur in almost any situation.

PSYCHOPATHOLOGY

Even a brief perusal of the *Diagnostic and Statistical Manual of Mental Disorders* (DSM-5; American Psychiatric Association, 2013) makes obvious the key role that emotions play in psychological maladjustment. Emotion-related symptoms are described for virtually all disorders included in the manual, with considerable overlap across categories. For example, a number of pathologies involve fear or anxiety, including obsessive–compulsive, somatic, avoidant, and dependent personality disorders, as well as the anxiety disorders. Likewise, a number of pathologies involve irritability or anger, including posttraumatic stress, disruptive mood dysregulation, and oppositional defiant, paranoid, and borderline personality disorders. Sadness is associated with reactive attachment disorder, as well as depression. Several researchers have proposed that shared emotion-related dysfunction may underlie the **comorbidity** of some forms of psychopathology (e.g., Rhee, Lahey, & Waldman, 2015).

Research Domain Criteria

Reflecting these considerations, the National Institute of Mental Health (NIMH) has initiated a newly recommended research approach, the **Research Domain Criteria (RDoC) framework** (Kozak & Cuthbert, 2016). Although not intended to replace current diagnostic procedures, its purpose is to promote the understanding of basic systems underlying psychological dysfunction and thereby improve both diagnosis and treatment. The RDoC identifies six domains or basic systems: (1) negative valence systems (e.g., fear, anxiety), (2) positive valence systems (e.g., reward prediction, reward valuation), (3) cognitive systems (e.g., attention, control, memory), (4) social processes (e.g., attachment, emotion recognition), (5) arousal/regulatory systems (e.g., sleep, circadian rhythms), and (6) sensorimotor systems (e.g., action initiation and inhibition, sense of agency vs. dissociative behavior, habit-based behaviors).

The RDoC approach suggests a focus on basic components and processes involved in emotion rather than discrete emotions per se (Aldao, Gee, De Los Reyes, & Seager, 2016). Reflecting this approach, Kring and Mote (2016) have identified four constructs that are relevant across multiple disorders that may include different specific emotions: (1) core affect (i.e., valence and arousal), (2) emotional clarity (e.g., awareness of one's own emotions), (3) emotion regulation, and (4) emotion disconnection (e.g., non-normative lack of coherence between feelings and expressions). Regarding core affect, negatively valenced emotions characterize many mental disorders. Regarding emotional clarity, **alexithymia** (i.e., difficulty in identifying and describing one's feelings) has been found in at least some studies to be associated with anxiety disorders, depression, borderline personality disorder, and eating disorders (Vine & Aldao, 2014). Emotion regulation is recognized as widely problematic, and use of several maladaptive strategies (e.g., rumination, avoidance) has been associated with anxiety, depression, eating, and substance disorders (Aldao, Nolen-Hoeksema, & Schweizer, 2010; see also Compas et al., 2017; Gross & Jazaieri, 2014; Sloan et al., 2017). Emotion disconnection characterizes both schizophrenia and criminal psychopathy, a type of antisocial personality disorder in which self-reported emotion may not be nonverbally manifested as it is in individuals without disorders (e.g., Kring & Elis, 2013). Given their relevance to multiple disorders, the constructs identified by Kring and Mote (2016) may each constitute a target for treatments that might be generalizable across different types of disorders.

Internalizing and Externalizing Problems

Anxiety and depression are two mental disorders in which emotion-related symptoms play a central role. However, exemplifying comorbidity among different forms of maladjustment, they sometimes are grouped together under the overarching heading of **internalizing problems**. In fact, many developmental studies use measurement instruments that can generate scores for internalizing symptoms as an alternative to distinguishing between anxiety and depression. For example, the **Child Behavior Checklist (CBCL;** Achenbach, 1991; Achenbach & Rescorla, 2000, 2001) is a widely used

assessment instrument that can be utilized to generate scores for both internalizing problems (i.e., anxious depression, withdrawn depression, and/
or somatic symptoms) and **externalizing problems** (i.e., rule breaking and
aggressive behavior). Clinical cutoff scores are provided to indicate when
internalizing or externalizing problems reach a level suggesting that clinical
evaluation and intervention may be warranted. However, the CBCL also is
often used to measure levels of problem behavior without reference to clinical diagnosis. Still, high scores have been found to predict DSM-diagnosed
disorders in adulthood (Reef, van Meurs, Verhulst, & van der Ende, 2010).

ANXIETY

Given the romantic stereotype of childhood as a time of carefree bliss, some
may be surprised to learn that anxiety disorders can be diagnosed in children even younger than 5 years of age. By one estimate, its prevalence in
this age group is 7–11% (Costello, Egger, & Angold, 2005). In older children, epidemiological estimates may be even higher. Approximately 27% of
children will receive an anxiety diagnosis sometime in their lives. Although
a certain amount of fear and anxiety is normal at any age, clinicians concur that "when fear and anxiety cause the individual undue distress, impair
functioning, and interfere with typical developmental tasks, they cross the
boundary from typical development to be considered more pathological"
(Kiel & Kalomiris, 2019, p. 666).

Can Temperament Contribute to Anxiety?

An important contributor to children's anxiety is thought to be temperament, particularly BI and negative reactivity. To illustrate, Mian, Wainwright, Briggs-Gowan, and Carter (2011) asked parents to rate their 3-year-
old children on both temperamental variables. When the children were 8
years old, they reported on their own anxiety symptoms in the context of
a child-friendly puppet procedure. Results showed that mother-reported
inhibition and negative emotionality were related to children's self-reported
anxiety. In reviewing the relationship between BI and anxiety, Klein and
Mumper (2018) concluded that there is consistent evidence that BI is a risk
factor for social anxiety disorder and probably other types of anxiety disorders as well (e.g., general anxiety disorder). Consistent with the proposed
linkage between temperament and anxiety, greater amygdala reactivity has

been associated with higher levels of anxiety, as well as with BI and negative affect in adolescents and adults (Pine, 2007).

Problems with Emotion Regulation

Individuals with anxiety also have difficulties with emotion regulation. In an illustrative study, Carthy, Horesh, Apter, Edge, and Gross (2010) presented pictures with threatening content (e.g., a dangerous animal) to 10- to 17-year-old adolescents who had been clinically diagnosed with an anxiety disorder and to a control group of same-age adolescents without anxiety. After viewing the pictures, adolescents with anxiety rated themselves as experiencing more negative affect than controls. In a subsequent portion of the study, all participants were instructed on using reappraisal to reduce their negative emotional responses (e.g., by imagining a happy outcome to the depicted event; by imagining that the depicted event was part of a movie rather than real). After instruction, they were presented with a set of images to be reappraised and were asked to describe aloud their reappraisal process as they engaged in it. Analysis of their responses indicated that adolescents with anxiety were less able to generate reappraisals than were controls— although when they did so, their reappraisals were as successful in lowering negative affect as those of the participants without anxiety.

Other studies have also focused on the emotion regulation of children and adolescents with anxiety. Children with anxiety appear less able to flexibly deploy their regulation strategies as appropriate to the particular situation (Suveg & Zeman, 2004). Another important difference may involve emotional self-awareness (Sendzik, Schäfer, Samson, Naumann, & Tuschen-Caffier, 2017). Without such awareness, children with anxiety may be less likely to recruit and deploy emotion regulation strategies that could defuse their anxiety. Lastly, children with anxiety are less confident in their abilities to control their negative emotions, and this belief may serve as a self-fulfilling prophecy (Weems, Silverman, Rapee, & Pina, 2003).

An Emotion Competence Perspective

Using Carolyn Saarni's (1999) **emotion competence** framework, Mathews, Koehn, Abtahi, and Kerns (2016) identified several areas of emotion functioning and conducted meta-analyses of findings in these areas as related to anxiety in childhood and adolescence. Results showed that greater anxiety in children was significantly related to (1) poorer understanding of others' emotions, (2) less awareness of one's own emotions, (3) more difficulties in expressing one's emotions to others, (4) less acceptance of one's own emotions, and (5) less satisfaction with one's emotional life. With respect to emotion regulation, children with anxiety used support seeking (considered an adaptive strategy) more frequently than their peers without anxiety but also used maladaptive strategies such as avoidance, venting of anger/hostility, rumination, and catastrophizing more often. Somewhat surprisingly, greater anxiety was not associated with less use of strategies exemplifying cognitive reappraisal (e.g., positive refocusing, cognitive restructuring). This may be because cognitive reappraisal tends to be underutilized even by individuals without disorders—possibly because it requires greater cognitive effort. Still, Mathews et al.'s (2016) findings suggest that discouraging the use of maladaptive emotion regulation strategies, as well as encouraging greater use of adaptive strategies, may constitute important goals for therapeutic intervention.

Socialization Influences

Some differences between children with and without anxiety in their emotional functioning may stem from their social experiences, that is, experiences with attachment, emotion socialization by parents, parents' own mental health, and culture (Kiel & Kalomiris, 2019). With respect to attachment, infants who exhibit insecure–resistant responses in the Strange Situation procedure (i.e., infants who are distressed and resist comforting) were originally predicted to be at risk for development of anxiety (Cassidy & Berlin, 1994). However, results of two meta-analytic investigations (Groh, Roisman, van IJzendoorn, Bakermans-Kranenburg, & Fearon, 2012; Madigan, Atkinson, Laurin, & Benoit, 2013) showed that avoidant attachment—rather than resistant attachment— is associated with higher levels of internalizing symptoms (including anxiety). Still, these analyses suggest that insecure attachment in some form may be an indicator of increased risk for anxiety during childhood.

With respect to parental socialization, a meta-analysis conducted by Pinquart (2017) found that internalizing problems in children and adolescents were associated with both authoritarian parenting (as described in Chapter 5) and psychological control (i.e., control via emotional manipulation, including love withdrawal, guilt, criticism, and shaming; Barber, 1996). Overcontrol in any form has been consistently linked to higher levels of internalizing problems (e.g., Edwards, Rapee, & Kennedy, 2010; Möller,

Nikolić, Majdandžić, & Bögels, 2016). Possibly parental overcontrol reflects anxiety on the part of parents themselves, and this anxiety is communicated to their children. In addition, by constraining their child's behaviors, such parents may interfere with the development of emotion regulation skills, particularly for children with BI (Lewis-Morrarty et al., 2012).

Regarding supportive parenting, Hurrell, Houwing, and Hudson (2017) reported that parents of children with anxiety engaged in less positive emotion socialization than did parents of children without anxiety. However, other studies have suggested a more complex relationship between child anxiety and behaviors generally thought to exemplify supportive or nonsupportive parenting. For example, Viana, Dixon, Stevens, and Ebesutani (2016) found several surprising relationships between children's anxiety, their bias toward interpreting events as threatening, and how their mothers responded to their negative emotions. In particular, for children with less of a negative bias, maternal minimization or punishment of their negative emotion was associated with greater anxiety. However, for children with greater negative bias, maternal minimization or punishment was related to less anxiety. Seeking to interpret these results, the investigators suggested that mothers' nonsupportive responses to the negative emotions of anxiety-prone children might serve as a reality check that could be helpful if experienced in the context of a generally heathy parent–child relationship. In any event, Viana et al.'s (2016) counterintuitive findings suggest that exploring children's interpretations (i.e., appraisals) of their parents' socialization behaviors would be instructive.

As described in Chapter 3, exposing children to emotional experiences also is considered a socialization behavior within Eisenberg's model (Eisenberg, Cumberland, & Spinrad, 1998; Eisenberg, Spinrad, & Cumberland, 1998). Allowing a child to be frequently exposed to high levels of interparental conflict would be considered an example of this type of behavior. According to a model developed by Cummings and his colleagues (e.g., Cummings & Davies, 1996; Davies & Cummings, 1994; Cummings & Miller-Graff, 2015), exposure to interparental conflict is a particularly important experience influencing children's overall emotional security, which in turn is related to adjustment problems. That is, while almost all parents argue without causing their children long-term emotional harm, excessive levels of conflict can be deleterious. At the same time, the influence of interparental conflict on emotional security is itself dependent upon several factors, including: (1) the child's initial emotional response to the conflict, (2) the child's evaluation of its potential impact on family relations, and (3) the appropriateness of the child's behavioral response to the conflict. For example, if the child becomes very upset, worries that her parents will divorce, and feels a responsibility to prevent this, then emotional damage may be incurred. Note that two of these factors involve the child's appraisal of the parental conflict he or she observes. In an investigation of 11- to 12-year-old children's responses to marital conflict, Harold, Shelton, Goeke-Morey, and Cummings (2004) found support for their model. All three factors were significantly related to an overall measure of the child's emotional security about parenting, which in turn was significantly related to both internalizing and externalizing problems. Consistent with the rationale underlying NIMH's RDoC framework, these findings also illustrate the frequent comorbidity of internalizing and externalizing problems.

Do Individuals with Anxiety Show Atypical Neurobiological Activity?

Given its role in detecting emotionally significant stimuli, it is not surprising to find that the amygdala plays an important role in anxiety, a disorder that is characterized by hypervigilance to environmental cues (Shackman & Fox, 2016). In an illustrative study, Fitzgerald et al. (2017) showed neutral and negative pictures to adult participants with and without anxiety in three conditions: (1) a baseline condition in which participants looked at neutral images, (2) a negative reactivity condition in which participants looked at negative images, and (3) a reappraisal condition in which participants were told to reappraise the negative images. Before the start of the procedures, participants were given training on reappraisal (i.e., thinking about the images in a way that reduced their negative emotional impact). Results showed that participants with anxiety reported more negative affect than did healthy controls when viewing the negative images in both the reactivity and the reappraisal conditions. Participants with anxiety also showed more amygdala reactivity than participants without anxiety in the reactivity condition, but no differences were found in the reappraisal condition. The authors interpreted their results as demonstrating that individuals with anxiety are more reactive than individuals without anxiety, as indicated by their higher negative affect ratings and greater amygdala activation in the reactivity condition. Results for amygdala activity in the reappraisal condition were more difficult to explain. Other studies have identified areas in the PFC that were found to be more active in participants without anxiety in comparison with participants with anxiety during reappraisal (Ball, Ramsawh, Campbell-Sills, Paulus, & Stein, 2013; Blair et al., 2012). However, the specific prefrontal areas identified in different studies do not always coincide.

Because identifying biomarkers specific to anxiety would be valuable, a task force of experts from the World Federation of Societies for Biological Psychiatry (Bandelow et al., 2016) reviewed and summarized the relevant neuroimaging literature. Unfortunately, the task force concluded that "despite a plethora of high-quality publications in the field, imaging research has not yet succeeded in reliably identifying neuroanatomical, functional or metabolic alterations, which have been unequivocally associated with . . . anxiety disorders" (p. 348). Still, the authors maintained optimism that further high-quality research will eventually produce a clearer picture of the neural correlates of anxiety.

A similar conclusion regarding HPA functioning was reached in a subsequent report by the same task force (Bandelow et al., 2017). Mixed results were obtained in studies examining baseline cortisol levels, as well as responses to stressors by participants diagnosed with general anxiety disorder. Still, a plausible pattern of findings has been obtained in some studies. For example, Dieleman et al. (2015) reported low levels of basal cortisol (i.e., cortisol measured during a baseline period preceding an experimental task), low pretask parasympathetic nervous system (PNS) activity, and high task-related SNS reactivity in 8- to 12-year-old children with anxiety disorders, a pattern also characteristic of responses to chronic stress. Still, in the face of other investigations with contradictory findings, further research is needed to clarify the picture of HPA functioning in the context of anxiety.

With respect to ANS functioning, some consistent results appear to have been obtained. In a meta-analytic investigation, Chalmers, Quintana, Abbott, and Kemp (2014) found that anxiety was associated with lower levels of heart rate variability. This conclusion held for several anxiety disorders considered as a single group and several of the disorders analyzed separately (i.e., general anxiety disorder, panic disorder, PTSD, and social anxiety disorder). Heart rate variability is a well-recognized measure of healthy ANS functioning that appears to be disrupted in individuals with anxiety.

DEPRESSION

Depression is a growing problem worldwide (Liu et al., 2020). In the United States, a large-scale epidemiological study found significant increases in depression between 2005 and 2015 for both men and women, particularly in the younger (12–25 years) and oldest (50 years and older) age groups (Weinberger et al., 2018). Although several subtypes of depression are described in DSM-5, they all include sad, empty, and/or irritable moods.

Can Temperament Contribute to Depression?

High levels of negative emotionality, low positive emotionality, and low effortful control (EC) have all been related to depressive symptomology (e.g., Dougherty, Klein, Durbin, Hayden, & Olino, 2010; Khazanov & Ruscio, 2016; Rudolph, Davis, & Monti, 2017). Of particular interest, several studies have found three-way interactions among these dimensions such that favorable levels for two of the three mitigates the risk associated with an unfavorable level of the third. For example, high levels of positive emotionality and EC have been found to protect against the increased risk of depression associated with high levels of negative emotionality in children and young adolescents (Van Beveren, Mezulis, Wante, & Braet, 2019), as well as in college students (Vasey et al., 2014).

Several models have described interactions between temperamental variables and environmental risk factors in the development of depressive symptoms (see review in Palmer, Lakhan-Pal, & Cicchetti, 2019). Two models currently receiving considerable scholarly attention are the diathesis-stress (i.e., vulnerability) model and the differential susceptibility model. Both posit that temperamental factors (in particular, negative emotionality) will exacerbate the effects of stress and/or poor parenting on the development of depression. In their narrative review of the literature, Compas, Connor-Smith, and Jaser (2004) offered support for this general proposition while not attempting to adjudicate between the different models.

Problems with Emotion Regulation

Researchers' attention also has turned to the study of emotion regulation difficulties associated with depression. For example, Gonçalves and colleagues (2019) conducted an investigation in which adolescents reported for 2 consecutive years on their depressive symptoms (e.g., feelings of sadness) and their self-perceived problems with emotion regulation (e.g., feelings of guilt and loss of control when they get upset). Emotion regulation difficulties reported in the 1st year were associated with depressive symptoms in both the 1st and 2nd years.

Other studies have focused on specific emotion regulation strategies. For example, D'Avanzato, Joormann, Siemer, and Gotlib (2013) investigated use of expressive suppression, cognitive reappraisal, and negative rumination by adults diagnosed with depression or social anxiety disorder in comparison with individuals without disorders. Individuals with depression or anxiety both reported using suppression and rumination more often and using cognitive reappraisal less often than the control participants. Comparing across disorders, participants with depression used rumination more often than participants with anxiety, who in turn used suppression and reappraisal more often than participants with depression. These findings are consistent with those of several meta-analyses of research with adults (Dryman & Heimberg, 2018; Liu & Thompson, 2017; Visted, Vøllestad, Nielsen, & Schanche, 2018). Across studies, adults with depression were found to use rumination and suppression more often than adults without depression and to use reappraisal less often. Additionally, individuals with depression were found to be less accepting of their own emotions.

In a meta-analysis involving children and adolescents (5–19 years), Compas et al. (2017) examined several specific strategies for emotion regulation and coping in relation to both internalizing and externalizing symptoms. Strategies included problem solving, cognitive reappraisal, acceptance, distraction, avoidance, and denial. Results showed that avoidance and denial were related to higher levels of internalizing for both children and adolescents, whereas suppression was related to internalizing only for adolescents. Avoidance was the only strategy related to externalizing symptoms. For those strategies considered to be adaptive (i.e., problem solving, cognitive reappraisal, acceptance), no significant association with either internalizing or externalizing symptoms was found. Using a somewhat different age group and set of inclusion criteria, Schäfer et al. (2017) conducted another meta-analytic investigation of adolescents' internalizing and externalizing symptoms in relation to their emotion regulation strategies. Replicating Compas et. al.'s (2017) findings, they examined avoidance, suppression, problem solving, reappraisal, and acceptance. In addition, they included rumination but did not include denial. Like Compas and colleagues (2017), Schäfer et al. (2017) reported that avoidance and suppression were significantly related to internalizing symptoms. However, in contrast to Compas et al. (2017), significant negative relationships were found between cognitive reappraisal, problem solving, and acceptance and both internalizing and externalizing symptoms. Thus there was disagreement between the two meta-analyses about the importance of adaptive regulation strategies for adolescents but general agreement regarding the negative impact of at least two strategies considered to be maladaptive.

Socialization Influences

Children's experiences with their parents can critically influence the development of depression. As part of his attachment theory, Bowlby (1980) posited that death or extended separation from a parent can lead to depression in infants and children. Other parenting variables can also be formative. For example, considerable literature has focused on the intergenerational transmission of depression, that is, the impact of parents' own depression on their children. To illustrate, Hammen and Brennan (2003) obtained measures of depressive symptoms in over 800 adolescents, along with information about their mothers' depression-related history. Data analyses showed that children of mothers with depression were twice as likely to develop clinically diagnosable depression as were children of mothers without depression. Exposure to just 1 month of major maternal depression or to 12 months of more minor depression resulted in an elevated risk for the children. However, not all studies have yielded such strong effects. In a meta-analysis that included 193 individual studies, Goodman and colleagues (2011) found only a small to medium effect size for the relationship between maternal depression and children's internalizing symptoms. Of additional interest, a similarly small to medium effect size was found for the relationship between maternal depression and externalizing symptoms.

Of course, children of parents without depression may also develop depression. Considerable literature based on Diana Baumrind's parenting typology (Baumrind, 1971) has shown that authoritarian parenting can lead to increased risk for depression (e.g., Lamborn, Mounts, Steinberg, & Dornbusch, 1991; Milevsky, Schlechter, Netter, & Keehn, 2007; Steinberg, Lamborn, Darling, Mounts, & Dornbusch, 1994). Psychological control also predicts increased depression and anxiety, particularly in adolescents (Rogers, Padilla-Walker, McLean, & Hurst, 2020). In a meta-analytic review, Yap, Pilkington, Ryan, and Jorm (2014) found that both forms of maladjustment were related to lack of parental warmth, more interparental conflict, parental overcontrol, and hostility. Depression was additionally associated with less autonomy granting, more authoritarian parenting, less monitoring, and more inconsistent discipline.

Do Children with Depression Show Atypical Neurobiological Activity?

Considerable research on the neurological underpinnings of depression has focused on emotion regulation. For example, Stephanou, Davey, Kerestes, Whittle, and Harrison (2017) studied brain activity in adolescents and young adults (15–25 years) with and without depression with a procedure similar to that used in Fitzgerald et al.'s (2017) study of anxiety as described above. Participants viewed neutral and negative emotion images in three conditions: (1) a baseline condition in which participants looked at neutral images, (2) a negative reactivity condition in which participants looked at negative images, and (3) a reappraisal condition in which participants were told to reappraise the negative images. As in Fitzgerald's study, participants were trained in how to use reappraisal. Results showed that participants with depression reported more negative affect than participants without depression only in the reappraisal condition. Correspondingly, group differences in neural responding were found in the reappraisal condition, including greater activation of both the amygdala and the ventromedial PFC (vmPFC) and less activation of the dorsal midline cortex in the group with depression. The investigators interpreted this pattern of neural responding as suggesting that individuals with depression react more strongly to the negative stimulus (as indicated by amygdala activation) but also become overly involved with considering its self-relevance (as indicated by vmPFC activation) at the expense of focusing on reinterpreting the meaning of the stimulus itself (as indicated by reduced activation of the dorsal midline cortical area). They note that their finding with respect to heightened amygdala activity in adolescents with depression is consistent with the findings of other studies in the adult literature.

In a narrative review of the adult literature, Park and colleagues (2019) identified multiple brain structures implicated in emotion regulation and summarized research showing differences between individuals with and without depression. These include increased amygdala reactivity in response to negative stimuli, increased reactivity in medial PFC (mPFC; associated with rumination), and increased activity in the dorsolateral PFC (dlPFC; associated with anticipation of negative stimuli) in individuals with depression. In addition, they reported atypical ventrolateral PFC (vlPFC) functioning. In individuals without depression, activation of the vlPFC generates activation of the vmPFC, which in turn results in decreased amygdala activity and increased nucleus accumbens (NAcc) activity (associated with experiencing pleasure and reward). In individuals with depression, vmPFC activation is instead associated with increased amygdala and decreased NAcc activity.

Fewer studies have investigated the ANS functioning of individuals with depression. As described in Chapter 2, low baseline levels of RSA and high RSA reactivity are generally considered indices of poor emotion regulation. In a narrative review of the extant literature for children and adults, Beauchaine (2001) reported that individuals with depression or anxiety both show lower baseline RSA and higher RSA reactivity than individuals without disorders. Consistent with these findings, Shannon, Beauchaine, Brenner, Neuhaus, and Gatzke-Kopp (2007) showed that 8- to 12-year-old children at risk for depression generated higher RSA reactivity during a laboratory task in which they were presented with a series of numbers on a computer screen and asked to press the corresponding key on the keyboard. In a rare study that included assessment of both ANS and HPA activity, El-Sheikh, Erath, Buckhalt, Granger, and Mize (2008) found that 8- to 9-year-old children with both high baseline cortisol levels and high SNS reactivity to stressful laboratory tasks showed more internalizing and externalizing symptoms than children with lower basal cortisol and SNS reactivity. Consistent with these findings, El-Sheikh, Arsiwalla, Hinnant, and Erath (2011) later showed that internalizing symptoms were associated with higher basal cortisol when accompanied by lower basal RSA (i.e., indicating less PNS control over SNS reactivity).

Focusing on the HPA system, adults diagnosed with depression show greater reactivity to stressors and a flatter diurnal trajectory when compared with individuals without depression (Gunnar, Doom, & Esposito, 2015; Palmer et al., 2019). With respect to children and adolescents, Lopez-Duran, Kovacs, and George (2009) conducted a meta-analysis of studies comparing HPA functioning between those diagnosed with major depressive disorder (MDD) and a set of controls without depression. One interesting analysis focused on studies that used a **dexamethasone suppression test** (DST). Dexamethasone is a form of synthetic cortisol, and its administration normally suppresses cortisol production via the negative feedback loop within the HPA system. Results showed that suppression was significantly reduced in participants with depression, indicating disruption of the normal feedback system and resulting in higher cortisol levels. Baseline levels of cortisol also were significantly higher for the children and adolescents with depression (although the effect size was small). Age did not moderate either relationship. These analyses illustrate the presence of hyperactivity in the HPA systems of adolescents and children, as well as adults, with depression.

DISRUPTIVE, AGGRESSIVE, AND ANTISOCIAL BEHAVIOR

DSM-5 (American Psychiatric Association, 2013) describes a number of disorders that involve disruptive, impulsive, and conduct-disordered behaviors, including aggression and antisocial activity (e.g., rule breaking, delinquency, violation of social norms, laws, and the rights of others). Among these are two disorders that have been well-studied in children: **oppositional defiant disorder (ODD)** and **conduct disorder (CD)**. Both have emotion-related components. ODD is characterized by angry/irritable mood, argumentative/defiant behavior, and vindictiveness—but not aggressive behavior. CD is characterized by aggression, destruction of property, theft, and truancy and may also be characterized by **callous unemotionality (CU)**, that is, disregard for others' feelings, shallow or lack of affect, and lack of remorse or guilt. To illustrate the difference between them, a child with ODD might throw a temper tantrum when a peer refuses to share his toy, whereas a child with CD/CU might dispassionately knock the other child down and steal the desired object. Both disorders fall into the transdiagnostic category of externalizing behaviors.

Temperament and Emotion Regulation

As might be expected given its diagnostic criteria, ODD has been associated with temperament and personality measures of negative affect. For example, Zastrow, Martel, and Widiger (2018) observed such a relationship in their study of 3- to 6-year-old children with or without symptoms of ODD as reported by their parents. Temperament was also assessed via parent report using Putnam and Rothbart's (2006) Children's Behavior Questionnaire (CBQ). In addition, the children participated in laboratory procedures taken from the Laboratory Temperament Assessment Battery (Lab-TAB; Goldsmith et al., 1999) that are designed to evoke frustration (i.e., instructions to draw an impossibly perfect circle), EC (i.e., a delay of gratification task), and exuberance (i.e., playtime with bubbles). An experimenter observed and interacted with the children during the laboratory procedures and subsequently rated them on several characteristics related to the personality dimensions of Agreeableness, Neuroticism, Extraversion, and Conscientiousness. Results showed that negative affect scores on the CBQ temperament measure were associated with three key manifestations of ODD (i.e., angry/irritable mood, argumentative/defiant behavior, and vindictiveness). Agreeableness was negatively related to angry/irritable mood, whereas surgency (a construct that includes approach motivation, high activity level, and positive affect) was positively related to argumentative/defiant behavior and vindictiveness. Exuberance during the bubble procedure also was associated with argumentative/defiant behavior. In a study of even younger children (18–35 months), Sánchez-Pérez, Putnam, Gartstein, and González-Salinas (2020) found that high levels of negative emotionality and low levels of inhibitory control and soothability were related to higher levels of ODD symptoms.

Better emotion regulation has been associated with lower levels of externalizing problems. This is not surprising in light of the methodology often used to measure emotion regulation. For example, Cavanagh, Quinn, Duncan, Graham, and Balbuena (2017) analyzed data from 5- to 17-year-old children whose parents or teachers completed the SNAP-IV, a DSM-based 90-item questionnaire designed to assess symptoms of ODD, CD, and other disorders. The measure also includes an emotion dysregulation scale with items that inquire about quarrelsomeness and defiance, as well as mood lability, irritability, and frustration. Using factor analysis, the investigators found that the 10 emotion dysregulation items grouped together with ODD items but were not associated with the CD items. Interestingly, many of the dysregulation items (e.g., irritability) may reflect emotional reactivity as much as emotion regulation. That is, it is unclear whether the items reflect the child's failure to attempt emotion regulation or failure of the attempt that he has made. Laboratory studies that assess emotion reactivity and regulation separately (e.g., Fitzgerald et al., 2017) would help to clarify this issue.

Callous Unemotionality (CU)

Callous lack of empathy characterizes individuals in one subtype of CD. Also known as callous unemotionality (CU), this characteristic is receiving increasing research attention. According to DSM-5 (American Psychiatric Association, 2013), individuals with CU are unconcerned about the feelings of others, are cold and uncaring, and are mostly concerned with how their actions affect themselves, even when they cause substantial harm to other persons. Given this conceptualization, it is not surprising to find that a meta-analysis by Waller and colleagues (2020) reported children with higher scores on measures of CU to also score lower on measures of empathy, guilt, and prosocial behavior than children with lower scores on CU measures.

Greater callous unemotionality is related to higher levels of conduct problems, even at a very early age. For example, Ezpeleta, Granero, de la Osa, and Domènech (2015) examined relations between 3-year-old children's scores on the Inventory of Callous–Unemotional Traits (Frick, 2004; Cardinale & Marsh, 2020) and several measures of social and psychological adjustment assessed 2 years later. Results showed that higher teacher ratings of CU at age 3 were related to higher parent ratings of externalizing and internalizing behaviors at age 5, to higher teacher ratings on measures of aggression, and to more mother-reported ODD-related symptoms. These results are consistent with those of Longman, Hawes, and Kohlhoff's (2016) meta-analysis of studies involving children younger than 5 years. These investigators found significant associations between CU and children's conduct problems. Of relevance to the issue of common method variance (discussed further in Chapter 9), effect sizes were greater when ratings of both variables were provided by the same informant (either teachers or parents) as opposed to different informants (teachers vs. parents). Whereas the effect size for same-informant ratings was medium to large, the effect size for different informant ratings was small to medium. Still, both methods provided evidence for a statistically significant relationship.

Socialization Influences

For over 50 years, Gerald Patterson and his colleagues investigated the development of aggressive and antisocial behavior in children and adolescents. Based on extensive and detailed observations in the home and at schools, Patterson (1982) early on described a process through which young children's aggression is socialized within the context of family interactions and then carried into school settings, where it is amplified in the context of peer interactions. The process begins when caregivers respond inappropriately to children's difficult behaviors, that is, with anger and hostility rather than calm and measured discipline. Children may then reciprocally respond to parent negativity with anger and hostility of their own. This escalates in a coercive cycle of reciprocal negativity that increases in intensity until one member of the pair backs down—thus reinforcing the other person's most recent negative behavior. For example, when a parent comments negatively about a young adolescent's choice of TV programs, the adolescent might respond with disrespectful language; this may in turn provoke the parent to threaten discipline that in turn provokes increased defiance on the part of the adolescent. In this way, the family serves as a training ground for aggression in children who then take the pattern of behavior they have learned with them to school (Ramsey, Patterson, & Walker, 1990). At school, the aggressive child may gravitate to peers who engage in similar behavior patterns. Now through a pattern of mutual reinforcement within the deviant peer group, the child's repertoire of antisocial behaviors expands and may reach levels that eventually incur a clinical diagnosis.

Results consistent with this description, as well as other elements of Patterson's model, have been obtained in many studies (e.g., Smith et al., 2014; Snyder, Cramer, Afrank, & Patterson, 2005). For example, Wakschlag and Keenan (2001) found that parenting stress and harsh behaviors, as well as low infant soothability, predicted the development of high levels of disruptive behavior in preschool children. Mence et al. (2014) found that parents' anger appraisal bias (i.e., tendency to interpret their toddlers' distress as anger), along with parents' tendency to become overwhelmed by their own emotions, also predicted harsh and overreactive discipline. With respect to emotion-related behaviors, Duncombe, Havighurst, Holland, and Frankling (2012) reported that parental negative emotional expressivity, as well as inconsistent discipline, predicted disruptive behavior problems in 5- to 9-year-old children. On the positive side, Dunsmore, Booker, and Ollendick (2013) found that supportive parenting (in this case, maternal emotion coaching, as described in Chapter 3) can mitigate the development of externalizing behaviors in emotionally labile 7- to 14-year-old children and adolescents.

Less research has been reported on relations between parenting and children's CU. However, some evidence for reciprocal influence has emerged. For example, Flom, White, Ganiban, and Saudino (2020) studied pairs of monozygotic and dizygotic twins at 2 and 3 years of age and found that CU at age 2 predicted increasingly negative parenting at age 3. At the same time, Kochanska, Kim, Boldt, and Yoon (2013) found that responsive parenting of 3-year-old children with high levels of CU resulted in decreasing levels of externalizing symptoms between 5 and 9 years. These findings suggest that children will benefit if parents can be helped to maintain optimal caring and disciplinary practices in the face of challenging child behavior.

Do Children with ODD/CD Show Atypical Neurobiological Activity?

Multiple studies have been reported in recent decades that involved neuro-imaging of children and adolescents with ODD and/or CD. Noordermeer, Luman, and Oosterlaan (2016) conducted a meta-analysis of investigations in which such participants engaged in procedures to evaluate their "hot" executive functioning, including emotion recognition, reward learning, and affective decision making. Results showed that amygdala activity was reduced in children and adolescents with ODD/CD when compared with controls without disorders. More recently, von Polier et al. (2020) conducted a neuroimaging study involving boys with CD who were instructed to empathize with persons shown in images they viewed while in the scanner. In addition, the boys completed a questionnaire measure assessing their empathic tendencies, and their parents completed a measure of their sons' CU traits. Results showed that boys with CD scored lower on empathy and higher on CU than boys without CD. Additionally, among both boys with CD and boys without CD, those who were rated higher on CU showed less amygdala activity. Together, these studies are consistent with the portrayal of CD as an antisocial category that does not involve emotional overreactivity but rather a lower level of emotional responsiveness, particularly when CD is accompanied by CU.

As noted earlier in this chapter, low resting RSA and high RSA reactivity have been proposed as transdiagnostic markers of psychopathology due to their association with poor emotion regulation (Beauchaine, 2015; Hinnant & El-Sheikh, 2009). However, relatively few studies have investigated relations between RSA and children's externalizing behavior problems. In one such investigation, Zhang, Fagan, and Gao (2017) measured RSA in 7- to 11-year-old children during a task in which emotion was evoked by having them watch a set of positive and negative film episodes. Parents completed the CBCL to provide measures of the children's externalizing and internalizing symptoms and also completed a measure of family adversity with items inquiring about divorce, criminality, illness, income, and so forth. CBCL data were also collected 1 year later. Data analyses showed that lower resting RSA at the initial session was related to increases in both externalizing and internalizing symptoms over the course of the following year for boys living in high-adversity families. Findings were stronger for externalizing than for internalizing behaviors. No significant results were found for girls nor for measures of RSA reactivity for either gender. Thus findings from this study were only partially consistent with the proposed relationship between RSA and psychopathology, including externalizing behaviors.

Externalizing and internalizing behaviors are conceptually related to different negative emotions (i.e., anger vs. fear or sadness), yet almost no research distinguishes among them. An exception is a study of 7- to 11-year-old children by Quiñones-Camacho and Davis (2018) in which regulation strategies associated with anger, fear, and sadness were investigated and resting RSA was measured. To assess their regulation strategies, children were interviewed and asked to describe a recent event that had made them angry, afraid, or sad. They were then asked to describe anything they had done to make themselves feel less bad. Responses were categorized into seven groups: problem solving, changing thoughts, changing goals, changing physiology, social support, religious activity, and acceptance, that is, "experiencing the emotion without trying to change it." Parents completed measures of the child's externalizing symptoms, depression, and anxiety-related symptoms. Data analyses showed that low resting RSA was related to externalizing symptoms but only for younger children. High resting RSA was significantly related to lower levels of anxiety but only for older children who reported larger strategy repertoires for dealing with fear. Thus further research is necessary to produce a coherent picture of relations between the RSA, regulation of specific emotions, and both externalizing and internalizing behaviors.

Early studies of HPA functioning in children and adolescents with antisocial behaviors suggested a relationship between low cortisol reactivity and externalizing behaviors (e.g., van Goozen, Fairchild, Snoek, & Harold, 2007). However, meta-analyses have yielded a more complex picture. For example, Alink and colleagues (2008) reported that externalizing behavior was significantly associated with lower basal (i.e., pretask baseline) cortisol in school-age children but higher basal cortisol levels in preschoolers and was not significantly related to basal cortisol in adolescents. In addition, no significant associations between cortisol reactivity and externalizing behavior were found in any age group. Similarly, little consistency in relations between externalizing behaviors and cortisol reactivity was reported in a more recent narrative review of studies with children and adolescents (Figueiredo et al., 2020).

In interpreting their mostly negative findings, both sets of investigators emphasized the potential influence of many moderating factors. These include type of antisocial or externalizing behavior (e.g., reactive aggression, proactive aggression, theft), comorbidity (e.g., co-occurrence with internalizing disorders), type of stressor used in reactivity studies (e.g., social evaluations, cognitive challenges), type of environmental stressors encountered in daily life (e.g., poverty, exposure to violence), measurement differences (e.g., parent report vs. observational measures of behavior, timing of cortisol assessment), gender, and age. These have proved difficult to disentangle from one another, perhaps resulting in failure to find consistent moderating effects for most of these variables. Still, as described above, Alink et al. (2008) did find significant relations between externalizing behaviors and basal cortisol levels that differed across age. Although the authors proposed several possible interpretations of these findings, one possibility can be offered that would be consistent with proposals about the effects of short-term versus long-term stress on HPA functioning. As previously noted, short-term stress is thought to generate hyperactivity of the HPA system, whereas persistent stress may lead to "burnout," that is, hypoactivity. Thus, if chronic stress contributes to externalizing behaviors in children, one might see a positive relationship between cortisol and aggression early on but a negative relationship at older ages.

Problems in Emotion Understanding

CU, ODD, and CD all have been related to deficits in emotion understanding. In their narrative review of the existing literature, Frick and White (2008) concluded that CU was related to impaired recognition of negative emotional expressions and less physiological reactivity to cues of distress in children and adolescents irrespective of whether or not they showed ODD or CD symptoms (see also Hartmann & Schwenck, 2020). In a study of 4- to 8-year-old children with ODD, O'Kearney, Salmon, Liwag, Fortune, & Dawel (2017) found that those with higher CU scores were less able to understand others' mixed emotion responses to an emotion-evoking event (e.g., learning to ride a bike) and were less able to accurately discern others' emotional reactions to a situation when those reactions differed from their own. Irrespective of their level of CU, boys with ODD also were less able to generate plausible causes for different emotional responses (i.e., happiness, sadness, anger, and fear) than those without ODD.

CULTURE AND PSYCHOPATHOLOGY

If cultures are conceptualized groups of people who share values, attitudes, and behaviors, then socioeconomics can create cultural differences within as well as across national boundaries. Within the United States, socioeconomically distinct neighborhoods may create different environments with corresponding differences in the adaptive value of particular personality and behavioral characteristics. As noted earlier, a well-known example involves aggression and neighborhood violence, whereby aggressive behaviors may be advantageous in a high-violence neighborhood but maladaptive elsewhere. At the same time, some behaviors (e.g., anxious behavior) may be maladaptive in almost all environmental contexts.

Clinical Treatment

DSM-5 (American Psychiatric Association, 2013) recognizes the importance of cultural considerations in the diagnosis and treatment of psychopathology. Clinicians are encouraged to assess cultural features that may affect patients' experience and behavior. Cultural factors affecting specific diagnoses also are described (albeit briefly). For example, the manual recognizes that individuals from different backgrounds may present their depression or anxiety in different ways (e.g., in terms of subjective feelings or somatic symptoms). Also acknowledged is the fact that behaviors that are considered symptoms of conduct disorder may be "near-normative" (p. 474) in high-risk environments. Many of these points are grounded in empirical research that stands at the intersection of culture, emotion, and psychopathology.

Exemplifying such research, studies of individuals with depression have found cultural differences in their emotional reactivity. To illustrate, Chentsova-Dutton and colleagues (2007) found that European Americans with depression reacted with decreased affect (i.e., less crying and less reported feelings of sadness) in comparison with individuals without depression when viewing a sad film. In contrast, Asian Americans with depression showed more crying than Asian American participants without depression and tended to report more sadness. These results are consistent with the authors' *cultural norm hypothesis*, which predicts that "depression reduces individuals' abilities to react in culturally ideal ways" (Chentsova-Dutton, Tsai, & Gotlib, 2010, p. 284).

Cultural differences between client and clinician may influence their relationship with each other. For example, as previously noted, Chinese Americans prefer lower intensities of positive affect than do European Americans (Tsai et al., 2006). Apropos of their interactions with health professionals, Sims and colleagues (2018) found that Chinese Americans and Hong Kong Chinese prefer physicians who are less emotionally expressive, whereas European Americans prefer those who are more emotionally expressive. Presumably these emotion-related differences could generalize to interactions with mental health care professionals as well.

Changing Cultural Norms and Behaviors

Cultural influences on social and emotional adjustment may also differ across historical time. One well-known example of this comes from Xinyin Chen's ongoing research on BI and shyness in mainland Chinese children (see Chen, 2019). In their analysis of data collected in 1990, Chen, Rubin, and Li (1995) found that 8- to 12-year-old shy children were considered well adjusted and were well liked by teachers and peers. However, as China moved to create a more capitalist economy, values with respect to children's personality and behaviors also changed. Thus, in recent decades, shy or inhibited children are less successful and experience more peer rejection and depression (Chen, Cen, Li, & He, 2005). Put more generally, cultural differences in the valuing of particular behaviors or dispositional characteristics will engender differences in their functional consequences and thus their relations to both social and personal adjustment.

A second example of historical change within and across cultures is the emergence in recent decades of a form of maladjustment known as **hikikomori** (Martinotti et al., 2020). Originally diagnosed in Japanese adolescents, hikikomori is a condition of severe social withdrawal in which sufferers may isolate themselves in their bedrooms for months at a time, often engaging in relentless Internet use. It often (although not always) includes clinical symptoms of anxiety (Malagón-Amor et al., 2018). Hikikomori was originally viewed as a culturally specific syndrome related to social and economic changes in Japan that created stress due (in part) to diminishing opportunities for job security that had traditionally been characteristic of employment in Japan (Norasakkunkit & Uchida, 2014). However, studies of youth have now identified behavioral syndromes roughly equivalent to hikikomori in a number of Asian and non-Asian countries, including Nigeria, Singapore, and the United States (Bowker et al., 2019). Consequently, the underlying causes of this syndrome are now in dispute, and its past and current prevalence are unknown (Li & Wong, 2015; Wu, Ooi, Wong, Catmur, & Lau, 2019). However, hikikomori's apparent emergence in modern times and current global reach exemplify the importance of considering historical as well as cultural factors when assessing an individual's social and emotional adjustment.

Are All Western Cultures the Same?

Most research in psychology is conducted under the assumption that all European countries share the same cultural orientation. However, an interesting study by Potthoff and colleagues (2016) suggests that this may not be the case with respect to emotion regulation. In an investigation of six European nations, Potthoff and colleagues (2016) found cultural differences in preferences for some specific regulation strategies. For example, participants from Spain, Italy, Portugal, and Hungary reported greater use of rumination and catastrophizing than participants from Germany and the Netherlands. However, the relationship between strategy use and participants' reports of depressive and anxiety symptoms was similar across cultural groups. Consistent relations between use of expressive suppression and depressive symptomology were also found by Mahali, Beshai, Feeney, and Mishra (2020) in a study of participants from four continents: North America, South America, Europe, and Asia. These findings suggest that some emotion-oriented intervention efforts may have value in a wide range of cultures. Still, the possibility of significant cultural differences in the value of certain regulation strategies should not be ignored. For example, as reported in Chapter 5, suppression has not been associated with poor adjustment in Hong Kong

Chinese individuals, an Asian culture that was not included in Malhali et al.'s (2020) study.

INTERVENTION PROGRAMS

Parenting Programs

Studies that show variability in parenting related to maladaptive child outcomes suggest the potential value of programs supporting the development of positive parenting skills. Although they may be embedded in somewhat different frameworks, developing a positive parent–child relationship and effective parenting skills are the goals of virtually all such intervention programs.

One example of a highly regarded parenting program is **Parent–Child Interaction Therapy (PCIT)** developed by Sheila Eyberg and her colleagues (Brinkmeyer & Eyberg, 2003) and designed for families having 2- to 7-year-old children with disruptive behavior problems. The program involves two phases, the first focusing on the development of an emotionally warm, positive relationship between parent and child and the second focusing on the development of effective behavior management skills. During the first phase, parents learn positive attention skills (e.g., demonstrating their attention to the child's nondisruptive behavior by describing and/or praising specific nondisruptive actions). In addition, they learn to ignore (i.e., not reinforce) the child's negative behaviors when this is feasible. During the second phase, parents learn effective discipline skills (e.g., giving clear instructions, praising compliance, using time-outs). During the training sessions, therapists explain the skills and coach the parents and children as they interact during practice episodes. Families also are also given brief homework assignments that involve practicing the skills at home.

Recently, several parenting programs have added optional components that target parents' and children's emotion functioning (England-Mason & Gonzalez, 2020). For example, PCIT-ED (Lenze, Pautsch, & Luby, 2011) adds eight sessions to the original PCIT program during which parents are trained to help preschool children identify, label, understand, and regulate their own emotions. Parents also explore their own feelings about the child and their own use of emotion regulation strategies. Consistent with current views of supportive parenting, parents are encouraged to allow children to express their emotions so that they may help the child learn to manage them. PCIT-ED is particularly designed to help alleviate child depression but might also enhance more general emotion functioning. In an initial small-scale study involving eight families who each had a preschool child diagnosed with depression, Lenze et al. (2011) found that the children's depressive symptoms decreased significantly over the course of treatment, and the effect size of the change was large. However, the children's performance on a facial expression recognition task—the study's only direct measure of their emotion processing—did not significantly improve. Still, in their narrative review of several emotion socialization interventions (including PCIT-ED), England-Mason and Gonzalez (2020) concluded that these programs appear promising but need further systematic evaluation.

Programs that have made efforts to measure treatment outcomes are considered to be **evidence-based**, and their effectiveness has been periodically evaluated. Using criteria developed by Chambless and Hollon (1998) based on an American Psychological Association Task Force report, Eyberg, Nelson, and Boggs (2008) identified a set of well-conducted evaluation studies that included features such as appropriate control or comparison conditions and random assignment. Depending on the number, quality, and results of their evaluation studies, programs could be designated as either well established, possibly efficacious, or probably efficacious. Although only one program was designated as well established (i.e., Parent Management Training—Oregon Model), PCIT met the criteria for probably efficacious, as did several other programs (e.g., Incredible Years Parent Training and Triple P: Positive Parenting Program).

Using a different approach, Mingebach, Kamp-Becker, Christiansen, and Weber (2018) conducted a meta-meta-analysis in which they combined results from several different meta-analytic evaluations of intervention programs for parents of children with externalizing behavior problems. Rather than seeking to rate the efficacy of individual programs, this study reported the overall effectiveness of all included programs considered as a single group. Results showed that parenting interventions overall had a moderately strong beneficial effect on various forms of child behavior, including prosocial behavior, other types of positive social behaviors, internalizing behaviors, and externalizing behaviors. Of particular value, the investigators also conducted separate analyses of studies in which the outcome measures involved parent reports versus objective observational data. For both types of measures, moderately strong significant effects were found.

Teacher-Oriented School-Based Programs

As noted earlier, children who develop disruptive behavior tendencies in the home will tend to carry those tendencies with them as they enter school.

Therefore, helping teachers manage such children within the classroom environment will benefit both the children themselves and the class as a whole. In addition, improving teachers' behavior management skills will reduce the likelihood that behavior problems will emerge in children who have not previously manifested such difficulties or whose behavior problems have not been previously recognized. Toward these goals, Karen Budd and her colleagues (Budd, Garbacz, & Carter, 2016; Gershenson, Lyon, & Budd, 2010) have developed a universal preventive intervention program based on PCIT but targeting classroom teachers (i.e., **Teacher–Child Interaction Training—Universal; TCIT-U**). One potential advantage of this universal approach is that it precludes the deviancy training effect that sometimes emerges when older children or adolescents with behavior problems are singled out and treated together in small groups (see Sawyer, Borduin, & Dopp, 2015, for a meta-analysis of such programs).

Like PCIT, TCIT-U emphasizes the development of teachers' positive attention skills and effective, consistent disciplinary skills. As in PCIT, one goal of the program is to enhance the positive emotional relationship between teachers and students. Teachers are trained in small groups, followed by individual coaching sessions that take place in the classroom, with further written feedback delivered after school. Teachers are also asked to practice skills in the classroom between coaching sessions. A climate of collaboration between teachers and researchers is emphasized. The effectiveness of TCIT-U has been recently evaluated in a pilot study that included two key components—random assignment of participating classrooms to either the intervention condition or a wait-list control condition and objective coding of videotaped samples of teachers' behaviors by coders who are blind to the teachers' status (Davidson et al., 2021). Results showed that the skills of TCIT-trained teachers (e.g., attending to and praising children's positive behaviors) increased over the course of the intervention in comparison with those of teachers in the control condition. In addition, teacher ratings indicated a small but significantly greater decrease in children's behavior problems in the intervention classrooms. Lastly, teacher satisfaction with the TCIT-U program was high.

Child-Oriented School-Based Programs

Several other universal prevention programs have been developed that target children's emotion-related knowledge and skills more directly. These **socio-emotional learning (SEL)** programs rest on evidence suggesting that competence in these areas is associated with more desirable social, behavioral, and academic outcomes (Domitrovich, Durlak, Staley, & Weissberg, 2017). Although several models of SEL have articulated specific components of socioemotional competence, Denham and Brown (2010) have perhaps most clearly distinguished between personal/prosocial skills and emotional skills. The latter include awareness of one's own emotions, managing one's emotions, understanding the emotions of others, and caring for others, whereas the former include cooperative behaviors and appropriate social decision making. These skills can develop spontaneously through dynamic interactions between children and their caregivers and peers. However, school-based universal SEL programs are designed to provide structured learning from which all children may benefit.

One widely used socioemotional learning program is **PATHS (Promoting Alternative Thinking Strategies;** Domitrovich, Greenberg, Cortes, & Kusche, 2004). PATHS is a teacher-delivered curriculum consisting of 44 core lessons that introduce the program's key concepts to children. These concepts fall within four domains: (1) self-control/emotion regulation, (2) attention, (3) communication, and (4) problem solving. Age-appropriate versions of the curriculum exist for preschool and elementary school students and include teaching emotion-related skills such as expression labeling and strategies for calming down. For preschool and kindergarten children, about 40% of the lessons involve understanding and communicating emotions. Teachers use a variety of materials to enable children to learn and practice various skills. For example, posters, storybooks, and stickers are used to teach children to "do turtle" (i.e., stop, breathe, say the problem, and tell how you feel). PATHS has been shown to increase kindergarten and elementary school children's social and emotional knowledge, reduce internalizing and externalizing behaviors, and increase emotion regulation and frustration tolerance (see Fishbein et al., 2016, for a brief review).

A second widely used SEL program is **RULER (Recognizing, Understanding, Labeling, Expressing, and Regulating emotion;** Hoffmann, Brackett, Bailey, & Willner, 2020). Developed at the Yale Center for Emotional Intelligence, RULER also aligns itself with Gross's process model of emotion and emotion regulation. At the same time, it shares many underlying principles, goals, and even some strategies with other SEL programs. For example, like PATHS, RULER emphasizes emotional awareness, labeling, and understanding as foundations for the development of emotion regulation skills. In addition, similar strategies for down-regulating emotions are recommended within the two programs (e.g., pausing to take a breath before deciding how to act). Each delineates a set of steps to take when a problematic emotion is activated. In RULER these are (1) identifying your feelings, (2) pausing to breathe, (3) considering your goals (i.e., imagining your best self), and (4) selecting and using an appropriate emotion regulation strategy. Several components of the RULER curriculum are designed to develop the skills necessary to engage in these steps. These include having students use a "mood meter" to identify their current emotion, after which they are encouraged to think about the cause of that emotion, whether they want to change the emotion, and if so, how to do it. Regulation strategies that fit within Gross's model (e.g., that involve situation selection, situation modification, attention deployment) are discussed. Students and teachers also discuss the meaning of words on the mood meter, recall times when they experienced one of the emotions, and have strategy sessions during which they discuss and role-play relevant emotion regulation strategies. As for PATHS, age-appropriate versions of the curriculum have been developed so that it may be used across a wide range of grades. In an evaluation study (Rivers, Brackett, Reyes, Elbertson, & Salovey, 2013), observer ratings of classrooms that had implemented RULER were higher for positive climate, emotional support from teachers, and teachers' regard for students' perspective when compared with similar classrooms that had not implemented the program. Additionally, RULER-trained teachers reported engaging in more emotion-focused interactions with students (e.g., acknowledging a student's improved behavior) and use of cooperative learning strategies (e.g., organized group activities for students) than did untrained teachers. Students in RULER classrooms rated their teachers higher in affiliation (e.g., respect for students), although the difference did not reach a conventional level of significance.

Overall Evaluation

Other school-based SEL programs (e.g., Positive Actions, Life Skills) have also yielded positive results. In a meta-analysis of 82 intervention studies evaluating a range of such programs, Taylor, Oberle, Durlak, and Weissberg (2017) found statistically significant benefits at follow-up (i.e., after 56 to 195 weeks) for (1) social and emotional skills (e.g., identifying emotions, perspective taking, self-control, interpersonal problem solving, conflict resolution, coping strategies, decision making), (2) attitudes toward self, others, and school (e.g., self-esteem, disapproval of violence and drugs, endorsing empathy), (3) positive social behaviors (e.g., teacher or student ratings of cooperation, helping others), (4) academic performance, (5) externalizing behaviors (e.g., aggression, bullying, disruptiveness), (6) internalizing symptoms (e.g., self-reported anxiety, depression, stress), and (7) self-reported drug use. However, effect sizes were minimal, that is, they exceeded 0.20 (the cutoff for a small effect) only for social and emotional skills and academic performance. Still, intervention researchers (including Taylor et al., 2017) have argued that even small effect sizes can translate into meaningful social and financial benefits for both those who respond to the program and society as a whole.

Age differences in the effectiveness of intervention programs were also reported in Taylor et al.'s (2017) study. When the investigators separately analyzed studies involving younger children (5–10 years), early adolescents (11–13 years), and older adolescents (14–18 years), effect sizes for younger children were found to be higher than those for the two older age groups. These findings suggest that early interventions are preferable to those that start later. However, some researchers have suggested ways of enhancing the effectiveness of programs targeting older children and adolescents. In particular, Yeager, Dahl, and Dweck (2018) have proposed modifications that better incorporate the adolescent's own perspective, that is, that implicitly acknowledge adolescents' age-typical goals of attaining social respect.

SUMMARY AND FINAL THOUGHTS

ACEs is a construct that covers a wide range of potentially damaging circumstances. Understanding individual differences in children's responses to adverse environments presents a challenge to researchers. Three models of environmental sensitivity have recently been proposed that may account for some differences: diathesis–stress, vantage sensitivity, and differential susceptibility. Negative emotionality during infancy may serve as a marker of differential susceptibility.

Maltreated children may become frustrated more easily than nonmaltreated children and use less adaptive emotion regulation strategies. Studies of their neural activity suggest greater amygdala reactivity that may require greater PFC activity to be successfully regulated. Maltreated children also show lower levels of SNS activation and lower cortisol responses to social stressors than nonmaltreated children. Maltreated children also are less able to identify emotional facial expressions than nonmaltreated children, and physically abused children have special difficulties with anger. Corresponding to their atypical experiences with others' anger, abused children appear biased to perceive it more often than other children in non-anger facial expressions and to expect anger to occur in a wider variety of situations.

Emotion plays a role in almost all forms of psychopathology. Rather than focusing on specific emotions, NIMH's RDoC framework recommends studying transdiagnostic constructs and processes such as deficits in emotional awareness and difficulties with emotion regulation. The hope is that this research-oriented framework will generate findings that are useful in designing treatments applicable to a range of disorders; however, it is not intended to replace current diagnostic practices.

Negative emotionality and BI have been associated with anxiety in children. Children with anxiety also have difficulties in many areas of emotion functioning, including emotional awareness, emotional expression, emotion regulation, and emotion understanding. Children with anxiety may have experienced insecure attachment and/or inappropriate parenting, including excessive control. Exposure to high levels of marital conflict can also result in emotional insecurity and lead to anxiety, as well as depression. Identifying biomarkers of anxiety has proved challenging, although some studies have shown greater amygdala activation and less PFC activation in individuals with anxiety compared with individuals without anxiety. In addition, some studies have shown low baseline cortisol levels and greater cortisol reactivity in participants with anxiety, whereas lower levels of heart rate variability have been found more consistently.

Depression can manifest itself in feelings of sadness, emptiness, or irritability. Temperamental contributors are high negative reactivity, low positivity, and low EC. Individuals with depression have been found to use more maladaptive emotion regulation strategies. Experiential contributors to depression are disrupted attachment (e.g., due to death of an attachment figure), maternal depression, and inappropriate parenting, including both authoritarian parenting and parenting characterized by psychological control. Although there is inconsistency across studies, a narrative review of neural activity in individuals with depression concluded that they show increased amygdala activity and increased activity in areas of the PFC associated with rumination and anticipation of negative stimuli. Individuals with depression also show higher daily cortisol levels, greater cortisol reactivity, and a pattern of RSA responses suggesting poorer emotion regulation.

ODD involves dispositional irritability that may first emerge in infancy or early childhood. The dysregulated emotional behavior seen in childhood and adolescence may reflect high levels of negative emotionality or emotion regulation difficulties or (most likely) both. One subtype of CD is characterized by CU. Children with higher levels of CU show lower levels of emotion understanding, less responsiveness to distress cues shown by other children, and less empathy, guilt, and prosocial behavior in comparison with children with lower levels of CU. Aggressiveness and antisocial behavior can develop within the context of family interactions that involve demonstrative modeling and reinforcement by parents. Other contributors are low soothability in infancy, parents' emotional reactivity, and family stress that can create parenting challenges. However, sensitive and responsive parenting can reduce levels of externalizing behaviors.

ODD/CD and CU have all been associated with reduced amygdala reactivity, including circumstances during which reactivity might be considered appropriate, for example, viewing empathy-evoking images. Low resting RSA may be related to poorer emotion regulation and higher levels of externalizing (as well as internalizing) psychopathology, but findings across studies are not consistent. Externalizing behaviors have been related to high levels of basal cortisol in preschoolers and low levels in school-age children and are unrelated to basal cortisol in adolescents. One possible interpretation of this pattern is that externalizing behavior is associated with chronic stress that may eventually result in hypocortisolism.

If psychopathology is conceptualized as maladjustment, then individuals' social and cultural context must be considered when determining whether their behavior is maladaptive. Emotional experiences and emotional problems may manifest themselves differently in persons from different cultural backgrounds. Behavioral tendencies may be related to adjustment difficulties in some cultures more than others, depending on whether they are more or less consistent with cultural norms or ideals. In addition, persons from different cultural backgrounds may have different emotional styles and preferences that can influence their interactions with each other, including interactions in health care and therapeutic settings. Although many studies focus on differences between Western and Asian cultures, substantial differences also may be seen among Western societies, for example, in their members' relative use of various emotion regulation strategies.

Some intervention programs have been developed to help parents and teachers more effectively manage children with behavior problems. For example, PCIT teaches parents specific strategies to deal with their child's disruptive behavior after an initial phase that focuses on developing a more emotionally positive relationship between parent and child. A recently developed version of the program includes sessions during which parents explore their own feelings toward the child and also are given lessons on how to increase their child's emotion understanding and emotion regulation capabilities. A universal version designed to help teachers manage student behavior in the classroom (i.e., TCIT-U) also has been developed.

Other universal intervention programs are designed to enhance the social and emotional development of all children and are also administered in a classroom setting. Two widely used programs of this type are PATHS and RULER. Both programs emphasize the development of the child's ability to recognize and understand both his or her own emotions and those of others. Additionally, emotion communication and regulation skills are taught. In point of fact, virtually all emotion-oriented intervention programs teach a similar set of emotion-related skills, though in somewhat different ways.

CHAPTER 9

Some Final Considerations

Writing a concise textbook on emotional development involves the enormous challenge of presenting a coherent picture of how development proceeds while simultaneously acknowledging the reality of mixed findings in many research areas. In the summary sections of each chapter, I have attempted to represent the current consensus regarding each topic under consideration. However, hints also are given that this consensus may change or that, more likely, it represents a somewhat oversimplified portrayal of development. Consider the reports of small effect sizes in virtually all of the many meta-analyses cited in this volume; these alone provide a strong clue that much remains to be learned about the topic under investigation. In some cases, moderator analyses have been helpful in enabling a better understanding of complex relations among the many factors influencing behavior and development. However, in many cases, these raise as many questions as they answer. On the positive side, such questions may spark some readers' particular interest, inspiring them to address one or more of these questions in their own future research.

In addition, readers may note that various topics of interest have received relatively little research attention thus far. Some of these are peer socialization of emotion, children's appraisals (i.e., interpretations) of potential emotion elicitors (e.g., fear elicitors), and paternal influences on emotional development. For example, peer behaviors that fall within Eisenberg's influential model of emotion socialization might be investigated. In addition, the importance of understanding emotional development within populations of particular interest (e.g., specific racial and ethnic groups, the LGBTQ community) is being increasingly recognized. Achieving this understanding will require greater research efforts.

Much contemporary research on emotion originated in cross-cultural studies that attempted to demonstrate the universality of emotional expressions and thus (presumably) the universal innateness of emotion itself. Although the universality of emotion itself appears undeniable, our conceptualization of its nature is evolving. Contemporary studies of cultural variation have raised questions about how best to conceptualize emotions themselves, for example, whether culture-specific emotions necessarily include one or more discrete biologically based (i.e., basic) emotions. Irrespective of these questions, these studies shed light on the socialization processes involved in emotional development. Lastly, they may challenge our assumptions about universally "healthy" emotional behaviors and encourage us to think about emotion as an adaptation to one's environmental circumstances.

One major question for future researchers to consider is whether they should focus on normative development or individual differences. Enthusiasm for producing a picture of normative development harks back to the halcyon days of Piaget's theory of universal cognitive stages. Those days are gone, having been replaced by an approach that focuses on processes rather than universal age-related cognitive competencies. With respect to emotional development, only a limited number of normative stage theories have been proposed, and most of these have focused on infancy. None have caught fire in the way that Piaget captured the hearts and minds of cognitive developmental researchers in the late 1960s. Furthermore, the feasibility of proposing normative stages for emotional development might be questionable because of the vast array of environmental influences that can create such variable outcomes. For Piaget, environmental experiences were also considered important for development, but those experiences were presumed to be universal because they were nonspecific (e.g., experiencing the opportunity to interact with objects of any sort). This may not be true for many aspects of emotional development.

Two alternatives to seeking normative developmental stages or milestones are represented in this book. One is to focus on processes, for example, the several forms of emotion socialization described in Chapter 3. The processes themselves need not be universal, and the researcher's goal would be to understand the circumstances under which they are employed and their associated developmental outcomes. In fact, many contemporary researchers take this approach, and their work is well represented herein (particularly in Chapters 2–6). The second alternative is to begin with a focus on outcomes, for example, higher or lower levels of internalizing or externalizing behaviors. In this case, the goal is to identify contributors to the outcomes of interest. This approach is particularly represented in Chapter 8. Adopting the second approach might be particularly appealing to those with clinical interests, whereas the first might be more appealing to those who take a more basic science approach to understanding emotional development. In either case, the challenge is the same, that is, how to understand the interactions among key processes or key contributors to particular outcomes. This will require both new models and new data. Furthermore, if new models are to be comprehensive (i.e., including a multiplicity of factors), they will require large amounts of data for effective evaluation. While there is ongoing progress in developing analytic methods appropriate for "big data," an additional challenge will be developing methods to collect big data of the kind needed to study emotional development.

Questionnaires constitute the most convenient means of collecting large amounts of data for easy analysis. As is true for any methodology, questionnaires have their advantages and disadvantages. These have been thoughtfully considered by some—but not all—researchers who have used them. For example, response biases of various types must be considered (e.g., memory biases, gender-labeling effects as described in Chapter 5). In addition, **common method variance** may be a concern if the same respondent completes measures of different variables whose relationship is being investigated (e.g., negative affect and externalizing behaviors both rated by the child's mother). At the same time, whether such method variance is a problem will depend upon the nature of the question being asked. For example, investigating relations between adolescents' perceptions of their parents' behavior and their self-perceived depressive symptoms may be just as valuable as investigating relations between more objective measures of parent behavior and adolescent self-reported depression. A third problem is that questionnaire measures cannot be used to study some phenomena, for example, spontaneous production of facial expressions. Behavioral observations are sometimes necessary.

Of course, behavioral observations also have significant limitations. Such observations typically involve only brief samples of behavior that may not be representative. Furthermore, behavioral observations can most conveniently be made in the context of laboratory procedures, and these may lack ecological validity. A third concern is that objectively coding behavioral data can be extremely labor intensive, and reliability among coders can be difficult to achieve. To address this problem, technologies for automatic behavioral coding are already available, although their current utility is limited (see Martinez, 2019). As an alternative to objective coding, obtaining emotion ratings from untrained observers may be a legitimate measurement strategy in some cases. For example, in studies of emotion communication, observer ratings may be preferred in light of growing recognition that emotional expression is multimodal and may not be fully captured by any existing objective coding system.

Studies using experience sampling methods (ESM) represent a laudable attempt to obtain ecologically valid measures of emotion functioning. However, they also have limitations. In particular, participants may be unable or unwilling to repeatedly interrupt their daily activities to complete a lengthy set of experimental measures. Therefore, very limited information has typically been gathered about the situational contexts surrounding participants' emotional responses.

Ideally, convergence is obtained between findings generated using ESM, questionnaires, and behavioral observations, thus engendering confidence in conclusions reached on the basis of any single type of study. However, in reality, only limited convergence is typically found. Although statistical methods have been developed to combine measures (e.g., modeling that involves the creation of latent variables), lack of strong convergence among measures may leave a lingering feeling of uncertainty and intellectual discomfort. Focusing on the larger picture, researchers often have given short shrift to this problem. However, a thoughtful consideration of differences among measures (i.e., attempts of reconcile them or to better understand their differences) would produce a more satisfactory understanding of the phenomenon they purport to measure. For example, future efforts to understand (and conceptually reconcile) differences between results from ESM and laboratory studies of emotion regulation would be of value. This may involve careful inspection of specific items in the measures that are employed.

Some readers of this book may be most interested in its relevance to clinical or community practice. Hopefully, these readers will find considerable material that can inform their work. Most obviously, the research on supportive and nonsupportive parenting, as well as the descriptions of current social and emotional intervention programs, will be particularly relevant. However, in a broader sense, this book is written under the assumption that having a general understanding of emotion and emotional development can aid in one's attempts to better address problems presented by clients and community members in ways that may not be immediately apparent. At the same time, as emphasized herein, our understanding of emotion and emotional development is evolving and at this time is still incomplete. Therefore, the material presented in this book must be considered in conjunction with training and experience that can only be provided in clinical, counseling, and community psychology programs. In the end, how much to rely on the theoretical versus practical components of one's education must be left to the judgment of the individual practitioner.

In conclusion, this book seeks to provide an introductory overview of a very extensive body of research that will continue to grow ever larger in future years. Although it may serve as an endpoint for some readers, I hope this book will inspire others to delve more deeply into the field of emotional development and possibly choose to contribute to increasing our knowledge and understanding thereof.

Glossary

Ability EI
: A conceptualization of emotional intelligence focusing on one's ability to perceive and reason about emotion apart from one's tendencies to act on such reasoning in a socially desirable manner. (Chapter 4)

Abuse
: With reference to childhood adversity, a category of maltreatment that may include harsh physical punishment, verbal threats, inappropriate sexual behaviors. (Chapter 7; Chapter 8)

Acceptingness
: A key feature of positive parenting conceptualized within infant attachment theory; defined as maintaining positive feelings about the infant while also realistically recognizing the challenges of parenting. (Chapter 2)

Accessibility
: A key feature of positive parenting conceptualized within infant attachment theory; defined as being continually aware of the infant's signals so as to enable appropriate responding. (Chapter 2)

Adverse childhood experiences (ACEs)
: Categories of childhood experiences thought to typically have detrimental effects on an individual's socioemotional adjustment both in childhood and beyond (e.g., maltreatment of the child, exposure to household violence). (Chapter 6; Chapter 8)

Affect
: Term used differently by different scholars to refer to a wide range of positive or negative feeling states that may include but also go beyond classic discrete emotions (e.g., afraid, inspired). (Chapter 1)

Affect balance score	Composite score designed to reflect the relative experience of positive versus negative affect (e.g., computed by subtracting the average rating across negative affect items from the average rating across positive affect items). (Chapter 6)
Affect programs	Conceptualized within classic discrete emotion theories as brain-based programs that generate a unique set of physiological, expressive, and phenomenological responses for each emotion when activated. (Chapter 1)
Affect valuation theory (AVT)	Proposal by Tsai that persons from collectivist cultures prefer lower intensity affective states, whereas persons from individualistic cultures prefer high-intensity states. (Chapter 5)
AFFEX	Izard's *System for Identifying Affect Expressions by Holistic Judgments*, a facial behavior coding system used to identify infants' expressions of emotion as proposed within differential emotions theory (DET). (Chapter 2)
Alexithymia	Difficulty in identifying, distinguishing among, and expressing one's emotions. (Chapter 8)
Allostasis	The body's physiological adaptation to meet environmental demands. (Chapter 1)
Anticipatory smile	Smile that is first directed at an object and then at one's social partner; considered an early form of affect sharing. (Chapter 2)
Anxious/preoccupied attachment	Adult attachment style considered roughly equivalent to the resistant/ambivalent style described for infants. (Chapter 6)
Appeal function	An emotional expression's implied request for a particular response from another person (e.g., sad expressions as appeals for comforting). (Chapter 1)
Appraisal	Within appraisal theories, evaluation of an object, event, or experience in terms of its overall significance, meaning, or value on a dimension described within the appraisal theory (e.g., goal relevance, expectedness, controllability); more generally, a person's interpretation of the circumstances he or she encounters. (Chapter 1)
Appraisal theories	Theories that focus on characterizing the appraisals that evoke specific emotions. (Chapter 1)

Attentional deployment	A category of emotion regulation strategies that involve modulating one's emotion by attending or disattending to particular features of the situation (e.g., closing one's eyes during the most graphic episodes of a movie). (Chapter 5)
Authoritarian parenting style	As conceptualized by Baumrind, parenting style involving little warmth but excessive control of children's behavior. (Chapter 5)
Authoritative parenting style	As conceptualized by Baumrind, parenting style involving both warmth and appropriate control over children's behavior. (Chapter 5)
Autonomic nervous system (ANS)	Portion of the nervous system that chiefly controls involuntary bodily function and responses (e.g., heart rate, respiration). (Chapter 1)
Avoidant attachment	Infant attachment style involving avoidance of the caregiver; these infants ignore or resist their caregivers when reunited after a brief separation during the Strange Situation procedure. (Chapter 2)
Basic (or discrete) emotion theories	Those theories positing a set of universal biologically based emotions, each with unique neurobiological, expressive, and feeling components. (Chapter 1)
Behavioral inhibition (BI)	Temperament characteristic conceptualized within Kagan's model as involving reluctance to approach novel stimuli; may be considered a form of fearfulness. (Chapter 2)
Benign masochism	Enjoyment of emotions in some situations that are normally experienced as negative (e.g., fear experienced while watching horror films). (Chapter 7)
Big Five/Five-Factor model	Widely used model conceptualizing personality in terms of five factors—that is, Conscientiousness, Intellect/Openness to Experience, Extraversion, Agreeableness, and Neuroticism—each factor having a number of constituent traits or facets. (Chapter 5)
Big Six emotions	Those emotions included within virtually all basic (or discrete) emotion theories, that is, happiness, surprise, anger, sadness, fear, disgust. (Chapter 1)

Broad-to-differentiated hypothesis	Proposal by Widen regarding the development of children's emotion concepts from a small set of broad categories that each include several different discrete emotions to a larger set of categories, each corresponding to a single discrete emotion. (Chapter 3)
Broaden-and-build theory (BBT)	Theory by Fredrickson proposing that positive emotions serve to broaden one's attention, thinking, and action, thus allowing for the building of social, cognitive, and physical resources that support adaptive functioning. (Chapter 7)
Callous unemotionality (CU)	Disregard for others' feelings, shallow or lack of affect, and lack of remorse or guilt. (Chapter 8)
Categorization	In relation to emotional expressions, the grouping together of expressions that represent the same emotion but may differ in perceptual features, for example, smiles with or without mouth opening. (Chapter 2)
Child Behavior Checklist (CBCL)	Widely used set of questionnaires for assessing children's and adolescents' behavioral and emotional difficulties, including internalizing problems, externalizing problems, and somatic complaints. (Chapter 3; Chapter 8)
Code-switching	As applied to emotion, the practice of adjusting one's emotions when interacting with members of one's own culture versus another culture. (Chapter 4)
Cognitive change	A category of emotion regulation strategies that involve accepting, reinterpreting, or reevaluating the emotion-eliciting situation; cognitive reappraisal is a member of this category. (Chapter 5)
Cognitive reappraisal	An often-studied emotion regulation strategy that involves changing one's thinking about an emotional event so as to change its emotional impact; for example, "looking on the bright side." (Chapter 3; Chapter 5)
Coherence	With reference to emotion, the view that discrete emotions each involve a distinct, coordinated, and co-occurring set of responses. (Chapter 5)
Collectivism	Within Hofstede's cultural dimensions theory, a set of cultural values that emphasizes allegiance to one's group, maintaining group harmony, and subordinating personal to group goals. (Chapter 3, Chapter 5)

Common method variance	Statistical variance due to measurement method, for example, ratings of both the independent and dependent variable by the same person rather than independent sources. (Chapter 5)
Comorbidity	As applied within psychology, co-occurrence between mental disorders. (Chapter 8)
Conduct disorder (CD)	Behavioral disorder characterized by aggression, destruction of property, theft, and/or serious rule breaking; may be accompanied by callous unemotionality (CU); see DSM-5 for further details. (Chapter 7; Chapter 8)
Contempt–anger–disgust (CAD) theory	Theory of morality and emotions that proposes contempt to be a response to violations of social standards, anger to be a response to violations of autonomy, and disgust to be a response to violations of physical or spiritual purity. (Chapter 7)
Contingent responding	An emotion socialization behavior in which a person reacts to the child's emotion, for example, with approval or disapproval. (Chapter 3)
Cooperativeness	A key feature of positive parenting conceptualized within infant attachment theory; defined as supporting the development of autonomy by not exerting excessive control over the infant's behavior. (Chapter 2)
Core affect	One's feeling state with respect to the dimension of valence (positivity/negativity) and level of arousal. (Chapter 1)
Cortisol awakening response (CAR)	Spike in cortisol production typically occurring shortly after awakening. (Chapter 2)
Cry face	One of the facial expressions typically produced during infant crying, may briefly occur during rapid eye movement (REM) sleep in very young infants. (Chapter 2)
Cultural dimensions theory	Hofstede's framework for conceptualizing differences across cultures in values and behavioral tendencies including six dimensions: individualism/collectivism, uncertainty avoidance, power distance, masculine/feminine, long term/short term, and indulgence/restraint. (Chapter 5)

Dedifferentiation	As applied to emotion-related neurobiology, similar levels of activation in specific brain areas during different forms of emotion regulation; seen more often in older than younger individuals. (Chapter 6)
Delay of gratification tasks	Laboratory procedures that evaluate children's ability to resist obtaining an immediate reward in favor of obtaining a greater reward after a period of waiting. (Chapter 3)
Demonstrative modeling	An emotion socialization behavior in which the child observes how another person behaves in an emotion-inducing situation. (Chapter 3)
Dexamethasone suppression test (DST)	Test used to identify disruption of functioning in the HPA system. (Chapter 8)
***Diagnostic and Statistical Manual of Mental Disorders* (DSM-5)**	Widely used manual for the assessment and diagnosis of mental disorders, published by the American Psychiatric Association. (Chapter 7; Chapter 8)
Dialect theory of emotional expression	Proposal by Elfenbein that cultural differences in emotional expression develop over time due to processes similar to those producing linguistic dialects. (Chapter 5)
Diathesis–stress model	Proposal that some individuals are more susceptible than others to adversity due to their biological predispositions or experiential history. (Chapter 8)
Differential emotions theory (DET)	Izard's basic (or discrete) emotion theory positing the emergence of affect programs during infancy that may constitute components of later developing emotion schemas. (Chapter 1)
Differential susceptibility model	Theory that some children are more susceptible than others to adversity but at the same time will benefit more than others from a high-quality environment. (Chapter 8)
Disappointing present procedure	Laboratory procedure used to evaluate children's ability to modify spontaneous expressions of disappointment by inhibiting negative expressive behavior or masking it by smiling. (Chapter 3)
Discrete emotion theories	*See* Basic emotion theories.
Discrimination	In relation to emotional expressions, perceiving that different configurations of facial movements are not identical. (Chapter 2)

Discussion of emotion	An emotion socialization behavior involving verbal transmission of information about emotion to the child, for example, during conversations or story reading. (Chapter 3)
Dismissing/avoidant attachment	Adult attachment style interpreted as being roughly equivalent to the avoidant attachment style described for infants. (Chapter 6)
Disorganized attachment	Infant attachment style interpreted as involving fear of the caregiver; the infant may avoid the caregiver's gaze or "freeze" in the midst of approaching the caregiver when reunited after a brief separation during the Strange Situation procedure. (Chapter 2)
Display rules	Cultural norms regarding the appropriate expression of emotion. (Chapter 1)
Distress reaction	With respect to emotional socialization, a form of contingent responding to a child's emotion in which the person becomes upset by the child's distress. (Chapter 3)
Distress to limitations	A subscale within Rothbart's Infant Behavior Questionnaire that is interpreted by some to be a measure of infant anger. (Chapter 7)
Distress to novelty	A subscale within Rothbart's Infant Behavior Questionnaire that is interpreted by some to be a measure of infant fearfulness. (Chapter 7)
Dot-probe paradigm	Laboratory procedure that may be used to assess attentional bias toward threat-related facial expressions in infants or adults. (Chapter 7)
Dual systems model	As applied to emotion-related neurobiology, model proposed by Steinberg positing two independent systems, that is, a socioemotional control system and a cognitive control system; as applied to decision making, models that posit both a deliberate analytic system and an emotion-related intuitive system. (Chapter 4; Chapter 6)
Duchenne smile	Smile that includes contraction of *orbicularis oculi* (i.e., contraction of the muscle surrounding the eye that produces cheek raising and crinkling at the eye corner); originally proposed to reflect genuine positive emotion. (Chapter 2)

Dynamical systems (DS) perspective	Theoretical framework that views complex systems (including emotions) as emerging from the self-organization of their components via synergistic links among components, as well as demands and constraints imposed by the environment. (Chapter 1)
Ecological validity	The extent to which experimental results or behavior observed in the laboratory are representative of behavior produced in real-world circumstances. (Chapter 4)
Effect size	A statistical measure used to interpret the magnitude of a relationship (or difference) found between two variables in terms of its meaningfulness, for example, as "small," "medium," or "large." (Chapter 2)
Effortful control (EC)	Widely studied temperament characteristic conceptualized within Rothbart's theory as involving the ability to voluntarily control one's attention and behavior, including the ability to change one's attention or behavior and to detect and correct performance errors. (Chapter 2)
Egocentric language	Self-talk used to help focus one's attention and guide one's behavior during a difficult task. (Chapter 1)
Electroencephalography (EEG)	A technology that can be used to measure electrical activity across the scalp in the form of brain waves. (Chapter 2)
Emotion competence	Framework for studying and encouraging emotion-related behaviors that are considered to contribute to adaptive functioning; emotion-related behaviors are viewed as skills that can be improved rather than innate abilities. (Chapter 8)
Emotion-focused reaction	With respect to emotion socialization, a form of contingent responding to a child's emotion in which a person tries to alleviate the child's distress. (Chapter 3)
Emotion knowledge	Sophisticated understanding of the mental states and experiential origins of an individual's emotional reactions, for example, his or her cultural background. (Chapter 2)
Emotion regulation	A widely used but controversial term for processes that involve monitoring, evaluating, and/or modifying emotional reactions. (Chapter 3)

Emotion-related socialization behaviors (ERSBs)	Behaviors of other persons through which children learn about emotion responding, that is, demonstrative modeling, contingent responding, discussion of emotion, and exposure to emotion-inducing experiences. (Chapter 3)
Emotion schema	Mental structures that involve associations between emotions and cognitions (e.g., thoughts and/or memories of experiences) as conceptualized within differential emotions theory (DET). (Chapter 1)
Emotion understanding	An umbrella term used herein to refer to emotion recognition and/or emotion knowledge. (Chapter 2)
Emotional go/no-go task	Laboratory procedure in which participants are instructed to press a button when presented with a particular emotional expression but refrain from responding to other emotional expressions. (Chapter 4)
Emotional intelligence (EI)	Conceptualization of emotion understanding as a form of intelligence or adaptive functioning that can be objectively measured in a manner analogous to the measurement of cognitive intelligence. (Chapter 4)
Emotional labor	As conceptualized by Hochschild, regulation of one's emotions to meet workplace demands by means of surface acting, deep acting, and emotion–rule dissonance. (Chapter 5)
Emotional roller coaster task	Laboratory procedure in which an adolescent and caregiver engage in discussions about times in when they felt each of several emotions. (Chapter 4)
Emotional self-awareness	Conscious awareness of the emotions or affect one is experiencing. (Chapter 8)
Empathy	A widely used term conceptualized differently by different scholars; defined herein as a process through which an emotion is generated when one perceives another's emotion and matches that feeling while retaining awareness that the source of one's emotion is that of the other person(s). (Chapter 7)
Endogenous smile	Smile produced by very young infants during rapid eye movement (REM) sleep; considered to reflect spontaneous activity of the subcortical nervous system. (Chapter 2)

Environmental sensitivity

Individual differences in persons' degree of responsiveness to their environmental circumstances as described in several models, including the diathesis–stress, vantage sensitivity, and differential susceptibility models. (Chapter 8)

Event-related potential (ERP)

Spikes of brain activity on various areas of the scalp measured using electroencephalography. (Chapter 2)

Evidence-based programs

Treatment and intervention programs that have been systematically evaluated in terms of effectiveness. (Chapter 8)

Exogenous smile

Smile produced by very young infants in response to an external stimulus such as stroking the cheek; not generally considered to reflect positive emotion. (Chapter 2)

Experience sampling methodology (ESM)

As applied to emotion research, procedures in which participants record episodes of emotional experience shortly after they occur, typically when remotely signaled via smartphone technology or at a predetermined time during the day. (Chapter 4)

Exposure to emotion-inducing experiences

An emotion socialization behavior in which the child is placed in situations that evoke emotion and thus may be provided with opportunities to learn how to respond. (Chapter 3)

Expressive encouragement

With respect to emotion socialization, a form of contingent responding to the child's emotional expression in which a person acknowledges and accepts the legitimacy of the child's emotion. (Chapter 3)

Expressive suppression

An emotion regulation strategy that involves inhibition of overt behavior reflecting an experienced emotion. (Chapter 4)

Externalizing behaviors

Problematic behaviors that involve acting upon other persons and/or objects in the world, for example, rule breaking, aggression. (Chapter 3; Chapter 8)

Facial feedback hypothesis

The proposal that voluntarily produced facial expressions generate feedback to the brain that itself generates other components of emotion, for example, an emotion-specific pattern of autonomic nervous system responding, and the subjective experience of the emotion. (Chapter 5)

Families of emotion regulation strategies	As conceptualized within Gross's model, categories of regulation strategies including situation selection, situation modification, attentional deployment, cognitive change, and response modulation. (Chapter 5)
Fear of missing out (FOMO)	Fear of being ignored or excluded from social activities or interactions, particularly those occurring via the Internet. (Chapter 4)
Fearful attachment	Adult attachment style considered to be roughly equivalent to the disorganized style described for infants. (Chapter 6)
Female advantage	Tendency for females to perform more favorably in some area of functioning, for example, emotion understanding. (Chapter 3)
Forced-choice method	Measurement strategy in which participants are required to choose among a fixed set of alternative responses to a test item. (Chapter 5)
Four Horsemen	As conceptualized within Gottman's model of couples' relationships, patterns of emotion communication that predict dissolution of the couple; that is, criticism, defensiveness, contempt, and stonewalling. (Chapter 5)
Functional magnetic resonance imaging (fMRI)	An imaging technology that can be used to produce images representing changes in blood flow associated with neural activity in various brain regions. (Chapter 2)
Functionalist/relational perspective	Developmental framework proposed by Campos that defines emotion as a process in which the individual attempts to establish, maintain, or change a significant relationship to some aspect of the external or internal environment; emphasizes flexibility in the specific behaviors that may be recruited to achieve an emotion-related goal. (Chapter 1)
Gender similarity hypothesis	The proposal that gender similarities outweigh gender differences in many areas and merit greater emphasis in the scholarly literature. (Chapter 2)
Glutamate amplifies noradrenergic effects (GANE) model	Proposal by Mather and colleagues regarding the neurobiological basis of emotion episodes characterized by extremely high arousal and narrowing of attentional focus. (Chapter 6)

Heterochronic development	As conceptualized within the dynamical systems framework, independent development of the components of a system that eventually become coordinated to form that system. (Chapter 1)
Hikikomori	A condition of severe social withdrawal. (Chapter 8)
Hostile attribution bias	Propensity to interpret ambiguous behaviors produced by another person as indications of their hostile intent. (Chapter 7)
Hypothalamic–pituitary–adrenal (HPA) system	Neurobiological system with many functions including the production of cortisol that both follows a daily rhythm and serves as a component of the stress response. (Chapter 1; Chapter 2)
Ideal affect	As conceptualized within Tsai's affect valuation theory, one's preferred level of affect intensity. (Chapter 6)
Imbalance model	As applied to emotion-related neurobiology, a model similar to the dual systems model but additionally focusing on interactions among components within the subcortical and cortical systems. (Chapter 4)
Incidental affect	Affect experienced during decision making that is not directly related to the decision-making process, for example, emotion produced by events earlier in the day. (Chapter 6)
Independent/ interdependent	Term corresponding to individualism/collectivism, commonly used to describe the psychological orientation of persons from cultures as categorized along that cultural dimension. (Chapter 3; Chapter 5)
Individualism/ collectivism	A dimension of cultural orientation representing the relative valuing of the individual versus the group; for example, valuing personal autonomy over subordination of personal goals to group goals. (Chapter 3; Chapter 5)
Ingroup advantage	As applied to emotion understanding, the ability to recognize and/or be responsive to the emotional expressions of persons from one's own ingroup, that is, the group of people with whom one identifies, such as members of one's own culture. (Chapter 7)
Instrumental action	A behavior intended and/or designed to achieve a goal. (Chapter 1)

Integral affect	Affect directly related to a decision-making process, for example, preference among the choices that are offered. (Chapter 6)
Intergenerational transmission	As applied to parenting, transmission of one's attachment and/or parenting style from one generation to another. (Chapter 5)
Internal working model (IWM)	The mental representation of one's attachment relationship; initially established in infants based on their positive or negative relations with their caregivers; establishes expectations about future social and emotional relations but also is modified as the result of those future relations. (Chapter 2)
Internalizing behaviors	Problematic behaviors that involve processes within the self, for example, depression, anxiety, somatic complaints. (Chapter 3; Chapter 8)
International core patterns (ICPs)	Patterns of facial and nonfacial behavior produced with significant frequency by members of different cultures who are asked to pose expressions for various emotions. (Chapter 5)
Joint storytelling task	Procedure during which mothers and children discuss stories about potentially distressing situations; used for assessing attachment-related maternal sensitivity in preschool and school-age children. (Chapter 3)
Locationist view	The view that neurobiological emotion programs are situated in different and nonoverlapping locations in the brain. (Chapter 5)
Magnetic resonance imaging (MRI)	An imaging technology that can be used to produce images of the anatomical structure of the brain. (Chapter 2)
Maltreatment	Treatment of another person that will predictably cause harm, including physical abuse of children (e.g., harsh physical punishment of or verbal threats), sexual abuse, and neglect (i.e., failure to provide proper physical care, social stimulation, and/or emotional support). (Chapter 7; Chapter 8)
Marshmallow task	A type of delay of gratification procedure that evaluates children's ability to resist obtaining a single marshmallow in favor of obtaining two marshmallows after a period of waiting. (Chapter 4)

MAX	Izard's *Maximally Discriminative Facial Movement Coding System* developed in conjunction with DET; used to describe infants' emotional and nonemotional facial expressions. (Chapter 2)
Meta-analysis	Statistical analysis that combines results from multiple studies in order to evaluate a body of research related to a particular question or issue (Preface)
Minimization	With respect to emotion socialization, a form of contingent responding in which a person dismisses or devalues a child's emotion. (Chapter 3)
Mirror-recognition task	Laboratory procedure to assess children's objective self-awareness as indicated by their response to their mirror image. (Chapter 7)
Moderation effect	A change in the relationship between two variables depending on the presence of a third (i.e., moderator) variable, for example, age differences in the effect of observing interparental conflict on children's emotional adjustment. (Chapter 3)
Mutual regulation model	Tronick's conceptualization of caregiver–infant interactions as involving reciprocal communication of affect and the reestablishment (i.e., regulation) of positive interactions after episodes of infant distress due to the infant's overarousal or caregiver's failure to engage with the infant. (Chapter 2)
Natural kinds	With reference to emotion, the view that emotions are discrete entities each having an innate biologically determined set of necessary and sufficient features that include a dedicated neural network or affect program. (Chapter 5)
Near-infrared spectroscopy (NIRS)	A technology that can be used to measure blood flow in various areas of the scalp representing neural activity in the cerebral cortex. (Chapter 2)
Negative reactivity	Temperament characteristic conceptualized within Rothbart's theory as involving sadness, anger/ frustration, fear, and slow recovery from these negative emotions. (Chapter 2)
Negativity bias	Tendency to focus on negative information more than positive information; proposed by some to be a universal human predisposition. (Chapter 7)

Neglect	With respect to childhood adversity, a category of maltreatment that involves failure to receive proper physical care, social stimulation, and/or emotional support. (Chapter 7; Chapter 8)
Neonate	Newborn infant up to approximately 1 month of age. (Chapter 1)
Objective self-awareness	Awareness of the self as a potential object of others' attention. (Chapter 1)
Oppositional defiant disorder (ODD)	Behavioral disorder characterized by angry/irritable mood, argumentative/defiant behavior, and vindictiveness; see the DSM-5 for further details. (Chapter 7; Chapter 8)
Orienting/regulation	An infant temperament characteristic conceptualized within Rothbart's theory as involving the showing of pleasure in quiet play, cuddliness, soothability, and the ability to attend to a single stimulus for an extended period of time. (Chapter 2)
Overlap procedure	Laboratory procedure that may be used to assess attentional bias toward threat-related facial expressions in infants and adults. (Chapter 7)
Parasocial attachment figures	Persons portrayed in the media to whom an individual may form an attachment without having reciprocal contact. (Chapter 6)
Parasympathetic nervous system (PNS)	A branch of the autonomic nervous system generally described as sustaining a lower state of arousal that allows the body to rest and recuperate. (Chapter 2)
PATHS (Promoting Alternative Thinking Strategies)	A socioemotional learning program administered by teachers in the classroom; designed to teach children skills related to emotion understanding, communication, and regulation. (Chapter 8)
PCIT (Parent–Child Interaction Therapy)	Program designed to teach positive attention skills and effective disciplinary skills to parents with children having disruptive behavior problems; PCIT-ED is a version that also includes teaching skills related to emotion understanding and regulation. (Chapter 8)
Permissive parenting style	As conceptualized by Baumrind, a parenting style involving high warmth but little control over children's behavior. (Chapter 5)

311

Personal distress	An empathy-related response in which a person is overwhelmed by the empathic distress they feel for another person. (Chapter 7)
Polyvagal theory	Theory advanced by Porges regarding the influence of the vagus nerve on the functioning of the autonomic nervous system during social interactions and emotion regulation. (Chapter 2)
Positive and Negative Affect Scales (PANAS)	Widely used self-report measure that assesses a set of both positive and negative affective states, for example, interest, excitement, distress, fear, strength, inspiration. (Chapter 6)
Positive psychology	Subfield within psychology that focuses on positive affect and the factors that contribute to and/or enhance it. (Chapter 7)
Positivity effect	Older persons' propensity to attend to and remember information related to positive affect more than information related to negative affect. (Chapter 6)
Proactive aggression	Aggression intended as a means to achieving a goal. (Chapter 7)
Problem-focused reaction	With respect to emotion socialization, a form of contingent responding to a child's emotion in which a person tries to help the child cope more effectively with the cause of his or her distress. (Chapter 3)
Prosocial behaviors	Behaviors or actions that are viewed as socially desirable or beneficial, for example, helping, sharing, cooperating. (Chapter 3)
Prototypic emotional facial expressions	Configurations of facial movements proposed to be universal expressions of basic (or discrete) emotions. (Chapter 1)
Psychological construction theories	Theories that view emotions as constructed from more basic psychological components that are not specific or unique to emotion (e.g., cognitive processes) and are not organized by innate affect programs. (Chapter 1)
Punitive reaction	With respect to emotion socialization, a form of contingent responding to a child's emotion in which a person punishes or threatens to punish the child. (Chapter 3)

Reactive aggression	Aggression produced in reaction to a perceived provocation. (Chapter 7)
Reappraisal	See Cognitive reappraisal. (Chapter 3)
Recognition	In relation to emotional expression, apprehending differences in the meaning of different emotional expressions, for example, their associated elicitors or action tendencies. (Chapter 2)
Referential communication	Communication between two persons about a third person, object, or event. (Chapter 2)
Research Domain Criteria (RDoC) framework	An approach to clinical research that focuses on understanding six basic systems of functioning that may be disrupted in one or several different mental disorders: (1) negative valence systems (e.g., fear, anxiety), (2) positive valence systems (e.g., reward prediction, reward valuation), (3) cognitive systems (e.g., attention, control, memory), (4) social processes (e.g., attachment, emotion recognition), (5) arousal/regulatory systems (e.g., sleep, circadian rhythms), and (6) sensorimotor systems (e.g., action initiation and inhibition, sense of agency vs. dissociative behavior, habit-based behaviors). (Chapter 8)
Resistant/ambivalent attachment	Infant attachment style involving anxious uncertainty about close relationships; these infants show distress and resist comforting by the caregiver when reunited after a brief separation during the Strange Situation procedure. (Chapter 2)
Respiratory sinus arrhythmia (RSA)	A measure of heart rate activity generally reflecting greater parasympathetic control; sometimes used as a measure of emotion regulation. (Chapter 2)
Response modulation	A category of emotion regulation strategies that involves altering the emotional responses that one might be spontaneously inclined to make; expressive suppression is an often-studied member of this category. (Chapter 5)
Reward system	Neurobiological system including a number of anatomical structures that respond with pleasure to presence of rewards. (Chapter 4)
RULER (Recognizing, Understanding, Labeling, Expressing, and Regulating Emotion)	A socioemotional learning program administered by teachers in the classroom; designed to teach children skills related to emotion understanding, communication, and regulation. (Chapter 8)

Schachter–Singer theory of emotion	Theory that conceptualizes emotions as a set of cognitions that one attributes to one's general state of physiological arousal, depending on the situational circumstances during which the arousal occurs. (Chapter 1)
Secure attachment style	Healthy attachment style indicated in infants by their secure base behavior and readiness to be comforted by the caregiver after a brief separation; indicated in adults by their positive attitude toward and positive expectations about emotional relationships. (Chapter 2; Chapter 6)
Secure base behavior	Attachment-related child behavior that demonstrates a willingness to explore a novel environment while periodically making visual or physical contact with a caregiver. (Chapter 2; Chapter 3)
Selection, optimization, and compensation (SOC) theory	A theory of aging that proposes that older adults focus on maintaining skills and resources and on preventing losses; includes the goal of maintaining positive emotion. (Chapter 6)
Self-conscious emotions	Emotions that require objective self-awareness, for example, embarrassment, guilt, shame. (Chapter 1)
Sensitivity	A key feature of positive parenting conceptualized within infant attachment theory; defined as noticing, correctly interpreting, and appropriately responding to the infant's signals, particularly signals of distress. (Chapter 2)
Situation modification	A category of emotion regulation strategies that involve altering some feature of the situation so as to modify one's expected emotional response, for example, instructing one's guests to avoid discussing politics at Thanksgiving dinner. (Chapter 5)
Situation selection	A category of emotion regulation strategies that involves exerting control over the type of emotion-eliciting situations to which one will be exposed, for example, avoiding predictably unpleasant events. (Chapter 5)
SOC–emotion regulation model (SOC-ER)	An extension of the selection, optimization, and compensation (SOC) theory of aging that focuses on optimal selection and utilization of emotion regulation strategies. (Chapter 6)

Social buffering effect	Reduction in an individual's stress response produced by the presence of an attachment figure. (Chapter 2)
Social construction theories	Constructivist theories that view emotions as constructed from more basic components (e.g., appraisals, expressions, instrumental actions) in accordance with social conventions that may vary from culture to culture. (Chapter 1)
Social referencing	The process of seeking information from another person to help determine how one should respond to an emotionally ambiguous event. (Chapter 2)
Social smiles	Smiles produced by infants starting at 6 to 8 weeks in response to human faces and voices; generally considered to reflect positive emotion. (Chapter 2)
Socioemotional learning (SEL) programs	School-based programs designed to enhance children's emotion-related knowledge and skills. (Chapter 8)
Socioemotional selectivity theory (SST)	A theory that proposes an age-related shift from future-oriented goals related to knowledge and achievement to present-oriented goals related to experiencing positive emotion in later adulthood. (Chapter 6)
SRGs	Socially dictated standards, rules, or goals. (Chapter 1)
Still-face paradigm	Laboratory procedure designed to investigate infant–caregiver interactions during the first half year; demonstrates infants' sensitivity to a caregiver's lack of normal facial expressivity. (Chapter 2)
Strange Situation procedure	Laboratory procedure designed to investigate attachment in infants or toddlers around 1–2 years of age; infants may be classified as securely attached or falling into one of several categories of insecure attachment: avoidant, resistant/ambivalent, or disorganized. (Chapter 2)
Strength and vulnerability integration (SVI) theory	A theory of aging that considers both the emotion regulation abilities and physiological challenges to those abilities faced by older individuals. (Chapter 6)
Subjective well-being (SWB)	One's self-perceived well-being conceptualized in terms of three components: positive affect, negative affect, and satisfaction with one's life. (Chapter 5)

Surgency	Infant temperament characteristic conceptualized within Rothbart's theory as involving positive emotion, rapid approach to potential rewards, and high activity level. (Chapter 2)
Sympathetic nervous system (SNS)	A branch of the autonomic nervous system generally described as preparing and sustaining bodily action (e.g., fight or flight). (Chapter 2)
Sympathy	As conceptualized by Eisenberg, an empathy-related response involving concern for another's distress. (Chapter 7)
TCIT-U (Teacher–Child Interaction Training–Universal)	School-based program designed to teach positive attention skills and effective disciplinary skills to teachers. (Chapter 8)
Temperament	One's characteristic behavioral and emotional tendencies; specified somewhat differently across different temperament theories. (Chapter 1)
Theory of constructed emotion	Theory proposed by Lisa Barrett that conceptualizes emotions as culturally labeled categories of experience including one's cognitive and neurobiological reactions within a particular situational context. (Chapter 1)
Transmission gap	As applied to intergenerational transmission of parenting, a deficiency (or gap) in scholars' understanding of the behavioral factors mediating the association between attachment and/or parenting styles across generations. (Chapter 5)
Valence	Dimension of feeling ranging from highly positive/pleasant to highly negative/unpleasant. (Chapter 1)
Vantage sensitivity model	Theory that some individuals will benefit more than others from a high-quality environment. (Chapter 8)
WEIRD	Acronym standing for "Western, educated, industrialized, rich and democratic," that is, those populations whose members have been the focus of study in most psychological investigations. (Chapter 2)

References

Abe, J. A. A. (2015). Differential emotions theory as a theory of personality development. *Emotion Review, 7*(2), 126–130.

Abend, R., de Voogd, L., Salemink, E., Wiers, R. W., Pérez-Edgar, K., Fitzgerald, A., . . . Bar-Haim, Y. (2018). Association between attention bias to threat and anxiety symptoms in children and adolescents. *Depression and Anxiety, 35*(3), 229–238.

Abraham, M. M., & Kerns, K. A. (2013). Positive and negative emotions and coping as mediators of mother–child attachment and peer relationships. *Merrill-Palmer Quarterly, 59*(4), 399–425.

Achenbach, T. (1991). *Manual for the Child Behavior Checklist/4–18 and 1991 Profile.* Available at ASEBA.org.

Achenbach, T., & Rescorla, L. (2000). *Manual for the ASEBA Preschool Forms and Profiles.* Available at ASEBA.org.

Achenbach, T., & Rescorla, L. (2001). *Manual for the ASEBA School-Age Forms and Profiles.* Available at ASEBA.org.

Adam, E. K. (2012). Emotion–cortisol transactions occur over multiple time scales in development: Implications for research on emotion and the development of emotional disorders. *Monographs of the Society for Research in Child Development, 77*(2), 17–27.

Adam, E. K., Hawkley, L., Kudielka, B. M., & Cacioppo, J. (2006). Day-to-day dynamics of experience–cortisol associations in a population-based sample of older adults. *Proceedings of the National Academy of Sciences of the USA, 103*(45), 1758–1763.

Adams, S., Kuebli, J., Boyle, P. A., & Fivush, R. (1995). Gender differences in parent–child conversations about past emotions: A longitudinal investigation. *Sex Roles, 33*(5–6), 309–323.

Adolphs, R. (2008). Fear, faces, and the human amygdala. *Current Opinion in Neurobiology, 18*(2), 166–172.

Adolphs, R. (2017). Reply to Barrett: Affective neuroscience needs objective criteria for emotions. *Social Cognitive and Affective Neuroscience, 12*(1), 32–33.

Ahnert, L., Gunnar, M. R., Lamb, M. E., & Barthel, M. (2004). Transition to child care:

Associations with infant–mother attachment, infant negative emotion, and cortisol elevations. *Child Development, 75*(3), 639–650.

Ainsworth, M. D. S., Blehar, M. C., Waters, E., & Wall, S. (1978). *Patterns of attachment: A psychological study of the Strange Situation.* Hillsdale, NJ: Erlbaum.

Aldao, A., Gee, D. G., De Los Reyes, A., & Seager, I. (2016). Emotion regulation as a transdiagnostic factor in the development of internalizing and externalizing psychopathology: Current and future directions. *Development and Psychopathology, 28*(4), 927–946.

Aldao, A., Nolen-Hoeksema, S., & Schweizer, S. (2010). Emotion-regulation strategies across psychopathology: A meta-analytic review. *Clinical Psychology Review, 30*(2), 217–237.

Alink, L. R. A., van IJzendoorn, M. H., Bakermans-Kranenburg, M. J., Mesman, J., Juffer, F., & Koot, H. M. (2008). Cortisol and externalizing behavior in children and adolescents: Mixed meta-analytic evidence for the inverse relation of basal cortisol and cortisol reactivity with externalizing behavior. *Developmental Psychobiology, 50*(5), 427–450.

Allard, E. S., & Kensinger, E. A. (2014). Age-related differences in neural recruitment during the use of cognitive reappraisal and selective attention as emotion regulation strategies. *Frontiers in Psychology, 5,* 296.

Allen, J. P., McElhaney, K. B., Land, D. J., Kuperminc, G. P., Moore, C. W., O'Beirne-Kelly, H., & Kilmer, S. L. (2003). A secure base in adolescence: Markers of attachment security in the mother–adolescent relationship. *Child Development, 74*(1), 292–307.

Allen, J. P., Moore, C., Kuperminc, G., & Bell, K. (1998). Attachment and adolescent psychosocial functioning. *Child Development, 69*(5), 1406–1419.

Allen, J. P, & Tan, J. S. (2016). The multiple facets of attachment in adolescence. In J. Cassidy & P. R. Shaver (Eds.), *Handbook of attachment* (3rd ed., pp. 399–415). New York: Guilford Press.

American Psychiatric Association. (2013). *Diagnostic and statistical manual of mental disorders* (5th ed.). Arlington, VA: Author.

American Psychological Association (2020). *APA dictionary of psychology.* Washington, DC: Author. Retrieved November 11, 2020, from *http://dictionary.apa.org.*

Anusic, I., & Schimmack, U. (2016). Stability and change of personality traits, self-esteem, and well-being: Introducing the meta-analytic stability and change model of retest correlations. *Journal of Personality and Social Psychology, 110*(5), 766–781.

Arnett, J. J. (1999). Adolescent storm and stress, reconsidered. *American Psychologist, 54*(5), 317–326.

Arnold, M. B. (1960). *Emotion and personality: Vol. I. Psychological aspects.* Oxford, UK: Columbia University Press.

Asaba, M., Ong, D. C., & Gweon, H. (2019). Integrating expectations and outcomes: Preschoolers' developing ability to reason about others' emotions. *Developmental Psychology, 55*(8), 1680–1693.

Atherton, O. E., Lawson, K. M., & Robins, R. W. (2020). The development of effortful control from late childhood to young adulthood. *Journal of Personality and Social Psychology, 119*(2), 417–456.

Atkins, D., Uskul, A. K., & Cooper, N. R. (2016). Culture shapes empathic responses to physical and social pain. *Emotion, 16*(5), 587–601.

Averill, J. R. (1983). Studies on anger and aggression: Implications for theories of emotion. *American Psychologist, 38*(11), 1145–1160.

Aviezer, H., Trope, Y., & Todorov, A. (2012). Body cues, not facial expressions, discriminate between intense positive and negative emotions. *Science, 338*(6111), 1225-1229.

Babkirk, S., Rios, V., & Dennis, T. A. (2015). The late positive potential predicts emotion regulation strategy use in school-aged children concurrently and two years later. *Developmental Science, 18*(5), 832-841.

Bailen, N. H., Green, L. M., & Thompson, R. J. (2019). Understanding emotion in adolescents: A review of emotional frequency, intensity, instability, and clarity. *Emotion Review, 11*(1), 63-73.

Bakermans-Kranenburg, M. J., Lotz, A., Alyousefi-van Dijk, K., & van IJzendoorn, M. (2019). Birth of a father: Fathering in the first 1,000 days. *Child Development Perspectives, 13*(4), 247-253.

Ball, T. M., Ramsawh, H. J., Campbell-Sills, L., Paulus, M. P., & Stein, M. B. (2013). Prefrontal dysfunction during emotion regulation in generalized anxiety and panic disorders. *Psychological Medicine, 43*(7), 1475-1486.

Baltes, P. B., & Baltes, M. M. (1990). Psychological perspectives on successful aging: The model of selective optimization with compensation. In P. B. Baltes & M. M. Baltes (Eds.), *Successful aging: Perspectives from the behavioral sciences* (pp. 1-34). New York: Cambridge University Press.

Band, E. B., & Weisz, J. R. (1988). How to feel better when it feels bad: Children's perspectives on coping with everyday stress. *Developmental Psychology, 24*(2), 247-253.

Bandelow, B., Baldwin, D., Abelli, M., Altamura, C., Dell'Osso, B., Domschke, K., . . . Riederer, P. (2016). Biological markers for anxiety disorders, OCD and PTSD—A consensus statement: Part I. Neuroimaging and genetics. *World Journal of Biological Psychiatry, 17*(5), 321-365.

Bandelow, B., Baldwin, D., Abelli, M., Bolea-Alamanac, B., Bourin, M., Chamberlain, S. R., . . . Riederer, P. (2017). Biological markers for anxiety disorders, OCD and PTSD: A consensus statement: Part II. Neurochemistry, neurophysiology and neurocognition. *World Journal of Biological Psychiatry, 18*(3), 162-214.

Barańczuk, U. (2019). The five factor model of personality and emotion regulation: A meta-analysis. *Personality and Individual Differences, 139*, 217-227.

Barber, B. K. (1996). Parental psychological control: Revisiting a neglected construct. *Child Development, 67*(6), 3296-3319.

Barlow, M. A., Wrosch, C., Gouin, J.-P., & Kunzmann, U. (2019). Is anger, but not sadness, associated with chronic inflammation and illness in older adulthood? *Psychology and Aging, 34*(3), 330-340.

Bar-On, R. (2000). Emotional and social intelligence: Insights from the Emotional Quotient Inventory. In R. Bar-On, J. D. Parker, & D. Goleman (Eds.), *Handbook of emotional intelligence* (pp. 363-388). San Francisco: Jossey-Bass.

Barrera, M. E., & Maurer, D. (1981). The perception of facial expressions by the three-month-old. *Child Development, 52*(1), 203-206.

Barrett, K. C., & Campos, J. J. (1987). Perspectives on emotional development: II. A functionalist approach to emotions. In J. D. Osofsky (Ed.), *Handbook of infant development* (2nd ed., pp. 555-578). Oxford, UK: Wiley.

Barrett, K. C., Zahn-Waxler, C., & Cole, P. M. (1993). Avoiders vs. amenders: Implications for the investigation of guilt and shame during toddlerhood? *Cognition and Emotion, 7*(6), 481-505.

Barrett, L. F. (2017a). *How emotions are made: The secret life of the brain.* Boston: Houghton Mifflin Harcourt.

Barrett, L. F. (2017b). The theory of constructed emotion: An active inference account of interoception and categorization. *Social Cognitive and Affective Neuroscience, 12*(1), 1–23.

Barrett, L. F., Adolphs, R., Marsella, S., Martinez, A. M., & Pollak, S. D. (2019). Emotional expressions reconsidered: Challenges to inferring emotion from human facial movements. *Psychological Science in the Public Interest, 20*(1), 1–68.

Barrett, L. F., & Gendron, M. (2016). The importance of context: Three corrections to Cordaro, Keltner, Tshering, Wangchuk, and Flynn (2016). *Emotion, 6*(6), 803–806.

Bartholomew, K., & Horowitz, L. M. (1991). Attachment styles among young adults: A test of a four-category model. *Journal of Personality and Social Psychology, 61*(2), 226–244.

Batson, C. D. (1998). Altruism and prosocial behavior. In D. T. Gilbert, S. T. Fiske, & G. Lindzey (Eds.), *The handbook of social psychology* (4th ed., Vols. 1–2, pp. 282–316). New York: McGraw-Hill.

Baumrind, D. (1971). Current patterns of parental authority. *Developmental Psychology, 4*(1, Pt. 2), 1–103.

Bayet, L., & Nelson, C. A. (2019). The perception of facial emotion in typical and atypical development. In V. LoBue, K. Pérez-Edgar, & K. Buss (Eds.), *Handbook of emotional development* (pp. 105–138). Cham, Switzerland: Springer.

Beauchaine, T. P. (2001). Vagal tone, development, and Gray's motivational theory: Toward an integrated model of autonomic nervous system functioning in psychopathology. *Development and Psychopathology, 13*(2), 183–214.

Beauchaine, T. P. (2015). Respiratory sinus arrhythmia: A transdiagnostic biomarker of emotion dysregulation and psychopathology. *Current Opinion in Psychology, 3*, 43–47.

Beier, J. S., Gross, J. T., Brett, B. E., Stern, J. A., Martin, D. R., & Cassidy, J. (2019). Helping, sharing, and comforting in young children: Links to individual differences in attachment. *Child Development, 90*(2), e273–e289.

Belden, A. C., Thomson, N. R., & Luby, J. L. (2008). Temper tantrums in healthy versus depressed and disruptive preschoolers: Defining tantrum behaviors associated with clinical problems. *Journal of Pediatrics, 152*(1), 117–122.

Belsky, J., & Fearon, R. M. P. (2002). Early attachment security, subsequent maternal sensitivity, and later child development: Does continuity in development depend upon continuity of caregiving? *Attachment and Human Development, 4*(3), 361–387.

Belsky, J., & Pluess, M. (2009). Beyond diathesis stress: Differential susceptibility to environmental influences. *Psychological Bulletin, 135*(6), 885–908.

Bennett, D. S., Sullivan, M. W., & Lewis, M. (2005). Young children's adjustment as a function of maltreatment, shame, and anger. *Child Maltreatment, 10*(4), 311–323.

Bennett, D. S., Sullivan, M. W., & Lewis, M. (2010). Neglected children, shame-proneness, and depressive symptoms. *Child Maltreatment, 15*(4), 305–314.

Bernard, K., Frost, A., Bennett, C. B., & Lindhiem, O. (2017). Maltreatment and diurnal cortisol regulation: A meta-analysis. *Psychoneuroendocrinology, 78*, 57–67.

Bernhold, Q. S., & Metzger, M. (2020). Older adults' parasocial relationships with favorite television characters and depressive symptoms. *Health Communication, 35*(2), 168–179.

Bernier, A., Carlson, S. M., & Whipple, N. (2010). From external regulation to self-regulation: Early parenting precursors of young children's executive functioning. *Child Development, 81*(1), 326–339.

Birdwhistell, R. L. (1970). *Kinesics and context: Essays on body motion communication*. Oxford, UK: Ballantine.

Blair, B. L., Perry, N. B., O'Brien, M., Calkins, S. D., Keane, S. P., & Shanahan, L. (2015). Identifying developmental cascades among differentiated dimensions of social competence and emotion regulation. *Developmental Psychology, 51*(8), 1062–1073.

Blair, K. S., Geraci, M., Smith, B. W., Hollon, N., DeVido, J., Otero, M., . . . Pine, D. S. (2012). Reduced dorsal anterior cingulate cortical activity during emotional regulation and top-down attentional control in generalized social phobia, generalized anxiety disorder, and comorbid generalized social phobia/generalized anxiety disorder. *Biological Psychiatry, 72*(6), 476–482.

Blanke, E. S., Brose, A., Kalokerinos, E. K., Erbas, Y., Riediger, M., & Kuppens, P. (2020). Mix it to fix it: Emotion regulation variability in daily life. *Emotion, 20*(3), 473–485.

Block, J., & Block, J. H. (2006). Venturing a 30-year longitudinal study. *American Psychologist, 61*(4), 315–327.

Boccia, M., & Campos, J. J. (1989). Maternal emotional signals, social referencing, and infants' reactions to strangers. *New Directions for Child Development, 44*, 25–49.

Bodner, E., & Cohen-Fridel, S. (2010). Relations between attachment styles, ageism and quality of life in late life. *International Psychogeriatrics, 22*(8), 1353–1361.

Boele, S., Graaff, J., Wied, M., Valk, I. E., Crocetti, E., & Branje, S. (2019). Linking parent–child and peer relationship quality to empathy in adolescence: A multilevel meta-analysis. *Journal of Youth and Adolescence, 48*(6), 1033–1055.

Boiger, M., Ceulemans, E., De Leersnyder, J., Uchida, Y., Norasakkunkit, V., & Mesquita, B. (2018). Beyond essentialism: Cultural differences in emotions revisited. *Emotion, 18*(8), 1142–1162.

Boiger, M., Uchida, Y., Norasakkunkit, V., & Mesquita, B. (2016). Protecting autonomy, protecting relatedness: Appraisal patterns of daily anger and shame in the United States and Japan. *Japanese Psychological Research, 58*(1), 28–41.

Boldt, L. J., Goffin, K. C., & Kochanska, G. (2020). The significance of early parent–child attachment for emerging regulation: A longitudinal investigation of processes and mechanisms from toddler age to preadolescence. *Developmental Psychology, 56*(3), 431–443.

Bolier, L., Haverman, M., Westerhof, G., Riper, H., Smit, F., & Bohlmeijer, E. (2013). Positive psychology interventions: A meta-analysis of randomized controlled studies. *BMC Public Health, 13*, 119.

Booth, A. T., Macdonald, J. A., & Youssef, G. J. (2018). Contextual stress and maternal sensitivity: A meta-analytic review of stress associations with the Maternal Behavior Q-Sort in observational studies. *Developmental Review, 48*, 145–177.

Bornstein, M. H., Putnick, D. L., Heslington, M., Gini, M., Suwalsky, J. T. D., Venuti, P., . . . Zingman de Galperín, C. (2008). Mother–child emotional availability in ecological perspective: Three countries, two regions, two genders. *Developmental Psychology, 44*(3), 666–680.

Bowker, J. C., Bowker, M. H., Santo, J. B., Ojo, A. A., Etkin, R. G., & Raja, R. (2019). Severe social withdrawal: Cultural variation in past hikikomori experiences of university students in Nigeria, Singapore, and the United States. *Journal of Genetic Psychology: Research and Theory on Human Development, 180*(4–5), 217–230.

Bowlby, J. (1969). *Attachment and loss: Vol. 1. Attachment.* New York: Basic Books.

Bowlby, J. (1973). *Attachment and loss: Vol. 2. Separation.* New York: Basic Books.

Bowlby, J. (1980). *Attachment and loss: Vol. 3. Loss.* New York: Basic Books.

Bowlby, J. (1988). *A secure base.* New York: Basic Books.

Brackett, M. A., Rivers, S. E., Bertoli, M., & Salovey, P. (2016). Emotional intelligence. In

L. F. Barrett, M. Lewis, & J. M. Haviland-Jones (Eds.), *Handbook of emotions* (4th ed., pp. 513–531). New York: Guilford Press.

Brackett, M. A., Warner, R. M., & Bosco, J. S. (2005). Emotional intelligence and relationship quality among couples. *Personal Relationships, 12*(2), 197–212.

Brady, B., Kneebone, I. I., & Bailey, P. E. (2019). Validation of the Emotion Regulation Questionnaire in older community-dwelling adults. *British Journal of Clinical Psychology, 58*(1), 110–122.

Braga, T., Cunha, O., & Maia, Â. (2018). The enduring effect of maltreatment on antisocial behavior: A meta-analysis of longitudinal studies. *Aggression and Violent Behavior, 40*, 91–100.

Braungart-Rieker, J. M., Hill-Soderlund, A. L., & Karrass, J. (2010). Fear and anger reactivity trajectories from 4 to 16 months: The roles of temperament, regulation, and maternal sensitivity. *Developmental Psychology, 46*(4), 791–804.

Braunstein, L. M., Gross, J. J., & Ochsner, K. N. (2017). Explicit and implicit emotion regulation: A multi-level framework. *Social Cognitive and Affective Neuroscience, 12*(10), 1545–1557.

Brennan, K. A., Clark, C. L., & Shaver, P. R. (1998). Self-report measurement of adult attachment: An integrative overview. In J. A. Simpson & W. S. Rholes (Eds.), *Attachment theory and close relationships* (pp. 46–76). New York: Guilford Press.

Brescoll, V. L., & Uhlmann, E. L. (2008). Can an angry woman get ahead? Status conferral, gender, and expression of emotion in the workplace. *Psychological Science, 19*(3), 268–275.

Bridges, K. M. B. (1930). A genetic theory of the emotions. *Pedagogical Seminary and Journal of Genetic Psychology, 37*, 514–527.

Bridges, K. M. B. (1932). Emotional development in early infancy. *Child Development, 3*, 324–341.

Briggs, E. C., Amaya-Jackson, L., Putnam, K. T., & Putnam, F. W. (2021). All adverse childhood experiences are not equal: The contribution of synergy to adverse childhood experience scores. *American Psychologist, 76*(2), 243–252.

Brinkmeyer, M. Y., & Eyberg, S. M. (2003). Parent–child interaction therapy for oppositional children. In A. E. Kazdin & J. R. Weisz (Eds.), *Evidence-based psychotherapies for children and adolescents* (pp. 204–223). New York: Guilford Press.

Brody, L., Hall, J. A., & Stokes, L. (2016). Gender and emotion: Theory, findings, and context. In L. F. Barrett, M. Lewis, & J. M. Haviland-Jones (Eds.), *Handbook of emotions* (4th ed., pp. 369–392). New York: Guilford Press.

Brooker, R. J., Buss, K. A., Lemery-Chalfant, K., Aksan, N., Davidson, R. J., & Goldsmith, H. H. (2014). Profiles of observed infant anger predict preschool behavior problems: Moderation by life stress. *Developmental Psychology, 50*(10), 2343–2352.

Browne, P., Carr, E., Fleischmann, M., Xue, B., & Stansfeld, S. A. (2019). The relationship between workplace psychosocial environment and retirement intentions and actual retirement: A systematic review. *European Journal of Ageing, 16*(1), 73–82.

Brownell, C. A., Svetlova, M., Anderson, R., Nichols, S. R., & Drummond, J. (2013). Socialization of early prosocial behavior: Parents' talk about emotions is associated with sharing and helping in toddlers. *Infancy, 18*(1), 91–119.

Buchanan, C. M., Eccles, J. S., & Becker, J. B. (1992). Are adolescents the victims of raging hormones? Evidence for activational effects of hormones on moods and behavior at adolescence. *Psychological Bulletin, 111*(1), 62–107.

Bucher, A., Voss, A., Spaniol, J., Hische, A., & Sauer, N. (2020). Age differences in emotion perception in a multiple target setting: An eye-tracking study. *Emotion, 20*(9), 1423-1434.

Budd, K. S., Garbacz, L. L., & Carter, J. S. (2016). Collaborating with public school partners to implement Teacher-Child Interaction Training (TCIT) as universal prevention. *School Mental Health, 8*(2), 207-221.

Buhle, J. T., Silvers, J. A., Wager, T. D., Lopez, R., Onyemekwu, C., Kober, H., . . . Ochsner, K. N. (2014). Cognitive reappraisal of emotion: A meta-analysis of human neuroimaging studies. *Cerebral Cortex, 24*(11), 2981-2990.

Buri, J. R. (1991). Parental Authority Questionnaire. *Journal of Personality Assessment, 57*(1), 110-119.

Burr, D. A., Castrellon, J. J., Zald, D. H., & Samanez-Larkin, G. R. (2021). Emotion dynamics across adulthood in everyday life: Older adults are more emotionally stable and better at regulating desires. *Emotion, 21*(3), 453-464.

Burris, J. L., Barry-Anwar, R. A., & Rivera, S. M. (2017). An eye tracking investigation of attentional biases towards affect in young children. *Developmental Psychology, 53*(8), 1418-1427.

Burris, J. L., Oleas, D., Reider, L., Buss, K. A., Pérez-Edgar, K., & LoBue, V. (2019). Biased attention to threat: Answering old questions with young infants. *Current Directions in Psychological Science, 28*(6), 534-539.

Burriss, L., Powell, D. A., & White, J. (2007). Psychophysiological and subjective indices of emotion as a function of age and gender. *Cognition and Emotion, 21*(1), 182-210.

Buss, K. A. (2011). Which fearful toddlers should we worry about? Context, fear regulation, and anxiety risk. *Developmental Psychology, 47*(3), 804-819.

Buss, K. A., Brooker, R. J., & Leuty, M. (2008). Girls most of the time, boys some of the time: Gender differences in toddlers' use of maternal proximity and comfort seeking. *Infancy, 13*(1), 1-29.

Buss, K. A., Davis, E. L., Ram, N., & Coccia, M. (2018). Dysregulated fear, social inhibition, and respiratory sinus arrhythmia: A replication and extension. *Child Development, 89*(3), e214-e228.

Butler, E. A., Lee, T. L., & Gross, J. J. (2007). Emotion regulation and culture: Are the social consequences of emotion suppression culture-specific? *Emotion, 7*(1), 30-48.

Bye, D., & Pushkar, D. (2009). How need for cognition and perceived control are differentially linked to emotional outcomes in the transition to retirement. *Motivation and Emotion, 33*(3), 320-332.

Cabello, R., Sorrel, M. A., Fernández-Pinto, I., Extremera, N., & Fernández-Berrocal, P. (2016). Age and gender differences in ability emotional intelligence in adults: A cross-sectional study. *Developmental Psychology, 52*(9), 1486-1492.

Cacioppo, J. T., Berntson, G. G., Bechara, A., Tranel, D., & Hawkley, L. C. (2011). Could an aging brain contribute to subjective well-being? The value added by a social neuroscience perspective. In A. Todorov, S. T. Fiske, & D. A. Prentice (Eds.), *Social neuroscience: Toward understanding the underpinnings of the social mind* (pp. 249-262). New York: Oxford University Press.

Calder, A. J., Young, A. W., Keane, J., & Dean, M. (2000). Configural information in facial expression perception. *Journal of Experimental Psychology: Human Perception and Performance, 26*(2), 527-551.

Calhoun, C. D., Helms, S. W., Heilbron, N., Rudolph, K. D., Hastings, P. D., & Prinstein,

M. J. (2014). Relational victimization, friendship, and adolescents' hypothalamic–pituitary–adrenal axis responses to an in vivo social stressor. *Development and Psychopathology, 26*(3), 605–618.

California Surgeon General's Clinical Advisory Committee. (2020). Adverse Childhood Experience Questionnaire for Adults. Available at *www.acesaware.org/wp-content/uploads/2020/02/ACE-Questionnaire-for-Adults-Identified-English.pdf.*

Calkins, S. D. (2002). Does aversive behavior during toddlerhood matter?: The effects of difficult temperament on maternal perceptions and behavior. *Infant Mental Health Journal, 23*(4), 381–402.

Campbell, A., Ruffman, T., Murray, J. E., & Glue, P. (2014). Oxytocin improves emotion recognition for older males. *Neurobiology of Aging, 35*(10), 2246–2248.

Campbell, J., & Gilmore, L. (2007). Intergenerational continuities and discontinuities in parenting styles. *Australian Journal of Psychology, 59*(3), 140–150.

Campos, J. J., & Barrett, K. C. (1985). Toward a new understanding of emotions and their development. In C. E. Izard, J. Kagan, & R. B. Zajonc (Eds.), *Emotions, cognition, and behavior* (pp. 229–263). New York: Cambridge University Press.

Campos, J. J., Barrett, K. C., Lamb, M., Goldsmith, H. H., & Stenberg, C. (1983). Socioemotional development. In P. Mussen (Series Ed.) & M. M. Haith & J. J. Campos (Vol. Eds.), *Handbook of child psychology: Vol. 2. Infancy and developmental psychobiology* (4th ed., pp. 784–915). Hoboken, NJ: Wiley.

Campos, J. J., Frankel, C. B., & Camras, L. (2004). On the nature of emotion regulation. *Child Development, 75*(2), 377–394.

Campos, J. J., Walle, E. A., Dahl, A., & Main, A. (2011). Reconceptualizing emotion regulation. *Emotion Review, 3*(1), 26–35.

Camras, L. A. (1992). Expressive development and basic emotions. *Cognition and Emotion, 6*(3–4), 269–283.

Camras, L. A. (2011). Differentiation, dynamical integration and functional emotional development. *Emotion Review, 3*(2), 138–146.

Camras, L. A. (2019). Facial expressions across the lifespan. In V. LoBue, K. Pérez-Edgar, & K. Buss (Eds.), *Handbook of emotional development* (pp. 83–103). Cham, Switzerland: Springer.

Camras, L. A., Castro, V. L., Halberstadt, A. G., & Shuster, M. M. (2017). Spontaneously produced facial expressions in infants and children. In J.-M. Fernández-Dols & J. A. Russell (Eds.), *The science of facial expression* (2nd ed., pp. 279–296). New York: Oxford University Press.

Camras, L. A., Chen, Y., Bakeman, R., Norris, K., & Cain, T. R. (2006). Culture, ethnicity, and children's facial expressions: A study of European American, mainland Chinese, Chinese American, and adopted Chinese girls. *Emotion, 6*(1), 103–114.

Camras, L. A., Fatani, S., Fraumeni, B., & Shuster, M. (2016). The development of facial expressions: Current perspectives on infant emotions. In L. F. Barrett, M. Lewis, & J. M. Haviland-Jones (Eds.), *Handbook of emotions* (4th ed., pp. 255–271). New York: Guilford Press.

Camras, L. A., Grow, J. G., & Ribordy, S. C. (1983). Recognition of emotional expression by abused children. *Journal of Clinical Child Psychology, 12*(3), 325–328.

Camras, L. A., Oster, H., Bakeman, R., Meng, Z., Ujiie, T., & Campos, J. J. (2007). Do infants show distinct negative facial expressions for fear and anger? Emotional expression in 11-month-old European American, Chinese, and Japanese Infants. *Infancy, 11*(2), 131–155.

Camras, L. A., Oster, H., Campos, J. J., Campos, R., Ujiie, T., Miyake, K., . . . Meng, Z. (1997). Observer judgments of emotion in American, Japanese, and Chinese infants. In K. C. Barrett (Ed.), *The communication of emotion: Current research from diverse perspectives* (pp. 89–105). San Francisco: Jossey-Bass.

Camras, L. A., Oster, H., Campos, J., Campos, R., Ujiie, T., Miyake, K., . . . Meng, Z. (1998). Production of emotional facial expressions in European American, Japanese, and Chinese infants. *Developmental Psychology, 34*(4), 616–628.

Camras, L. A., Ribordy, S., Hill, J., Martino, S., Sachs, V., Spaccarelli, S., & Stefani, R. (1990). Maternal facial behavior and the recognition and production of emotional expression by maltreated and nonmaltreated children. *Developmental Psychology, 26*(2), 304–312.

Camras, L. A., & Shutter, J. M. (2010). Emotional facial expressions in infancy. *Emotion Review, 2*(2), 120–129.

Camras, L. A., Sullivan, J., & Michel, G. (1993). Do infants express discrete emotions? Adult judgments of facial, vocal, and body actions. *Journal of Nonverbal Behavior, 17*(3), 171–186.

Camras, L. A., Sun, K., Fraumeni, B. R., & Li, Y. (2017). Interpretations of parenting by mainland Chinese and U.S. American children. *Parenting: Science and Practice, 17*(4), 262–280.

Camras, L. A., Sun, K., Li, Y., & Wright, M. F. (2012). Do Chinese and American children's interpretations of parenting moderate links between perceived parenting and child adjustment? *Parenting: Science and Practice, 12*(4), 306–327.

Cannon, W. B. (1927). The James–Lange theory of emotion: A critical examination and an alternative theory. *American Journal of Psychology, 39*, 106–124.

Cardinale, E. M., & Marsh, A. A. (2020). The reliability and validity of the Inventory of Callous Unemotional Traits: A meta-analytic review. *Assessment, 27*(1), 57–71.

Carlson, S. M., & Wang, T. S. (2007). Inhibitory control and emotion regulation in preschool children. *Cognitive Development, 22*(4), 489–510.

Caron, A. J., Caron, R. F., & MacLean, D. J. (1988). Infant discrimination of naturalistic emotional expressions: The role of face and voice. *Child Development, 59*(3), 604–616.

Caron, R. F., Caron, A. J., & Myers, R. S. (1982). Abstraction of invariant face expressions in infancy. *Child Development, 53*(4), 1008–1015.

Carstensen, L. L. (2019). Integrating cognitive and emotion paradigms to address the paradox of aging. *Cognition and Emotion, 33*(1), 119–125.

Carstensen, L. L., Isaacowitz, D. M., & Charles, S. T. (1999). Taking time seriously: A theory of socioemotional selectivity. *American Psychologist, 54*(3), 165–181.

Carstensen, L. L., Shavit, Y. Z., & Barnes, J. T. (2020). Age advantages in emotional experience persist even under threat from the COVID-19 pandemic. *Psychological Science, 31*(11), 1374–1385.

Carstensen, L. L., Turan, B., Scheibe, S., Ram, N., Ersner-Hershfield, H., Samanez-Larkin, G. R., . . . Nesselroade, J. R. (2011). Emotional experience improves with age: Evidence based on over 10 years of experience sampling. *Psychology and Aging, 26*(1), 21–33.

Carthy, T., Horesh, N., Apter, A., Edge, M. D., & Gross, J. J. (2010). Emotional reactivity and cognitive regulation in anxious children. *Behaviour Research and Therapy, 48*(5), 384–393.

Casey, B. J. (2015). Beyond simple models of self-control to circuit-based accounts of adolescent behavior. *Annual Review of Psychology, 66*, 295–319.

Casey, B. J., & Caudle, K. (2013). The teenage brain: Self control. *Current Directions in Psychological Science, 22*(2), 82–87.

Casey, B. J., Heller, A. S., Gee, D. G., & Cohen, A. O. (2019). Development of the emotional brain. *Neuroscience Letters, 693*, 29–34.

Caspi, A., & Silva, P. A. (1995). Temperamental qualities at age three predict personality traits in young adulthood: Longitudinal evidence from a birth cohort. *Child Development, 66*(2), 486–498.

Cassano, M., Perry-Parrish, C., & Zeman, J. (2007). Influence of gender on parental socialization of children's sadness regulation. *Social Development, 16*(2), 210–231.

Cassidy, J. (1994). Emotion regulation: Influences of attachment relationships. *Monographs of the Society for Research in Child Development, 59*(2–3), 228–283.

Cassidy, J., & Berlin, L. J. (1994). The insecure/ambivalent pattern of attachment: Theory and research. *Child Development, 65*(4), 971–981.

Castro, V. L., Camras, L. A., Halberstadt, A. G., & Shuster, M. (2018). Children's prototypic facial expressions during emotion-eliciting conversations with their mothers. *Emotion, 18*(2), 260–276.

Castro, V. L., Cheng, Y., Halberstadt, A. G., & Grühn, D. (2016). EUReKA! A conceptual model of emotion understanding. *Emotion Review, 8*(3), 258–268.

Castro, V. L., Halberstadt, A. G., & Garrett-Peters, P. T. (2018). Changing tides: Mothers' supportive emotion socialization relates negatively to third-grade children's social adjustment in school. *Social Development, 27*(3), 510–525.

Castro, V. L., & Nelson, J. A. (2018). Social development quartet: When is parental supportiveness a good thing? The dynamic value of parents' supportive emotion socialization across childhood. *Social Development, 27*(3), 461–465.

Cavanagh, M., Quinn, D., Duncan, D., Graham, T., & Balbuena, L. (2017). Oppositional defiant disorder is better conceptualized as a disorder of emotional regulation. *Journal of Attention Disorders, 21*(5), 381–389.

Cervantes, R. C., & Cordova, D. (2011). Life experiences of Hispanic adolescents: Developmental and language considerations in acculturation stress. *Journal of Community Psychology, 39*(3), 336–352.

Chaby, L., Luherne-du Boullay, V., Chetouani, M., & Plaza, M. (2015). Compensating for age limits through emotional crossmodal integration. *Frontiers in Psychology, 6*, 691.

Chalmers, J. A., Quintana, D. S., Abbott, M. J. A., & Kemp, A. H. (2014). Anxiety disorders are associated with reduced heart rate variability: A meta-analysis. *Frontiers in Psychiatry, 5*, 80.

Chambless, D. L., & Hollon, S. D. (1998). Defining empirically supported therapies. *Journal of Consulting and Clinical Psychology, 66*(1), 7–18.

Chao, R., & Tseng, V. (2002). Parenting of Asians. In M. H. Bornstein (Ed.), *Handbook of parenting: Vol. 4. Social conditions and applied parenting* (2nd ed., pp. 59–93). Mahwah, NJ: Erlbaum.

Chaplin, T. M., & Aldao, A. (2013). Gender differences in emotion expression in children: A meta-analytic review. *Psychological Bulletin, 139*(4), 735–765.

Charles, S. T. (2010). Strength and vulnerability integration: A model of emotional well-being across adulthood. *Psychological Bulletin, 136*(6), 1068–1091.

Charles, S. T., & Luong, G. (2013). Emotional experience across adulthood: The theoretical model of strength and vulnerability integration. *Current Directions in Psychological Science, 22*(6), 443–448.

Charles, S. T., Mather, M., & Carstensen, L. L. (2003). Aging and emotional memory: The forgettable nature of negative images for older adults. *Journal of Experimental Psychology: General, 132*(2), 310-324.

Charles, S. T., Reynolds, C. A., & Gatz, M. (2001). Age-related differences and change in positive and negative affect over 23 years. *Journal of Personality and Social Psychology, 80*(1), 136-151.

Cheah, C. S. L., Yu, J., Liu, J., & Coplan, R. (2019). Children's cognitive appraisal moderates associations between psychologically controlling parenting and children's depressive symptoms. *Journal of Adolescence, 76*, 109-119.

Chen, F. M., Lin, H. S., & Li, C. H. (2012). The role of emotion in parent-child relationships: Children's emotionality, maternal meta-emotion, and children's attachment security. *Journal of Child and Family Studies, 21*(3), 403-410.

Chen, S. H., & Zhou, Q. (2019). Longitudinal relations of cultural orientation and emotional expressivity in Chinese American immigrant parents: Sociocultural influences on emotional development in adulthood. *Developmental Psychology, 55*(5), 1111-1123.

Chen, X. (2000). Growing up in a collectivist culture: Socialization and socioemotional development in Chinese children. In A. L. Comunian & U. P. Gielen (Eds.), *International perspectives on human development* (pp. 331-353). Lengerich, Germany: Pabst Science.

Chen, X. (2019). Culture and shyness in childhood and adolescence. *New Ideas in Psychology, 53*, 58-66.

Chen, X., Cen, G., Li, D., & He, Y. (2005). Social functioning and adjustment in Chinese children: The imprint of historical time. *Child Development, 76*(1), 182-195.

Chen, X., Rubin, K. H., & Li, Z.-Y. (1995). Social functioning and adjustment in Chinese children: A longitudinal study. *Developmental Psychology, 31*(4), 531-539.

Chentsova-Dutton, Y. E., Chu, J. P., Tsai, J. L., Rottenberg, J., Gross, J. J., & Gotlib, I. H. (2007). Depression and emotional reactivity: Variation among Asian Americans of East Asian descent and European Americans. *Journal of Abnormal Psychology, 116*(4), 776-785.

Chentsova-Dutton, Y. E., Tsai, J. L., & Gotlib, I. H. (2010). Further evidence for the cultural norm hypothesis: Positive emotion in depressed and control European American and Asian American women. *Cultural Diversity and Ethnic Minority Psychology, 16*(2), 284-295.

Choi, K. S., Stewart, R., & Dewey, M. (2013). Participation in productive activities and depression among older Europeans: Survey of Health, Ageing and Retirement in Europe (SHARE). *International Journal of Geriatric Psychiatry, 28*(11), 1157-1165.

Chopik, W. J., Edelstein, R. S., & Grimm, K. J. (2019). Longitudinal changes in attachment orientation over a 59-year period. *Journal of Personality and Social Psychology, 116*(4), 598-611.

Chou, K.-L., Lee, T. M. C., & Ho, A. H. Y. (2007). Does mood state change risk taking tendency in older adults? *Psychology and Aging, 22*(2), 310-318.

Cicchetti, D. (2016). Socioemotional, personality, and biological development: Illustrations from a multilevel developmental psychopathology perspective on child maltreatment. *Annual Review of Psychology, 67*, 187-211.

Clarke-Stewart, K. A., Goossens, F. A., & Allhusen, V. D. (2001). Measuring infant-mother attachment: Is the Strange Situation enough? *Social Development, 10*(2), 143-169.

Cohen, J. (1988). *Statistical power analysis for the behavioral sciences.* Hillsdale, NJ: Erlbaum.

Cohen, J. (1992). A power primer. *Psychological Bulletin, 112*(1), 155-159.

Cole, P. M. (1986). Children's spontaneous control of facial expression. *Child Development, 57*(6), 1309-1321.

Cole, P. M., Martin, S. E., & Dennis, T. A. (2004). Emotion regulation as a scientific construct: Methodological challenges and directions for child development research. *Child Development, 75*(2), 317-333.

Cole, P. M., & Tamang, B. L. (1998). Nepali children's ideas about emotional displays in hypothetical challenges. *Developmental Psychology, 34*(4), 640-646.

Cole, P. M., Tamang, B., & Shrestha, S. (2006). Cultural variations in the socialization of young children's anger and shame. *Child Development, 77*(5), 1237-1251.

Cole, P. M., Tan, P. Z., Hall, S. E., Zhang, Y., Crnic, K. A., Blair, C. B., & Li, R. (2011). Developmental changes in anger expression and attention focus: Learning to wait. *Developmental Psychology, 47*(4), 1078-1089.

Collishaw, S., Pickles, A., Messer, J., Rutter, M., Shearer, C., & Maughan, B. (2007). Resilience to adult psychopathology following childhood maltreatment: Evidence from a community sample. *Child Abuse and Neglect, 31*(3), 211-229.

Compas, B. E., Connor-Smith, J., & Jaser, S. S. (2004). Temperament, stress reactivity, and coping: Implications for depression in childhood and adolescence. *Journal of Clinical Child and Adolescent Psychology, 33*(1), 21-31.

Compas, B. E., Jaser, S. S., Bettis, A. H., Watson, K. H., Gruhn, M. A., Dunbar, J. P., . . . Thigpen, J. C. (2017). Coping, emotion regulation, and psychopathology in childhood and adolescence: A meta-analysis and narrative review. *Psychological Bulletin, 143*(9), 939-991.

Condry, J., & Condry, S. (1976). Sex differences: A study of the eye of the beholder. *Child Development, 47*(3), 812-819.

Cong, Y.-Q., Junge, C., Aktar, E., Raijmakers, M., Franklin, A., & Sauter, D. (2019). Preverbal infants perceive emotional facial expressions categorically. *Cognition and Emotion, 33*(3), 391-403.

Consedine, N. S., & Magai, C. (2003). Attachment and emotion experience in later life: The view from emotions theory. *Attachment and Human Development, 5*(2), 165-187.

Consedine, N. S., & Magai, C. (2006, July). *Patterns of attachment and attachment change in later life: Preliminary results from a longitudinal study of 415 older adults.* Paper presented at the Third Biennial Conference of the International Association for Relationship Research, Crete, Greece.

Cooke, J. E., Kochendorfer, L. B., Stuart-Parrigon, K. L., Koehn, A. J., & Kerns, K. A. (2019). Parent-child attachment and children's experience and regulation of emotion: A meta-analytic review. *Emotion, 19*(6), 1103-1126.

Cordaro, D. T., Keltner, D., Tshering, S., Wangchuk, D., & Flynn, L. M. (2016). The voice conveys emotion in ten globalized cultures and one remote village in Bhutan. *Emotion, 16*(1), 117-128.

Cordaro, D. T., Sun, R., Keltner, D., Kamble, S., Huddar, N., & McNeil, G. (2018). Universals and cultural variations in 22 emotional expressions across five cultures. *Emotion, 18*(1), 75-93.

Costa, P. T., & McCrae, R. R. (1992). Normal personality assessment in clinical practice: The NEO Personality Inventory. *Psychological Assessment, 4*(1), 5-13.

Costa, P. T., Jr., McCrae, R. R., & Löckenhoff, C. E. (2019). Personality across the life span. *Annual Review of Psychology, 70*, 423-448.

Costa, P. T., Jr., Terracciano, A., & McCrae, R. R. (2001). Gender differences in personality traits across cultures: Robust and surprising findings. *Journal of Personality and Social Psychology, 81*(2), 322-331.

Costello, E. J., Egger, H. L., & Angold, A. (2005). The developmental epidemiology of anxiety disorders: Phenomenology, prevalence, and comorbidity. *Child and Adolescent Psychiatric Clinics of North America, 14*(4), 631–648.

Cowen, A. S., Elfenbein, H. A., Laukka, P., & Keltner, D. (2019). Mapping 24 emotions conveyed by brief human vocalization. *American Psychologist, 74*(6), 698–712.

Cowen, A. S., Laukka, P., Elfenbein, H. A., Liu, R., & Keltner, D. (2019). The primacy of categories in the recognition of 12 emotions in speech prosody across two cultures. *Nature Human Behavior, 3*(4), 369–382.

Craig, B. M., & Lipp, O. V. (2018). The influence of multiple social categories on emotion perception. *Journal of Experimental Social Psychology, 75*, 27–35.

Crick, N. R., & Dodge, K. A. (1994). A review and reformulation of social information-processing mechanisms in children's social adjustment. *Psychological Bulletin, 115*(1), 74–101.

Cui, L., Morris, A. S., Harrist, A. W., Larzelere, R. E., Criss, M. M., & Houltberg, B. J. (2015). Adolescent RSA responses during an anger discussion task: Relations to emotion regulation and adjustment. *Emotion, 15*(3), 360–372.

Cummings, E. M., & Davies, P. (1996). Emotional security as a regulatory process in normal development and the development of psychopathology. *Development and Psychopathology, 8*(1), 123–139.

Cummings, E. M., El-Sheikh, M., Kouros, C. D., & Buckhalt, J. A. (2009). Children and violence: The role of children's regulation in the marital aggression–child adjustment link. *Clinical Child and Family Psychology Review, 12*(1), 3–15.

Cummings, E. M., & Miller-Graff, L. E. (2015). Emotional security theory: An emerging theoretical model for youths' psychological and physiological responses across multiple developmental contexts. *Current Directions in Psychological Science, 24*(3), 208–213.

Curtis, V., de Barra, M., & Aunger, R. (2011). Disgust as an adaptive system for disease avoidance behaviour. *Philosophical Transactions of the Royal Society of London: Series B. Biological Sciences, 366*(1563), 389–401.

Dagan, O., & Sagi-Schwartz, A. (2018). Early attachment network with mother and father: An unsettled issue. *Child Development Perspectives, 12*(2), 115–121.

Damasio, A. (1994). *Descartes' error: Emotion, reason, and the human brain.* New York: Putnam.

Darwin, C. (1998). *The expression of the emotions in man and animals* (3rd ed., with introduction, afterword, and commentaries by P. Ekman). New York: Oxford University Press. (Original work published 1872)

D'Avanzato, C., Joormann, J., Siemer, M., & Gotlib, I. H. (2013). Emotion regulation in depression and anxiety: Examining diagnostic specificity and stability of strategy use. *Cognitive Therapy and Research, 37*(5), 968–980.

Davidov, M., Zahn-Waxler, C., Roth-Hanania, R., & Knafo, A. (2013). Concern for others in the first year of life: Theory, evidence, and avenues for research. *Child Development Perspectives, 7*(2), 126–131.

Davidson, B., Davis, E., Cadenas, H., Barnett, M., Sanchez, B., Gonzalez, J., & Jent, J. (2021). Universal teacher–child interaction training in early special education: A pilot cluster-randomized control trial. *Behavior Therapy, 52*(2), 379–393.

Davies, P. T., & Cummings, E. M. (1994). Marital conflict and child adjustment: An emotional security hypothesis. *Psychological Bulletin, 116*(3), 387–411.

Davis, M. (1992). The role of the amygdala in fear and anxiety. *Annual Review of Neuroscience, 15*, 353–375.

De Bellis, M. D., & Hooper, S. R. (2012). Neural substrates for processing task-irrelevant emotional distracters in maltreated adolescents with depressive disorders: A pilot study. *Journal of Traumatic Stress, 25*(2), 198–202.

De France, K., & Hollenstein, T. (2017). Assessing emotion regulation repertoires: The Regulation of Emotion Systems Survey. *Personality and Individual Differences, 119,* 204–215.

De France, K., & Hollenstein, T. (2019). Emotion regulation and relations to well-being across the lifespan. *Developmental Psychology, 55*(8), 1768–1774.

De Leersnyder, J., Kim, H., & Mesquita, B. (2020). My emotions belong here and there: Extending the phenomenon of emotional acculturation to heritage cultural contexts. *Cognition and Emotion, 34*(8), 1573–1590.

De Vaus, J., Hornsey, M. J., Kuppens, P., & Bastian, B. (2018). Exploring the East–West divide in prevalence of affective disorder: A case for cultural differences in coping with negative emotion. *Personality and Social Psychology Review, 22*(3), 285–304.

De Wolff, M., & van IJzendoorn, M. H. (1997). Sensitivity and attachment: A meta-analysis on parental antecedents of infant attachment. *Child Development, 68*(4), 571–591.

Decety, J. (2011). Dissecting the neural mechanisms mediating empathy. *Emotion Review, 3*(1), 92–108.

Decety, J., & Michalska, K. (2020). A developmental neuroscience perspective on empathy. In J. Rubenstein & P. Rakic (Eds.), *Neural circuit and cognitive development* (2nd ed., pp. 485–522). London: Academic Press.

DeCicco, J. M., O'Toole, L. J., & Dennis, T. A. (2014). The late positive potential as a neural signature for cognitive reappraisal in children. *Developmental Neuropsychology, 39*(7), 497–515.

DeLoache, J. S., & LoBue, V. (2009). The narrow fellow in the grass: Human infants associate snakes and fear. *Developmental Science, 12*(1), 201–207.

Denham, S. A. (1986). Social cognition, prosocial behavior, and emotion in preschoolers: Contextual validation. *Child Development, 57*(1), 194–201.

Denham, S. A. (2019). Emotional competence during childhood and adolescence. In V. LoBue, K. Pérez-Edgar, & K. Buss (Eds.), *Handbook of emotional development* (pp. 493–541). Cham, Switzerland: Springer.

Denham, S. A., & Brown, C. (2010). "Plays nice with others": Social-emotional learning and academic success. *Early Education and Development, 21*(5), 652–680.

Denham, S. A., & Grout, L. (1993). Socialization of emotion: Pathway to preschoolers' emotional and social competence. *Journal of Nonverbal Behavior, 17*(3), 205–227.

Dewey, J. (1971). The theory of emotion. In J. A. Boyle (Ed.), *John Dewey: The early works* (pp. 152–169). Carbondale: Southern Illinois University Press. (Original work published 1894)

DiBiase, R., & Lewis, M. (1997). The relation between temperament and embarrassment. *Cognition and Emotion, 11*(3), 259–271.

Dickerson, S. S., & Kemeny, M. E. (2004). Acute stressors and cortisol responses: A theoretical integration and synthesis of laboratory research. *Psychological Bulletin, 130*(3), 355–391.

Dickson, K. L., Walker, H., & Fogel, A. (1997). The relationship between smile type and play type during parent–infant play. *Developmental Psychology, 33*(6), 925–933.

Dieleman, G. C., Huizink, A. C., Tulen, J. H. M., Utens, E. M. W. J., Creemers, H. E., van der Ende, J., & Verhulst, F. C. (2015). Alterations in HPA-axis and autonomic nervous system functioning in childhood anxiety disorders point to a chronic stress hypothesis. *Psychoneuroendocrinology, 51,* 135–150.

Diener, E. (1984). Subjective well-being. *Psychological Bulletin, 95*(3), 542–575.

Diener, E., Diener, C., Choi, H., & Oishi, S. (2018). Revisiting "Most people are happy"— and discovering when they are not. *Perspectives on Psychological Science, 13*(2), 166–170.

Diener, E., Seligman, M. E., Choi, H., & Oishi, S. (2018). Happiest people revisited. *Perspectives on Psychological Science, 13*(2), 176–184.

DiGirolamo, M. A., & Russell, J. A. (2017). The emotion seen in a face can be a methodological artifact: The process of elimination hypothesis. *Emotion, 17*(3), 538–546.

Do, K. T., Sharp, P. B., & Telzer, E. H. (2020). Modernizing conceptions of valuation and cognitive-control deployment in adolescent risk taking. *Current Directions in Psychological Science, 29*(1), 102–109.

Dodge, K. A., & Coie, J. D. (1987). Social-information-processing factors in reactive and proactive aggression in children's peer groups. *Journal of Personality and Social Psychology, 53*(6), 1146–1158.

Doebel, S., Michaelson, L. E., & Munakata, Y. (2020). Good things come to those who wait: Delaying gratification likely does matter for later achievement (A commentary on Watts, Duncan, & Quan, 2018). *Psychological Science, 31*(1), 97–99.

Dollar, J. M., & Calkins, S. (2019). The development of anger. In V. LoBue, K. Pérez-Edgar, & K. Buss (Eds.), *Handbook of emotional development* (pp. 199–226). Cham, Switzerland: Springer.

Dollar, J. M., Calkins, S. D., Berry, N. T., Perry, N. B., Keane, S. P., Shanahan, L., & Wideman, L. (2020). Developmental patterns of respiratory sinus arrhythmia from toddlerhood to adolescence. *Developmental Psychology, 56*(4), 783–794.

Domitrovich, C. E., Durlak, J. A., Staley, K. C., & Weissberg, R. P. (2017). Social-emotional competence: An essential factor for promoting positive adjustment and reducing risk in school children. *Child Development, 88*(2), 408–416.

Domitrovich, C. E., Greenberg, M., Cortes, R., & Kusche, C. (2004). *The Preschool/Kindergarten PATHS curriculum.* Deerfield, MA: Channing-Bete.

Dondi, M., Gervasi, M., Valente, A., Vacca, T., Borana, G., Bellis, I., . . . Oster, H. (2014). *Spontaneous facial expressions of distress in fetuses.* Paper presented at the 14th European Conference on Facial Expression, Lisboa, Portugal.

Dong, Q., Yang, B., & Ollendick, T. H. (1994). Fears in Chinese children and adolescents and their relations to anxiety and depression. *Child Psychology and Psychiatry and Allied Disciplines, 35*(2), 351–363.

Dougherty, L. R., Klein, D. N., Durbin, C. E., Hayden, E. P., & Olino, T. M. (2010). Temperamental positive and negative emotionality and children's depressive symptoms: A longitudinal prospective study from age three to age ten. *Journal of Social and Clinical Psychology, 29*(4), 462–488.

Dryman, M. T., & Heimberg, R. G. (2018). Emotion regulation in social anxiety and depression: A systematic review of expressive suppression and cognitive reappraisal. *Clinical Psychology Review, 65,* 17–42.

Dudeney, J., Sharpe, L., & Hunt, C. (2015). Attentional bias towards threatening stimuli in children with anxiety: A meta-analysis. *Clinical Psychology Review, 40,* 66–75.

Duncombe, M. E., Havighurst, S. S., Holland, K. A., & Frankling, E. J. (2012). The contribution of parenting practices and parent emotion factors in children at risk for disruptive behavior disorders. *Child Psychiatry and Human Development, 43*(5), 715–733.

Dunn, J., Bretherton, I., & Munn, P. (1987). Conversations about feeling states between mothers and their young children. *Developmental Psychology, 23*(1), 132–139.

Dunn, J., & Brown, J. (1994). Affect expression in the family, children's understanding of emotions, and their interactions with others. *Merrill-Palmer Quarterly, 40*(1), 120–137.

Dunn, J., Brown, J., & Beardsall, L. (1991). Family talk about feeling states and children's later understanding of others' emotions. *Developmental Psychology, 27*(3), 448–455.

Dunsmore, J. C., Booker, J. A., & Ollendick, T. H. (2013). Parental emotion coaching and child emotion regulation as protective factors for children with oppositional defiant disorder. *Social Development, 22*(3), 444–466.

Duran, C. A. K., & Grissmer, D. W. (2020). Choosing immediate over delayed gratification correlates with better school-related outcomes in a sample of children of color from low-income families. *Developmental Psychology, 56*(6), 1107–1120.

Durán, J. I., Reisenzein, R., & Fernández-Dols, J.-M. (2017). Coherence between emotions and facial expressions: A research synthesis. In J.-M. Fernández-Dols & J. A. Russell (Eds.), *The science of facial expression* (pp. 107–129). New York: Oxford University Press.

Dweck, C. S., & Leggett, E. L. (1988). A social-cognitive approach to motivation and personality. *Psychological Review, 95*(2), 256–273.

Dykas, M. J., Woodhouse, S. S., Cassidy, J., & Waters, H. S. (2006). Narrative assessment of attachment representations: Links between secure base scripts and adolescent attachment. *Attachment and Human Development, 8*(3), 221–240.

Dykas, M. J., Ziv, Y., & Cassidy, J. (2008). Attachment and peer relations in adolescence. *Attachment and Human Development, 10*(2), 123–141.

Ebner, N. C., Freund, A. M., & Baltes, P. B. (2006). Developmental changes in personal goal orientation from young to late adulthood: From striving for gains to maintenance and prevention of losses. *Psychology and Aging, 21*(4), 664–678.

Ebner, N. C., He, Y., & Johnson, M. K. (2011). Age and emotion affect how we look at a face: Visual scan patterns differ for own-age versus other-age emotional faces. *Cognition and Emotion, 25*(6), 983–997.

Ebner, N. C., Johnson, M. K., & Fischer, H. (2012). Neural mechanisms of reading facial emotions in young and older adults. *Frontiers in Psychology, 3*, 223.

Edwards, S. L., Rapee, R. M., & Kennedy, S. (2010). Prediction of anxiety symptoms in preschool-aged children: Examination of maternal and paternal perspectives. *Journal of Child Psychology and Psychiatry, 51*(3), 313–321.

Eichorn, D. H., Clausen, J. A., Haan, N., Honzik, M. P., & Mussen, P. H. (1981). *Present and past in middle life.* New York: Academic Press.

Eisenberg, N., Cumberland, A., & Spinrad, T. L. (1998). Parental socialization of emotion. *Psychological Inquiry, 9*(4), 241–273.

Eisenberg, N., Cumberland, A., Spinrad, T. L., Fabes, R. A., Shepard, S. A., Reiser, M., . . . Guthrie, I. K. (2001). The relations of regulation and emotionality to children's externalizing and internalizing problem behavior. *Child Development, 72*(4), 1112–1134.

Eisenberg, N., Fabes, R. A., Guthrie, I. K., Murphy, B. C., Maszk, P., Holmgren, R., & Suh, K. (1996). The relations of regulation and emotionality to problem behavior in elementary school children. *Development and Psychopathology, 8*(1), 141–162.

Eisenberg, N., Hofer, C., Sulik, M. J., & Spinrad, T. L. (2014). Self-regulation, effortful control, and their socioemotional correlates. In J. J. Gross (Ed.), *Handbook of emotion regulation* (2nd ed., pp. 157–172). New York: Guilford Press.

Eisenberg, N., Smith, C. L., & Spinrad, T. L. (2014). Effortful control: Relations with emotion regulation, adjustment, and socialization in childhood. In K. D. Vohs & R.

F. Baumeister (Eds.), *Handbook of self-regulation: Research, theory, and applications* (2nd ed., pp. 263–283). New York: Guilford Press.

Eisenberg, N., Spinrad, T. L., & Cumberland, A. (1998). The socialization of emotion: Reply to commentaries. *Psychological Inquiry, 9*(4), 317–333.

Eisenberg, N., Spinrad, T. L., & Eggum, N. D. (2010). Emotion-related self-regulation and its relation to children's maladjustment. *Annual Review of Clinical Psychology, 6,* 495–525.

Eisenberg, N., Spinrad, T. L., Taylor, Z. E., & Liew, J. (2019). Relations of inhibition and emotion-related parenting to young children's prosocial and vicariously induced distress behavior. *Child Development, 90*(3), 846–858.

Eisenberg, N., VanSchyndel, S. K., & Hofer, C. (2015). The association of maternal socialization in childhood and adolescence with adult offsprings' sympathy/caring. *Developmental Psychology, 51*(1), 7–16.

Ekman, P. (1971). Universals and cultural differences in facial expressions of emotion. *Nebraska Symposium on Motivation, 19,* 207–283.

Ekman, P., & Cordaro, D. (2011). What is meant by calling emotions basic. *Emotion Review, 3*(4), 364–370.

Ekman, P., Davidson, R. J., & Friesen, W. V. (1990). The Duchenne smile: Emotional expression and brain physiology: II. *Journal of Personality and Social Psychology, 58*(2), 342–353.

Ekman, P., & Friesen, W. V. (1969). The repertoire of nonverbal behavior: Categories, origins, usage, and coding. *Semiotica, 1*(1), 49–98.

Ekman, P., & Friesen, W. V. (1971). Constants across cultures in the face and emotion. *Journal of Personality and Social Psychology, 17*(2), 124–129.

Ekman, P., & Friesen, W. V. (1975). *Unmasking the face: A guide to recognizing emotions from facial clues.* Oxford, UK: Prentice-Hall.

Ekman, P., Friesen, W. V., & Hager, J. (2002). *Facial Action Coding System* (2nd ed.). Salt Lake City, UT: Research Nexus.

Ekman, P., Sorenson, E. R., & Friesen, W. V. (1969). Pan-cultural elements in facial displays of emotion. *Science, 164*(3875), 86–88.

El-Sheikh, M., Arsiwalla, D. D., Hinnant, J. B., & Erath, S. A. (2011). Children's internalizing symptoms: The role of interactions between cortisol and respiratory sinus arrhythmia. *Physiology and Behavior, 103*(2), 225–232.

El-Sheikh, M., Erath, S. A., Buckhalt, J. A., Granger, D. A., & Mize, J. (2008). Cortisol and children's adjustment: The moderating role of sympathetic nervous system activity. *Journal of Abnormal Child Psychology, 36*(4), 601–611.

Eldesouky, L., & English, T. (2018). Another year older, another year wiser? Emotion regulation strategy selection and flexibility across adulthood. *Psychology and Aging, 33*(4), 572–585.

Eldesouky, L., & English, T. (2019). Individual differences in emotion regulation goals: Does personality predict the reasons why people regulate their emotions? *Journal of Personality, 87*(4), 750–766.

Elfenbein, H. A. (2017). Emotional dialects in the language of emotion. In J.-M. Fernández-Dols & J. A. Russell (Eds.), *The science of facial expression* (pp. 479–496). New York: Oxford University Press.

Elfenbein, H. A., & Ambady, N. (2002). On the universality and cultural specificity of emotion recognition: A meta-analysis. *Psychological Bulletin, 128*(2), 203–235.

Elfenbein, H. A., Beaupré, M., Lévesque, M., & Hess, U. (2007). Toward a dialect theory:

Cultural differences in the expression and recognition of posed facial expressions. *Emotion, 7*(1), 131–146.

Elliott, M. L., Knodt, A. R., Caspi, A., Moffitt, T. E., & Hariri, A. R. (2021). Need for psychometric theory in neuroscience research and training: Reply to Kragel et al. (2021). *Psychological Science, 32*(4), 627–629.

Elliott, M. L., Knodt, A. R., Ireland, D., Morris, M. L., Poulton, R., Ramrakha, S., . . . Hariri, A. R. (2020). What is the test–retest reliability of common task-functional MRI measures? New empirical evidence and a meta-analysis. *Psychological Science, 31*(7), 792–806.

Ellis, B. J., Bianchi, J., Griskevicius, V., & Frankenhuis, W. E. (2017). Beyond risk and protective factors: An adaptation-based approach to resilience. *Perspectives on Psychological Science, 12*(4), 561–587.

Ellis, R., Seal, M., Simmons, J., Whittle, S., Schwartz, O., Byrne, M., & Allen, N. (2017). Longitudinal trajectories of depression symptoms in adolescence: Psychosocial risk factors and outcomes. *Child Psychiatry and Human Development, 48,* 554–571.

Else-Quest, N. M., Higgins, A., Allison, C., & Morton, L. C. (2012). Gender differences in self-conscious emotional experience: A meta-analysis. *Psychological Bulletin, 138*(5), 947–981.

Else-Quest, N. M., Hyde, J. S., Goldsmith, H. H., & Van Hulle, C. A. (2006). Gender differences in temperament: A meta-analysis. *Psychological Bulletin, 132*(1), 33–72.

Emde, R. N., & Koenig, K. L. (1969). Neonatal smiling and rapid eye movement states. *Journal of the American Academy of Child Psychiatry, 8*(1), 57–67.

England-Mason, G., & Gonzalez, A. (2020). Intervening to shape children's emotion regulation: A review of emotion socialization parenting programs for young children. *Emotion, 20*(1), 98–104.

English, T., Lee, I. A., John, O. P., & Gross, J. J. (2017). Emotion regulation strategy selection in daily life: The role of social context and goals. *Motivation and Emotion, 41*(2), 230–242.

Evans, D. E., & Rothbart, M. K. (2007). Developing a model for adult temperament. *Journal of Research in Personality, 41*(4), 868–888.

Eyberg, S. M., Nelson, M. M., & Boggs, S. R. (2008). Evidence-based psychosocial treatments for children and adolescents with disruptive behavior. *Journal of Clinical Child and Adolescent Psychology, 37*(1), 215–237.

Ezpeleta, L., Granero, R., de la Osa, N., & Domènech, J. M. (2015). Clinical characteristics of preschool children with oppositional defiant disorder and callous–unemotional traits. *PLOS ONE, 10*(9), e0139346.

Fabes, R. A., Poulin, R. E., Eisenberg, N., & Madden-Derdich, D. A. (2002). The Coping with Children's Negative Emotions Scale (CCNES): Psychometric properties and relations with children's emotional competence. *Marriage and Family Review, 34*(3–4), 285–310.

Fabris, M. A., Marengo, D., Longobardi, C., & Settanni, M. (2020). Investigating the links between fear of missing out, social media addiction, and emotional symptoms in adolescence: The role of stress associated with neglect and negative reactions on social media. *Addictive Behaviors, 106.*

Falk, A., Kosse, F., & Pinger, P. (2020). Re-revisiting the marshmallow test: A direct comparison of studies by Shoda, Mischel, and Peake (1990) and Watts, Duncan, and Quan (2018). *Psychological Science, 31*(1), 100–104.

Farroni, T., Menon, E., Rigato, S., & Johnson, M. H. (2007). The perception of facial expressions in newborns. *European Journal of Developmental Psychology, 4*(1), 2–13.

Fearon, R. P., Bakermans-Kranenburg, M. J., van IJzendoorn, M. H., Lapsley, A.-M., & Roisman, G. I. (2010). The significance of insecure attachment and disorganization in the development of children's externalizing behavior: A meta-analytic study. *Child Development, 81*(2), 435–456.

Felitti, V. J., Anda, R. F., Nordenberg, D., Williamson, D. F., Spitz, A. M., Edwards, V., . . . Marks, J. S. (1998). Relationship of childhood abuse and household dysfunction to many of the leading causes of death in adults: The Adverse Childhood Experiences (ACE) Study. *American Journal of Preventive Medicine, 14*(4), 245–258.

Fernald, A. (1993). Approval and disapproval: Infant responsiveness to vocal affect in familiar and unfamiliar languages. *Child Development, 64*(3), 657–674.

Fernández-Dols, J.-M., & Crivelli, C. (2013). Emotion and expression: Naturalistic studies. *Emotion Review, 5*(1), 24–29.

Fernández-Dols, J.-M., & Russell, J. A. (2017). Introduction. In J.-M. Fernández-Dols & J. A. Russell (Eds.), *The science of facial expression* (pp. 3–14). New York: Oxford University Press.

Field, T., Hernandez-Reif, M., Diego, M., Feijo, L., Vera, Y., Gil, K., & Sanders, C. (2007). Still-face and separation effects on depressed mother–infant interactions. *Infant Mental Health Journal, 28*(3), 314–323.

Field, T. M., Woodson, R., Greenberg, R., & Cohen, D. (1982). Discrimination and imitation of facial expressions by neonates. *Science, 218*(4568), 179–181.

Figueiredo, P., Ramião, E., Azeredo, A., Moreira, D., Barroso, R., & Barbosa, F. (2020). Relation between basal cortisol and reactivity cortisol with externalizing problems: A systematic review. *Physiology and Behavior, 225*.

Fishbein, D. H., Domitrovich, C., Williams, J., Gitukui, S., Guthrie, C., Shapiro, D., & Greenberg, M. (2016). Short-term intervention effects of the PATHS curriculum in young low-income children: Capitalizing on plasticity. *Journal of Primary Prevention, 37*(6), 493–511.

Fitzgerald, J. M., Phan, K. L., Kennedy, A. E., Shankman, S. A., Langenecker, S. A., & Klumpp, H. (2017). Prefrontal and amygdala engagement during emotional reactivity and regulation in generalized anxiety disorder. *Journal of Affective Disorders, 218*, 398–406.

Fivush, R. (1991). Gender and emotion in mother–child conversations about the past. *Journal of Narrative and Life History, 1*(4), 325–341.

Flom, M., White, D., Ganiban, J., & Saudino, K. J. (2020). Longitudinal links between callous–unemotional behaviors and parenting in early childhood: A genetically informed design. *Journal of the American Academy of Child and Adolescent Psychiatry, 59*(3), 401–409.

Fogel, A., Hsu, H.-C., Shapiro, A. F., Nelson-Goens, G. C., & Secrist, C. (2006). Effects of normal and perturbed social play on the duration and amplitude of different types of infant smiles. *Developmental Psychology, 42*(3), 459–473.

Fogel, A., Nwokah, E., Dedo, J. Y., Messinger, D., Dickson, K. L., Matusov, E., & Holt, S. A. (1992). Social process theory of emotion: A dynamic systems approach. *Social Development, 1*(2), 122–142.

Fogel, A., & Thelen, E. (1987). Development of early expressive and communicative action: Reinterpreting the evidence from a dynamic systems perspective. *Developmental Psychology, 23*(6), 747–761.

Fölster, M., Hess, U., & Werheid, K. (2014). Facial age affects emotional expression decoding. *Frontiers in Psychology, 5*, 30.

Ford, B. Q., & Troy, A. S. (2019). Reappraisal reconsidered: A closer look at the costs of an acclaimed emotion-regulation strategy. *Current Directions in Psychological Science, 28*(2), 195–203.

Foul, Y. A., Eitan, R., & Aviezer, H. (2018). Perceiving emotionally incongruent cues from faces and bodies: Older adults get the whole picture. *Psychology and Aging, 33*(4), 660–666.

Fox, N. A., Henderson, H. A., Rubin, K. H., Calkins, S. D., & Schmidt, L. A. (2001). Continuity and discontinuity of behavioral inhibition and exuberance: Psychophysiological and behavioral influences across the first four years of life. *Child Development, 72*(1), 1–21.

Fox, N. A., Snidman, N., Haas, S. A., Degnan, K. A., & Kagan, J. (2015). The relations between reactivity at 4 months and behavioral inhibition in the second year: Replication across three independent samples. *Infancy, 20*(1), 98–114.

Fraley, R. C., Waller, N. G., & Brennan, K. A. (2000). An item response theory analysis of self-report measures of adult attachment. *Journal of Personality and Social Psychology, 78*(2), 350–365.

Franz, C. E., Spoon, K., Thompson, W., Hauger, R. L., Hellhammer, D. H., Jacobson, K. C., . . . Kremen, W. S. (2013). Adult cognitive ability and socioeconomic status as mediators of the effects of childhood disadvantage on salivary cortisol in aging adults. *Psychoneuroendocrinology, 38*(10), 2127–2139.

Fredrickson, B. L. (1998). What good are positive emotions? *Review of General Psychology, 2*(3), 300–319.

Fredrickson, B. L. (2013). Positive emotions broaden and build. In E. A. Plant & P. Devine (Eds.), *Advances in experimental social psychology* (Vol. 47, pp. 1–53). Burlington, VT: Academic Press.

Fredrickson, B. L., & Branigan, C. (2005). Positive emotions broaden the scope of attention and thought-action repertoires. *Cognition and Emotion, 19*(3), 313–332.

Fredrickson, B. L., & Cohn, M. A. (2008). Positive emotions. In M. Lewis, J. M. Haviland-Jones, & L. F. Barrett (Eds.), *Handbook of emotions* (3rd ed., pp. 777–796). New York: Guilford Press.

Fredrickson, B. L., Cohn, M. A., Coffey, K. A., Pek, J., & Finkel, S. M. (2008). Open hearts build lives: Positive emotions, induced through loving-kindness meditation, build consequential personal resources. *Journal of Personality and Social Psychology, 95*(5), 1045–1062.

Fredrickson, B. L., & Levenson, R. W. (1998). Positive emotions speed recovery from the cardiovascular sequelae of negative emotions. *Cognition and Emotion, 12*(2), 191–220.

Freedman, V. A., Cornman, J. C., Carr, D., & Lucas, R. E. (2019). Late life disability and experienced wellbeing: Are economic resources a buffer? *Disability and Health Journal, 12*(3), 481–488.

Frenkel, T. I., Fox, N. A., Pine, D. S., Walker, O. L., Degnan, K. A., & Chronis-Tuscano, A. (2015). Early childhood behavioral inhibition, adult psychopathology and the buffering effects of adolescent social networks: A twenty-year prospective study. *Journal of Child Psychology and Psychiatry, 56*(10), 1065–1073.

Freud, S. (1930). *Civilization and its discontents*. Oxford, UK: Hogarth Press

Frick, P. J. (2004). The Inventory of Callous–Unemotional Traits. Retrieved from http://labs.uno.edu/developmental-psychopathology/ICU.html.

Frick, P. J., & White, S. F. (2008). Research review: The importance of callous–unemotional traits for developmental models of aggressive and antisocial behavior. *Journal of Child Psychology and Psychiatry, 49*(4), 359–375.

Fulkerson, A. L., & Waxman, S. R. (2007). Words (but not tones) facilitate object categorization: Evidence from 6- and 12-month-olds. *Cognition, 105*(1), 218-228.

Fung, H. (1999). Becoming a moral child: The socialization of shame among young Chinese children. *Ethos, 27*(2), 180-209.

Fung, H. H., Carstensen, L. L., & Lang, F. R. (2001). Age-related patterns in social networks among European Americans and African Americans: Implications for socioemotional selectivity across the life span. *International Journal of Aging and Human Development, 52*(3), 185-206.

Fung, H. H., Gong, X., Ngo, N., & Isaacowitz, D. M. (2019). Cultural differences in the age-related positivity effect: Distinguishing between preference and effectiveness. *Emotion, 19*(8), 1414-1424.

Gaffey, A. E., Bergeman, C. S., Clark, L. A., & Wirth, M. M. (2016). Aging and the HPA axis: Stress and resilience in older adults. *Neuroscience and Biobehavioral Reviews, 68*, 928-945.

Gallegos, J. M., Vescio, T. K., & Shields, S. A. (2019). Perceived morality determines the acceptability of stereotypic feminine emotional displays in men. *Psychology of Men and Masculinities, 20*(4), 623-636.

Gallo, E. A. G., Munhoz, T. N., de Mola, C. L., & Murray, J. (2018). Gender differences in the effects of childhood maltreatment on adult depression and anxiety: A systematic review and meta-analysis. *Child Abuse and Neglect, 79*, 107-114.

Garnefski, N., Legerstee, J., Kraaij, V., van den Kommer, T., & Teerds, J. (2002). Cognitive coping strategies and symptoms of depression and anxiety: A comparison between adolescents and adults. *Journal of Adolescence, 25*(6), 603-611.

Garner, P. W., Dunsmore, J. C., & Southam-Gerrow, M. (2008). Mother-child conversations about emotions: Linkages to child aggression and prosocial behavior. *Social Development, 17*(2), 259-277.

Garrison, J. (2003). Dewey's theory of emotions: The unity of thought and emotion in naturalistic functional "co-ordination" of behavior. *Transactions of the Charles S. Peirce Society, 39*(3), 405-443.

Gartstein, M. A., & Rothbart, M. K. (2003). Studying infant temperament via the Revised Infant Behavior Questionnaire. *Infant Behavior and Development, 26*(1), 64-86.

Gaspar, A., & Esteves, F. G. (2012). Preschooler's faces in spontaneous emotional contexts: How well do they match adult facial expression prototypes? *International Journal of Behavioral Development, 36*(5), 348-357.

Gee, D. G., Humphreys, K. L., Flannery, J., Goff, B., Telzer, E. H., Shapiro, M., . . . Tottenham, N. (2013). A developmental shift from positive to negative connectivity in human amygdala-prefrontal circuitry. *Journal of Neuroscience, 33*(10), 4584-4593.

Gendron, M., Hoemann, K., Crittenden, A. N., Mangola, S., Ruark, G. A., & Barrett, L. F. (2020). Emotion perception in Hadza hunter-gatherers. *Nature Research: Scientific Reports, 10*, 3867.

Gershenson, R. A., Lyon, A. R., & Budd, K. S. (2010). Promoting positive interactions in the classroom: Adapting parent-child interaction therapy as a universal prevention program. *Education and Treatment of Children, 33*(2), 261-287.

Gerstorf, D., Ram, N., Estabrook, R., Schupp, J., Wagner, G. G., & Lindenberger, U. (2008). Life satisfaction shows terminal decline in old age: Longitudinal evidence from the German Socio-Economic Panel Study (SOEP). *Developmental Psychology, 44*(4), 1148-1159.

Gilliom, M., Shaw, D. S., Beck, J. E., Schonberg, M. A., & Lukon, J. L. (2002). Anger regulation in disadvantaged preschool boys: Strategies, antecedents, and the development of self-control. *Developmental Psychology, 38*(2), 222-235.

Gilmore, J. H., Shi, F., Woolson, S. L., Knickmeyer, R. C., Short, S. J., Lin, W., . . . Shen, D. (2012). Longitudinal development of cortical and subcortical gray matter from birth to 2 years. *Cerebral Cortex, 22*(11), 2478-2485.

Gold, J., Sullivan, M. W., & Lewis, M. (2011). The relation between abuse and violent delinquency: The conversion of shame to blame in juvenile offenders. *Child Abuse and Neglect, 35*(7), 459-467.

Goldberg, S., & Lewis, M. (1969). Play behavior in the year-old infant: Early sex differences. *Child Development, 40*(1), 21-31.

Goldenberg, A., & Gross, J. J. (2020). Digital emotion contagion. *Trends in Cognitive Sciences, 24*(4), 316-328.

Goldsmith, H. H., Buss, A. H., Plomin, R., Rothbart, M. K., Thomas, A., Chess, S., . . . McCall, R. B. (1987). What is temperament? Four approaches. *Child Development, 58*(2), 505-529.

Goldsmith, H. H., & Campos, J. J. (1982). Toward a theory of infant temperament. In R. Emde & R. Harmon (Eds.), *The development of attachment and affiliative systems* (pp. 161-193). New York: Plenum Press.

Goldsmith, H. H., & Campos, J. J. (1986). Fundamental issues in the study of early temperament: The Denver Twin Temperament Study. In M. Lamb & A. Brown (Eds.), *Advances in developmental psychology* (pp. 231-283). Hillsdale, NJ: Erlbaum.

Goldsmith, H. H., Reilly, J., Lemery, K., Longley, S., & Prescott, A. (1999). *The Laboratory Temperament Assessment Battery: Preschool Version*. Madison, WI: University of Wisconsin.

Goldsmith, H. H., & Rothbart, M. K. (1996). *Prelocomotor and Locomotor Laboratory Temperament Assessment Battery (LAB-TAB, v.3)*. Madison, WI: University of Wisconsin.

Goleman, D. (1995). *Emotional intelligence: Why it can matter more than IQ*. New York: Bantam Books.

Gonçalves, S. F., Chaplin, T. M., Turpyn, C. C., Niehaus, C. E., Curby, T. W., Sinha, R., & Ansell, E. B. (2019). Difficulties in emotion regulation predict depressive symptom trajectory from early to middle adolescence. *Child Psychiatry and Human Development, 50*(4), 618-630.

Goodman, S. H., Rouse, M. H., Connell, A. M., Broth, M. R., Hall, C. M., & Heyward, D. (2011). Maternal depression and child psychopathology: A meta-analytic review. *Clinical Child and Family Psychology Review, 14*(1), 1-27.

Gopnik, A., & Wellman, H. M. (2012). Reconstructing constructivism: Causal models, Bayesian learning mechanisms, and the theory theory. *Psychological Bulletin, 138*(6), 1085-1108.

Gottman, J., & Gottman, J. (2017). The natural principles of love. *Journal of Family Theory and Review, 9*(1), 7-26.

Gottman, J. M., Katz, L. F., & Hooven, C. (1996). Parental meta-emotion philosophy and the emotional life of families: Theoretical models and preliminary data. *Journal of Family Psychology, 10*(3), 243-268.

Gottman, J. M., Katz, L. F., & Hooven, C. (1997). *Meta-emotion: How families communicate emotionally*. Hillsdale, NJ: Erlbaum.

Gottman, J. M., & Levenson, R. W. (2002). A two-factor model for predicting when a couple will divorce: Exploratory analyses using 14-year longitudinal data. *Family Process, 41*(1), 83-96.

Grabell, A. S., Huppert, T. J., Fishburn, F. A., Li, Y., Jones, H. M., Wilett, A. E., . . . Perlman, S. B. (2018). Using facial muscular movements to understand young children's emotion regulation and concurrent neural activation. *Developmental Science, 21*(5), 1–10.

Granat, A., Gadassi, R., Gilboa-Schechtman, E., & Feldman, R. (2017). Maternal depression and anxiety, social synchrony, and infant regulation of negative and positive emotions. *Emotion, 17*(1), 11–27.

Green, J., & Gustafson, G. (2016). Crying. In H. Montgomery (Ed.), *Oxford bibliographies in childhood studies.* New York: Oxford University Press.

Groh, A. M., Roisman, G. I., van IJzendoorn, M. H., Bakermans-Kranenburg, M. J., & Fearon, R. P. (2012). The significance of insecure and disorganized attachment for children's internalizing symptoms: A meta-analytic study. *Child Development, 83*(2), 591–610.

Grolnick, W. S., Bridges, L. J., & Connell, J. P. (1996). Emotion regulation in two-year-olds: Strategies and emotional expression in four contexts. *Child Development, 67*(3), 928–941.

Grommisch, G., Koval, P., Hinton, J. D. X., Gleeson, J., Hollenstein, T., Kuppens, P., & Lischetzke, T. (2020). Modeling individual differences in emotion regulation repertoire in daily life with multilevel latent profile analysis. *Emotion, 20*(8), 1462–1474.

Gross, J. J. (2013). Emotion regulation: Taking stock and moving forward. *Emotion, 13*(3), 359–365.

Gross, J. J. (2015a). Emotion regulation: Current status and future prospects. *Psychological Inquiry, 26*(1), 1–26.

Gross, J. J. (2015b). The extended process model of emotion regulation: Elaborations, applications, and future directions. *Psychological Inquiry, 26*(1), 130–137.

Gross, J. J., & Barrett, L. F. (2011). Emotion generation and emotion regulation: One or two depends on your point of view. *Emotion Review, 3*(1), 8–16.

Gross, J. J., & Jazaieri, H. (2014). Emotion, emotion regulation, and psychopathology: An affective science perspective. *Clinical Psychological Science, 2*(4), 387–401.

Gross, J. J., & John, O. P. (2003). Individual differences in two emotion regulation processes: Implications for affect, relationships, and well-being. *Journal of Personality and Social Psychology, 85*(2), 348–362.

Gross, J. J., John, O. P., & Richards, J. M. (2000). The dissociation of emotion expression from emotion experience: A personality perspective. *Personality and Social Psychology Bulletin, 26*(6), 712–726.

Gross, J. J., & Levenson, R. W. (1993). Emotional suppression: Physiology, self-report, and expressive behavior. *Journal of Personality and Social Psychology, 64*(6), 970–986.

Gross, J. T., & Cassidy, J. (2019). Expressive suppression of negative emotions in children and adolescents: Theory, data, and a guide for future research. *Developmental Psychology, 55*(9), 1938–1950.

Grossmann, I., Karasawa, M., Kan, C., & Kitayama, S. (2014). A cultural perspective on emotional experiences across the life span. *Emotion, 14*(4), 679–692.

Grossmann, T. (2010). The development of emotion perception in face and voice during infancy. *Restorative Neurology and Neuroscience, 28*(2), 219–236.

Grühn, D., Smith, J., & Baltes, P. B. (2005). No aging bias favoring memory for positive material: Evidence from a heterogeneity-homogeneity list paradigm using emotionally toned words. *Psychology and Aging, 20*(4), 579–588.

Gulley, L. D., Hankin, B. L., & Young, J. F. (2016). Risk for depression and anxiety in youth: The interaction between negative affectivity, effortful control, and stressors. *Journal of Abnormal Child Psychology, 44*(2), 207–218.

Gullone, E. (2000). The development of normal fear: A century of research. *Clinical Psychology Review, 20*(4), 429–451.

Gullone, E., Hughes, E. K., King, N. J., & Tonge, B. (2010). The normative development of emotion regulation strategy use in children and adolescents: A 2-year follow-up study. *Journal of Child Psychology and Psychiatry, 51*(5), 567–574.

Gullone, E., & King, N. J. (1992). Psychometric evaluation of a revised fear survey schedule for children and adolescents. *Child Psychology and Psychiatry and Allied Disciplines, 33*(6), 987–998.

Gunnar, M., & Quevedo, K. (2007). The neurobiology of stress and development. *Annual Review of Psychology, 58*, 145–173.

Gunnar, M. R. (2017). Social buffering of stress in development: A career perspective. *Perspectives on Psychological Science, 12*(3), 355–373.

Gunnar, M. R., & Adam, E. (2012). The hypothalamic–pituitary–adrenocortical system and emotion: Current wisdom and future directions. *Monographs of the Society for Research in Child Development, 77*(2), 109–119.

Gunnar, M. R., & Donzella, B. (2002). Social regulation of the cortisol levels in early human development. *Psychoneuroendocrinology, 27*(1–2), 199–220.

Gunnar, M. R., Doom, J. R., & Esposito, E. A. (2015). Psychoneuroendocrinology of stress: Normative development and individual differences. In M. E. Lamb & R. M. Lerner (Eds.), *Handbook of child psychology and developmental science: Vol. 3. Socioemotional processes* (7th ed., pp. 106–151). Hoboken, NJ: Wiley.

Gunnar, M. R., Sebanc, A. M., Tout, K., Donzella, B., & van Dulmen, M. M. H. (2003). Peer rejection, temperament, and cortisol activity in preschoolers. *Developmental Psychobiology, 43*(4), 346–358.

Gunnar, M. R., Talge, N. M., & Herrera, A. (2009). Stressor paradigms in developmental studies: What does and does not work to produce mean increases in salivary cortisol. *Psychoneuroendocrinology, 34*(7), 953–967.

Gunnar, M. R., Wewerka, S., Frenn, K., Long, J. D., & Griggs, C. (2009). Developmental changes in hypothalamus–pituitary–adrenal activity over the transition to adolescence: Normative changes and associations with puberty. *Development and Psychopathology, 21*(1), 69–85.

Guthrie, I. K., Eisenberg, N., Fabes, R. A., Murphy, B. C., Holmgren, R., Mazsk, P., & Suh, K. (1997). The relations of regulation and emotionality to children's situational empathy-related responding. *Motivation and Emotion, 21*(1), 87–108.

Gutchess, A. (2019). *Cognitive and social neuroscience of aging*. Cambridge, UK: Cambridge University Press.

Hackman, D. A., O'Brien, J. R., & Zalewski, M. (2018). Enduring association between parenting and cortisol: A meta-analysis. *Child Development, 89*(5), 1485–1503.

Hadiwijaya, H., Klimstra, T. A., Vermunt, J. K., Branje, S. J. T., & Meeus, W. H. J. (2017). On the development of harmony, turbulence, and independence in parent-adolescent relationships: A five-wave longitudinal study. *Journal of Youth and Adolescence, 46*(8), 1772–1788.

Haines, S. J., Gleeson, J., Kuppens, P., Hollenstein, T., Ciarrochi, J., Labuschagne, I., . . . Koval, P. (2016). The wisdom to know the difference: Strategy–situation fit in emotion regulation in daily life is associated with well-being. *Psychological Science, 27*(12), 1651–1659.

Haken, H. (1983). *Synergetics of complex systems in physics, chemistry, and biological motion.* New York: Springer-Verlag.

Halberstadt, A. G., Denham, S. A., & Dunsmore, J. C. (2001). Affective social competence. *Social Development, 10*(1), 79–119.

Halberstadt, A. G., & Eaton, K. L. (2002). A meta-analysis of family expressiveness and children's emotion expressiveness and understanding. *Marriage and Family Review, 34*(1-2), 35–62.

Halberstadt, A. G., & Lozada, F. T. (2011). Emotion development in infancy through the lens of culture. *Emotion Review, 3*(2), 158–168.

Halberstadt, A. G., Thompson, J. A., Parker, A. E., & Dunsmore, J. C. (2008). Parents' emotion-related beliefs and behaviours in relation to children's coping with the 11 September 2001 terrorist attacks. *Infant and Child Development, 17*, 557–580.

Hall, G. S. (1904). *Adolescence.* New York: Appleton Press.

Hall, J. A. (1978). Gender effects in decoding nonverbal cues. *Psychological Bulletin, 85*(4), 845–857.

Hall, J. A. (1984). *Nonverbal sex differences: Communication accuracy and expressive style.* Baltimore: Johns Hopkins University Press.

Hamann, S. (2012). Mapping discrete and dimensional emotions onto the brain: Controversies and consensus. *Trends in Cognitive Sciences, 16*(9), 458–466.

Hamby, S., Elm, J. H. L., Howell, K. H., & Merrick, M. T. (2021). Recognizing the cumulative burden of childhood adversities transforms science and practice for trauma and resilience. *American Psychologist, 76*(2), 230–242.

Hammen, C., & Brennan, P. A. (2003). Severity, chronicity, and timing of maternal depression and risk for adolescent offspring diagnoses in a community sample. *Archives of General Psychiatry, 60*(3), 253–258.

Hampton-Anderson, J. N., Carter, S., Fani, N., Gillespie, C. F., Henry, T. L., Holmes, E., . . . Kaslow, N. J. (2021). Adverse childhood experiences in African Americans: Framework, practice, and policy. *American Psychologist, 76*(2), 314–325.

Harmon-Jones, E., Gable, P. A., & Peterson, C. K. (2010). The role of asymmetric frontal cortical activity in emotion-related phenomena: A review and update. *Biological Psychology, 84*(3), 451–462.

Harold, G. T., Shelton, K. H., Goeke-Morey, M. C., & Cummings, E. M. (2004). Marital conflict, child emotional security about family relationships and child adjustment. *Social Development, 13*(3), 350–376.

Harris, P., de Rosnay, M., & Pons, F. (2016). Understanding emotion. In L. F. Barrett, M. Lewis, & J. M. Haviland-Jones (Eds.), *Handbook of emotions* (4th ed., pp. 293–306). New York: Guilford Press.

Harris, P., de Rosnay, M., & Ronfard, S. (2013). The mysterious emotional life of Little Red Riding Hood. In K. Lagattuta (Ed.), *Children and emotion: New insights into developmental affective science* (pp. 106–118). Basel, Switzerland: Karger.

Harris, P. L., Johnson, C. N., Hutton, D., Andrews, G., & Cooke, T. (1989). Young children's theory of mind and emotion. *Cognition and Emotion, 3*(4), 379–400.

Hartmann, D., & Schwenck, C. (2020). Emotion processing in children with conduct problems and callous–unemotional traits: An investigation of speed, accuracy, and attention. *Child Psychiatry and Human Development, 51*(5), 721–733.

Hastings, P. D., & Kahle, S. (2019). Get bent into shape: The non-linear, multi-system, contextually-embedded psychophysiology of emotional development. In V. LoBue, K. Pérez-Edgar, & K. Buss (Eds.), *Handbook of emotional development* (pp. 27–55). Cham, Switzerland: Springer.

Haviland, J. M., & Lelwica, M. (1987). The induced affect response: 10-week-old infants' responses to three emotion expressions. *Developmental Psychology, 23*(1), 97–104.

Hawes, D. J., Lechowicz, M., Roach, A., Fisher, C., Doyle, F. L., Noble, S., & Dadds, M. R. (2021). Capturing the developmental timing of adverse childhood experiences: The Adverse Life Experiences Scale. *American Psychologist, 76*(2), 253–267.

Hayes, G. S., McLennan, S. N., Henry, J. D., Phillips, L. H., Terrett, G., Rendell, P. G., . . . Labuschagne, I. (2020). Task characteristics influence facial emotion recognition age-effects: A meta-analytic review. *Psychology and Aging, 35*(2), 295–315.

Hazan, C., & Shaver, P. (1987). Romantic love conceptualized as an attachment process. *Journal of Personality and Social Psychology, 52*(3), 511–524.

Hedges, L., & Olkin, I. (1985). *Statistical methods for meta-analysis*. Orlando, FL: Academic Press.

Hein, T. C., & Monk, C. S. (2017). Research review: Neural response to threat in children, adolescents, and adults after child maltreatment: A quantitative meta-analysis. *Journal of Child Psychology and Psychiatry, 58*(3), 222–230.

Hendricks, M. A., & Buchanan, T. W. (2016). Individual differences in cognitive control processes and their relationship to emotion regulation. *Cognition and Emotion, 30*(5), 912–924.

Henker, B., Whalen, C. K., Jamner, L. D., & Delfino, R. J. (2002). Anxiety, affect, and activity in teenagers: Monitoring daily life with electronic diaries. *Journal of the American Academy of Child and Adolescent Psychiatry, 41*(6), 660–670.

Henrich, J., Heine, S. J., & Norenzayan, A. (2010). Beyond WEIRD: Towards a broad-based behavioral science. *Behavioral and Brain Sciences, 33*(2–3), 111–135.

Hepach, R., Vaish, A., & Tomasello, M. (2013). Young children sympathize less in response to unjustified emotional distress. *Developmental Psychology, 49*(6), 1132–1138.

Hernández, M. M., Eisenberg, N., Valiente, C., Spinrad, T. L., VanSchyndel, S. K., Diaz, A., . . . Southworth, J. (2017). Observed emotions as predictors of quality of kinder-gartners' social relationships. *Social Development, 26*(1), 21–39.

Hernández, M. M., Eisenberg, N., Valiente, C., VanSchyndel, S. K., Spinrad, T. L., Silva, K. M., . . . Southworth, J. (2016). Emotional expression in school context, social relationships, and academic adjustment in kindergarten. *Emotion, 16*(4), 553–566.

Hertenstein, M. J., & Campos, J. J. (2004). The retention effects of an adult's emotional displays on infant behavior. *Child Development, 75*(2), 595–613.

Hesse, E. (2016). The Adult Attachment Interview: Protocol, method of analysis, and empirical studies: 1985–2015. In J. Cassidy & P. R. Shaver (Eds.), *Handbook of attachment* (3rd ed., pp. 553–557). New York: Guilford Press.

Hilgard, E. R. (1980). Consciousness in contemporary psychology. *Annual Review of Psychology, 31*, 1–26.

Hinnant, J. B., & El-Sheikh, M. (2009). Children's externalizing and internalizing symptoms over time: The role of individual differences in patterns of RSA responding. *Journal of Abnormal Child Psychology, 37*(8), 1049–1061.

Hochschild, A. (1983). *The managed heart: Commercialization of human feeling*. Berkeley: University of California Press.

Hodel, A. S. (2018). Rapid infant prefrontal cortex development and sensitivity to early environmental experience. *Developmental Review, 48*, 113–144.

Hoemann, K., Crittenden, A. N., Msafiri, S., Liu, Q., Li, C., Roberson, D., . . . Barrett, L. (2019). Context facilitates performance on a classic cross-cultural emotion perception task. *Emotion, 19*(7), 1292–1313.

Hoemann, K., Xu, F., & Barrett, L. F. (2019). Emotion words, emotion concepts, and emotional development in children: A constructionist hypothesis. *Developmental Psychology, 55*(9), 1830–1849.

Hoffman, M. L. (2000). *Empathy and moral development: Implications for caring and justice.* New York: Cambridge University Press.

Hoffman, M. L. (2008). Empathy and prosocial behavior. In M. Lewis, J. M. Haviland-Jones, & L. F. Barrett (Eds.), *Handbook of emotions* (3rd ed., pp. 440–455). New York: Guilford Press.

Hoffmann, J. D., Brackett, M. A., Bailey, C. S., & Willner, C. J. (2020). Teaching emotion regulation in schools: Translating research into practice with the RULER approach to social and emotional learning. *Emotion, 20*(1), 105–109.

Hofstede, G. (2001). *Culture's consequences* (2nd ed.). Newbury Park, CA: Sage.

Hofstede, G. (2011). Dimensionalizing cultures: The Hofstede model in context. Online Readings in Psychology and Culture, 2(1). Retrieved from *https://scholarworks.gvsu.edu/orpc/vol2/iss1/8*.

Hollenstein, T., & Lanteigne, D. (2018). Emotion regulation dynamics in adolescence. In P. M. Cole & T. Hollenstein (Eds.), *Emotion regulation: A matter of time* (pp. 158–176). New York: Routledge.

Holodynski, M. (2004). The miniaturization of expression in the development of emotional self-regulation. *Developmental Psychology, 40*(1), 16–28.

Holodynski, M., & Friedlmeier, W. (2006). *Development of emotions and emotion regulation.* New York: Springer Science + Business Media.

Holodynski, M., & Seeger, D. (2019). Expressions as signs and their significance for emotional development. *Developmental Psychology, 55*(9), 1812–1829.

Hong, Y., Chiu, C., Dweck, C. S., Lin, D. M. S., & Wan, W. (1999). Implicit theories, attributions, and coping: A meaning system approach. *Journal of Personality and Social Psychology, 77*(3), 588–599.

Hostinar, C. E., Johnson, A. E., & Gunnar, M. R. (2015). Parent support is less effective in buffering cortisol stress reactivity for adolescents compared to children. *Developmental Science, 18*(2), 281–297.

Hubbard, J. A., Smithmyer, C. M., Ramsden, S. R., Parker, E. H., Flanagan, K. D., Dearing, K. F., . . . Simons, R. F. (2002). Observational, physiological, and self-report measures of children's anger: Relations to reactive versus proactive aggression. *Child Development, 73*(4), 1101–1118.

Hudson, A., & Jacques, S. (2014). Put on a happy face! Inhibitory control and socioemotional knowledge predict emotion regulation in 5- to 7-year-olds. *Journal of Experimental Child Psychology, 123*, 36–52.

Hülsheger, U. R., & Schewe, A. F. (2011). On the costs and benefits of emotional labor: A meta-analysis of three decades of research. *Journal of Occupational Health Psychology, 16*(3), 361–389.

Hunter, E. M., Phillips, L. H., & MacPherson, S. E. (2010). Effects of age on cross-modal emotion perception. *Psychology and Aging, 25*(4), 779–787.

Hurrell, K. E., Houwing, F. L., & Hudson, J. L. (2017). Parental meta-emotion philosophy and emotion coaching in families of children and adolescents with an anxiety disorder. *Journal of Abnormal Child Psychology, 45*(3), 569–582.

Hutcherson, C. A., & Gross, J. J. (2011). The moral emotions: A social-functionalist account of anger, disgust, and contempt. *Journal of Personality and Social Psychology, 100*(4), 719–737.

Hutchinson, J., & Barrett, L. F. (2019). The power of predictions: An emerging paradigm for psychological research. *Current Directions in Psychological Science, 28*(3), 280–291.

Huttenlocher, P. R. (1994). Synaptogenesis in human cerebral cortex. In G. Dawson & K. W. Fischer (Eds.), *Human behavior and the developing brain* (pp. 137–152). New York: Guilford Press.

Hyde, J. S. (2014). Gender similarities and differences. *Annual Review of Psychology, 65*, 373–398.

Ice, G. H., Katz-Stein, A., Himes, J., & Kane, R. L. (2004). Diurnal cycles of salivary cortisol in older adults. *Psychoneuroendocrinology, 29*(3), 355–370.

Ilan, S. D., Tamuz, N., & Sheppes, G. (2019). The fit between emotion regulation choice and individual resources is associated with adaptive functioning among young children. *Cognition and Emotion, 33*(3), 597–605.

Infurna, M. R., Reichl, C., Parzer, P., Schimmenti, A., Bifulco, A., & Kaess, M. (2016). Associations between depression and specific childhood experiences of abuse and neglect: A meta-analysis. *Journal of Affective Disorders, 190*, 47–55.

Inhelder, B., & Piaget, J. (1958). *The growth of logical thinking from childhood to adolescence.* New York: Basic Books.

Isaacowitz, D. M., & Choi, Y. (2012). Looking, feeling, and doing: Are there age differences in attention, mood, and behavioral responses to skin cancer information? *Health Psychology, 31*(5), 650–659.

Isaacowitz, D. M., Wadlinger, H. A., Goren, D., & Wilson, H. R. (2006). Selective preference in visual fixation away from negative images in old age? An eye-tracking study. *Psychology and Aging, 21*(1), 40–48.

Israelashvili, J., Hassin, R. R., & Aviezer, H. (2019). When emotions run high: A critical role for context in the unfolding of dynamic, real-life facial affect. *Emotion, 19*(3), 558–562.

Izard, C. E. (1971). *The face of emotion.* East Norwalk, CT: Appleton-Century-Crofts.

Izard, C. E. (1977). *Human emotions.* New York: Plenum Press.

Izard, C. E. (1991). *The psychology of emotions.* New York: Plenum Press.

Izard, C. E. (1995). *The maximally discriminative facial movement coding system (MAX).* Newark, DE: University of Delaware Instruction Resources Center.

Izard, C. E. (1997). Emotions and facial expressions: A perspective from differential emotions theory. In J. A. Russell & J. M. Fernández-Dols (Eds.), *The psychology of facial expression* (pp. 57–77). New York: Cambridge University Press.

Izard, C. E. (2007). Basic emotions, natural kinds, emotion schemas, and a new paradigm. *Perspectives on Psychological Science, 2*(3), 260–280.

Izard, C. E. (2009). Emotion theory and research: Highlights, unanswered questions, and emerging issues. *Annual Review of Psychology, 60*, 1–25.

Izard, C. E. (2011). Forms and functions of emotions: Matters of emotion–cognition interactions. *Emotion Review, 3*(4), 371–378.

Izard, C. E., & Abe, J. A. A. (2004). Developmental changes in facial expressions of emotions in the Strange Situation during the second year of life. *Emotion, 4*(3), 251–265.

Izard, C. E., Dougherty, L. R., & Hembree, E. (1983). *A system for identifying affect expressions by holistic judgments (AFFEX).* Newark: University of Delaware Instructional Resource Center.

Izard, C. E., Fantauzzo, C. A., Castle, J. M., Haynes, O. M., Rayias, M. F., & Putnam, P. H. (1995). The ontogeny and significance of infants' facial expressions in the first 9 months of life. *Developmental Psychology, 31*(6), 997–1013.

Izard, C. E., Hembree, E. A., Dougherty, L. M., & Spizzirri, C. C. (1983). Changes in facial expressions of 2- to 19-month-old infants following acute pain. *Developmental Psychology, 19*(3), 418-426.

Izard, C. E., Hembree, E. A., & Huebner, R. R. (1987). Infants' emotion expressions to acute pain: Developmental change and stability of individual differences. *Developmental Psychology, 23*(1), 105-113.

Izard, C. E., Libero, D. Z., Putnam, P., & Haynes, O. M. (1993). Stability of emotion experiences and their relations to traits of personality. *Journal of Personality and Social Psychology, 64*(5), 847-860.

Izard, C. E., & Malatesta, C. Z. (1987). Perspectives on emotional development: I. Differential emotions theory of early emotional development. In J. D. Osofsky (Ed.), *Handbook of infant development* (2nd ed., pp. 494-554). Oxford, UK: Wiley.

Izard, C. E., Youngstrom, E. A., Fine, S. E., Mostow, A. J., & Trentacosta, C. J. (2006). Emotions and developmental psychopathology. In D. Cicchetti & D. J. Cohen (Eds.), *Developmental psychopathology: Vol. 1. Theory and method* (2nd ed., pp. 244-292). Hoboken, NJ: Wiley.

Jaffe, J., Beebe, B., Feldstein, S., Crown, C., & Jasnow, M. (2001). Rhythms of dialogue in infancy. *Monographs of the Society for Research in Child Development, 66*(2), 1-131.

Jakobs, E., Manstead, A. S. R., & Fischer, A. H. (2001). Social context effects on facial activity in a negative emotional setting. *Emotion, 1*(1), 51-69.

James, W. (1884). What is an emotion? *Mind, 9,* 188-205.

James, W. (1950). *The principles of psychology.* New York: Dover. (Original work published 1890)

Jasini, A., De Leersnyder, J., Phalet, K., & Mesquita, B. (2019). Tuning in emotionally: Associations of cultural exposure with distal and proximal emotional fit in acculturating youth. *European Journal of Social Psychology, 49*(2), 352-365.

Jebb, A. T., Morrison, M., Tay, L., & Diener, E. (2020). Subjective well-being around the world: Trends and predictors across the life span. *Psychological Science, 31*(3), 293-305.

Jeronimus, B. F., Riese, H., Oldehinkel, A. J., & Ormel, J. (2017). Why does frustration predict psychopathology? Multiple prospective pathways over adolescence: A TRAILS study. *European Journal of Personality, 31*(1), 85-103.

Jewell, T., Gardner, T., Susi, K., Watchorn, K., Coopey, E., Simic, M., . . . Eisler, I. (2019). Attachment measures in middle childhood and adolescence: A systematic review of measurement properties. *Clinical Psychology Review, 68,* 71-82.

Johnson, A. M., Hawes, D. J., Eisenberg, N., Kohlhoff, J., & Dudeney, J. (2017). Emotion socialization and child conduct problems: A comprehensive review and meta-analysis. *Clinical Psychology Review, 54,* 65-80.

Johnson, M. H., Senju, A., & Tomalski, P. (2015). The two-process theory of face processing: Modifications based on two decades of data from infants and adults. *Neuroscience and Biobehavioral Reviews, 50,* 169-179.

Johnson, V. C., Olino, T. M., Klein, D. N., Dyson, M. W., Bufferd, S. J., Durbin, C. E., . . . Hayden, E. P. (2016). A longitudinal investigation of predictors of the association between age 3 and age 6 behavioural inhibition. *Journal of Research in Personality, 63,* 51-61.

Jones-Mason, K., Alkon, A., Coccia, M., & Bush, N. R. (2018). Autonomic nervous system functioning assessed during the still-face paradigm: A meta-analysis and systematic review of methods, approach and findings. *Developmental Review, 50*(Part B), 113-139.

Jopp, D., & Rott, C. (2006). Adaptation in very old age: Exploring the role of resources, beliefs, and attitudes for centenarians' happiness. *Psychology and Aging, 21*(2), 266–280.

Joseph, D. L., & Newman, D. A. (2010). Emotional intelligence: An integrative meta-analysis and cascading model. *Journal of Applied Psychology, 95*(1), 54–78.

Kagan, J. (1974). Discrepancy, temperament and infant distress. In M. Lewis & L. Rosenblum (Eds.), *The origins of fear* (pp. 229–248). New York: Wiley.

Kagan, J. (1997). Temperament and the reactions to unfamiliarity. *Child Development, 68*(1), 139–143.

Kagan, J., Reznick, J. S., & Snidman, N. (1988). Biological bases of childhood shyness. *Science, 240*(4849), 167–171.

Kagan, J., & Snidman, N. (1991). Infant predictors of inhibited and uninhibited profiles. *Psychological Science, 2*(1), 40–44.

Kagan, J., Snidman, N., Arcus, D., & Reznick, J. S. (1994). *Galen's prophecy: Temperament in human nature.* New York: Basic Books.

Kahn, R. E., Ermer, E., Salovey, P., & Kiehl, K. A. (2016). Emotional intelligence and callous–unemotional traits in incarcerated adolescents. *Child Psychiatry and Human Development, 47*(6), 903–917.

Kahneman, D. (2003). A perspective on judgment and choice: Mapping bounded rationality. *American Psychologist, 58*(9), 697–720.

Katz, L. F., Maliken, A. C., & Stettler, N. M. (2012). Parental meta-emotion philosophy: A review of research and theoretical framework. *Child Development Perspectives, 6*(4), 417–422.

Keller, H. (2013). Attachment and culture. *Journal of Cross-Cultural Psychology, 44,* 175–194.

Keller, H. (2017). Culture and development: A systematic relationship. *Perspectives on Psychological Science, 12*(5), 833–840.

Keller, H., & Otto, H. (2009). The cultural socialization of emotion regulation during infancy. *Journal of Cross-Cultural Psychology, 40*(6), 996–1011.

Kelso, J. A. S. (1995). *Dynamic patterns: The self-organization of brain and behavior.* Cambridge, MA: MIT Press.

Kerns, K. A., & Brumariu, L. (2016). Attachment in middle childhood. In J. Cassidy & P. R. Shaver (Eds.), *Handbook of attachment: Theories, research, and clinical applications* (3rd ed., pp. 349–365). New York: Guilford Press.

Khazanov, G. K., & Ruscio, A. M. (2016). Is low positive emotionality a specific risk factor for depression? A meta-analysis of longitudinal studies. *Psychological Bulletin, 142*(9), 991–1015.

Kiel, E. J., & Kalomiris, A. (2019). Emotional development and anxiety. In V. LoBue, K. Pérez-Edgar, & K. A. Buss (Eds.), *Handbook of emotional development* (pp. 665–694). New York: Springer.

Kieras, J. E., Tobin, R., Graziano, W., & Rothbart, M. K. (2005). You can't always get what you want: Effortful control and children's responses to undesirable gifts. *Psychological Science, 16*(5), 391–396.

Kim, S., Healey, M. K., Goldstein, D., Hasher, L., & Wiprzycka, U. J. (2008). Age differences in choice satisfaction: A positivity effect in decision making. *Psychology and Aging, 23*(1), 33–38.

Kim, S., & Kochanska, G. (2012). Child temperament moderates effects of parent–child mutuality on self-regulation: A relationship-based path for emotionally negative infants. *Child Development, 83*(4), 1275–1289.

Kim, S., Thibodeau, R., & Jorgensen, R. S. (2011). Shame, guilt, and depressive symptoms: A meta-analytic review. *Psychological Bulletin, 137*(1), 68–96.

Kirschbaum, C., Pirke, K.-M., & Hellhammer, D. H. (1993). The "Trier Social Stress Test": A tool for investigating psychobiological stress responses in a laboratory setting. *Neuropsychobiology, 28*(1–2), 76–81.

Kitayama, S., Berg, M. K., & Chopik, W. J. (2020). Culture and well-being in late adulthood: Theory and evidence. *American Psychologist, 75*(4), 567–576.

Kitayama, S., Markus, H. R., Matsumoto, H., & Norasakkunkit, V. (1997). Individual and collective processes in the construction of the self: Self-enhancement in the United States and self-criticism in Japan. *Journal of Personality and Social Psychology, 72*(6), 1245–1267.

Kitayama, S., Mesquita, B., & Karasawa, M. (2006). Cultural affordances and emotional experience: Socially engaging and disengaging emotions in Japan and the United States. *Journal of Personality and Social Psychology, 91*(5), 890–903.

Klein, D. N., & Mumper, E. (2018). Behavioral inhibition as a precursor to psychopathology. In K. Pérez-Edgar & N. A. Fox (Eds.), *Behavioral inhibition* (pp. 263–282). Cham, Switzerland: Springer.

Kliewer, W. (2006). Violence exposure and cortisol responses in urban youth. *International Journal of Behavioral Medicine, 13*(2), 109–120.

Klimes-Dougan, B., Brand, A. E., Zahn-Waxler, C., Usher, B., Hastings, P. D., Kendziora, K., & Garside, R. B. (2007). Parental emotion socialization in adolescence: Differences in sex, age and problem status. *Social Development, 16*(2), 326–342.

Klimes-Dougan, B., & Zeman, J. (2007). Introduction to the special issue on emotion socialization in childhood and adolescence. *Social Development, 16*(2), 203–209.

Knack, J. M., Jensen-Campbell, L. A., & Baum, A. (2011). Worse than sticks and stones? Bullying is associated with altered HPA axis functioning and poorer health. *Brain and Cognition, 77*(2), 183–190.

Knothe, J. M., & Walle, E. A. (2018). Parental communication about emotional contexts: Differences across discrete categories of emotion. *Social Development, 27*(2), 247–261.

Kobak, R. R., Cole, H. E., Ferenz-Gillies, R., Fleming, W. S., & Gamble, W. (1993). Attachment and emotion regulation during mother–teen problem solving: A control theory analysis. *Child Development, 64*(1), 231–245.

Kochanska, G. (1991). Socialization and temperament in the development of guilt and conscience. *Child Development, 62*(6), 1379–1392.

Kochanska, G. (1995). Children's temperament, mother's discipline, and security of attachment: Multiple pathways to emerging internalization. *Child Development, 66*(3), 597–615.

Kochanska, G., & Aksan, N. (2006). Children's conscience and self-regulation. *Journal of Personality, 74*(6), 1587–1617.

Kochanska, G., Kim, S., Boldt, L. J., & Yoon, J. E. (2013). Children's callous–unemotional traits moderate links between their positive relationships with parents at preschool age and externalizing behavior problems at early school age. *Journal of Child Psychology and Psychiatry, 54*(11), 1251–1260.

Kochanska, G., Murray, K. T., & Harlan, E. T. (2000). Effortful control in early childhood: Continuity and change, antecedents, and implications for social development. *Developmental Psychology, 36*(2), 220–232.

Kondo-Ikemura, K., Behrens, K. Y., Umemura, T., & Nakano, S. (2018). Japanese mothers' prebirth Adult Attachment Interview predicts their infants' response to the Strange

Situation procedure: The Strange Situation in Japan revisited three decades later. *Developmental Psychology, 54*(11), 2007-2015.

Kopp, C. B. (1989). Regulation of distress and negative emotions: A developmental view. *Developmental Psychology, 25*(3), 343-354.

Koss, K. J., & Gunnar, M. R. (2018). Annual research review: Early adversity, the hypothalamic–pituitary–adrenocortical axis, and child psychopathology. *Journal of Child Psychology and Psychiatry, 59*(4), 327-346.

Köster, M., Kayhan, E., Langeloh, M., & Hoehl, S. (2020). Making sense of the world: Infant learning from a predictive processing perspective. *Perspectives on Psychological Science, 15*(3), 562-571.

Kozak, M. J., & Cuthbert, B. N. (2016). The NIMH Research Domain Criteria initiative: Background, issues, and pragmatics. *Psychophysiology, 53*(3), 286-297.

Kragel, P. A., Han, X., Kraynak, T. E., Gianaros, P. J., & Wager, T. D. (2021). Functional MRI can be highly reliable, but it depends on what you measure: A commentary on Elliott et al. (2020). *Psychological Science, 32*(4), 622-626.

Kramer, A., Guillory, J., & Hancock, J. (2014). Experimental evidence of massive-scale emotional contagion through social networks. *Proceedings of the National Academy of Sciences of the USA, 111*(24), 8788-8790.

Krassnei, A. M., Gartstein, M. A., Park, C., Dragan, W. Ł., Lecannelier, F., & Putnam, S. P. (2017). East–west, collectivist–individualist: A cross-cultural examination of temperament in toddlers from Chile, Poland, South Korea, and the US. *European Journal of Developmental Psychology, 14*(4), 449-464.

Kraut, R. E., & Johnston, R. E. (1979). Social and emotional messages of smiling: An ethological approach. *Journal of Personality and Social Psychology, 37*(9), 1539-1553.

Kring, A. M., & Elis, O. (2013). Emotion deficits in people with schizophrenia. *Annual Review of Clinical Psychology, 9*, 409-433.

Kring, A. M., & Mote, J. (2016). Emotion disturbances as transdiagnostic processes in psychopathology. In L. F. Barrett, M. Lewis, & J. M. Haviland-Jones (Eds.), *Handbook of emotions* (4th ed., pp. 653-669). New York: Guilford Press.

Kumari, M., Badrick, E., Chandola, T., Adler, N. E., Epel, E., Seeman, T., . . . Marmot, M. G. (2010). Measures of social position and cortisol secretion in an aging population: Findings from the Whitehall II Study. *Psychosomatic Medicine, 72*(1), 27-34.

Kunzmann, U., Richter, D., & Schmukle, S. C. (2013). Stability and change in affective experience across the adult life span: Analyses with a national sample from Germany. *Emotion, 13*(6), 1086-1095.

Kunzmann, U., Rohr, M., Wieck, C., Kappes, C., & Wrosch, C. (2017). Speaking about feelings: Further evidence for multidirectional age differences in anger and sadness. *Psychology and Aging, 32*(1), 93-103.

Kupperbusch, C., Levenson, R. W., & Ebling, R. (2003). Predicting husbands' and wives' retirement satisfaction from the emotional qualities of marital interaction. *Journal of Social and Personal Relationships, 20*(3), 335-354.

La Guardia, J. G., Ryan, R. M., Couchman, C. E., & Deci, E. L. (2000). Within-person variation in security of attachment: A self-determination theory perspective on attachment, need fulfillment, and well-being. *Journal of Personality and Social Psychology, 79*(3), 367-384.

LaBarbera, J., Izard, C. E., Vietze, P., & Parisi, S. (1976). Four- and six-month-old infants' visual responses to joy, anger, and neutral expressions. *Child Development, 47*, 535-538.

Laceulle, O. M., Nederhof, E., Karreman, A., Ormel, J., & van Aken, M. A. G. (2012). Stressful events and temperament change during early and middle adolescence: The TRAILS study. *European Journal of Personality, 26*(3), 276–284.

Lagacé-Séguin, D. G., & Coplan, R. J. (2005). Maternal emotional styles and child social adjustment: Assessment, correlates, outcomes and goodness of fit in early childhood. *Social Development, 14*(4), 613–636.

Lagattuta, K. (2005). When you shouldn't do what you want to do: Young children's understanding about desires, rules, and emotions. *Child Development, 76*(2), 713–733.

Lagattuta, K. H., & Kramer, H. J. (2021). Advanced emotion understanding: Children's and adults' knowledge that minds generalize from prior emotional events. *Emotion, 21*(1), 1–16.

Lagattuta, K. H., & Wellman, H. M. (2001). Thinking about the past: Early knowledge about links between prior experience, thinking, and emotion. *Child Development, 72*(1), 82–102.

Laible, D. (2004). Mother–child discourse in two contexts: Links with child temperament, attachment security, and socioemotional competence. *Developmental Psychology, 40*(6), 979–992.

Lamborn, S. D., Mounts, N. S., Steinberg, L., & Dornbusch, S. M. (1991). Patterns of competence and adjustment among adolescents from authoritative, authoritarian, indulgent, and neglectful families. *Child Development, 62*(5), 1049–1065.

Lamm, C., Decety, J., & Singer, T. (2011). Meta-analytic evidence for common and distinct neural networks associated with directly experienced pain and empathy for pain. *NeuroImage, 54*(3), 2492–2502.

Lange, C. (1992). The emotions (I. Haupt, Trans.). In E. Dunlap (Ed.), *The emotions* (pp. 33–90). Baltimore: Williams & Wilkins. (Original work published 1885)

Larson, R., Csikszentmihalyi, M., & Graef, R. (1980). Mood variability and the psychosocial adjustment of adolescents. *Journal of Youth and Adolescence, 9*(6), 469–490.

Larson, R., & Lampman-Petraitis, C. (1989). Daily emotional states as reported by children and adolescents. *Child Development, 60*(5), 1250–1260.

Larson, R. W., Moneta, G., Richards, M. H., & Wilson, S. (2002). Continuity, stability, and change in daily emotional experience across adolescence. *Child Development, 73*(4), 1151–1165.

Laukka, P., & Elfenbein, H. A. (2021). Cross-cultural emotion recognition and in-group advantage in vocal expression: A meta-analysis. *Emotion Review, 13*(1), 3–11.

Lavelli, M., Carra, C., Rossi, G., & Keller, H. (2019). Culture-specific development of early mother–infant emotional co-regulation: Italian, Cameroonian, and West African immigrant dyads. *Developmental Psychology, 55*(9), 1850–1867.

Lazarus, R. (1966). *Psychological stress and the coping process.* New York: McGraw-Hill.

Lazarus, R. (1991). *Emotion and adaptation.* New York: Oxford University Press.

Lazarus, R., & Folkman, S. (1984). *Stress, appraisal, and coping.* New York: Oxford University Press.

Lee, H. Y., Jamieson, J. P., Reis, H. T., Beevers, C. G., Josephs, R. A., Mullarkey, M. C., . . . Yeager, D. S. (2020). Getting fewer "likes" than others on social media elicits emotional distress among victimized adolescents. *Child Development, 91*(6), 2141–2159.

Lee, V., Cheal, J. L., & Rutherford, M. D. (2015). Categorical perception along the happy-angry and happy-sad continua in the first year of life. *Infant Behavior and Development, 40*, 95–102.

Leerkes, E. M., & Bailes, L. G. (2019). Emotional development within the family context.

In V. LoBue, K. Pérez-Edgar, & K. Buss (Eds.), *Handbook of emotional development* (pp. 627–661). Cham, Switzerland: Springer.

Leerkes, E. M., Bailes, L. G., & Augustine, M. E. (2020). The intergenerational transmission of emotion socialization. *Developmental Psychology, 56*(3), 390–402.

Leger, K. A., Charles, S. T., Turiano, N. A., & Almeida, D. M. (2016). Personality and stressor-related affect. *Journal of Personality and Social Psychology, 111*(6), 917–928.

Leitzke, B. T., Hilt, L. M., & Pollak, S. D. (2015). Maltreated youth display a blunted blood pressure response to an acute interpersonal stressor. *Journal of Clinical Child and Adolescent Psychology, 44*(2), 305–313.

Lemerise, E. A., & Arsenio, W. F. (2000). An integrated model of emotion processes and cognition in social information processing. *Child Development, 71*(1), 107–118.

Lenhart, A. (2015). Teens, social media and technology. Retrieved from *www.pewresearch. org/internet/2015/04/09/teens-social-media-technology-2015*.

Lenhart, A., Madden, M., Smith, A., Purcell, K., & Zickuhr, K. (2011). Teens, kindness and cruelty on social network sites. Retrieved from *www.pewresearch.org/internet/2011/11/09/teens-kindness-and-cruelty-on-social-network-sites*.

Lennarz, H. K., Hollenstein, T., Lichtwarck-Aschoff, A., Kuntsche, E., & Granic, I. (2019). Emotion regulation in action: Use, selection, and success of emotion regulation in adolescents' daily lives. *International Journal of Behavioral Development, 43*(1), 1–11.

Lenze, S. N., Pautsch, J., & Luby, J. (2011). Parent–child interaction therapy emotion development: A novel treatment for depression in preschool children. *Depression and Anxiety, 28*(2), 153–159.

Leppänen, J. M., Cataldo, J. K., Enlow, M. B., & Nelson, C. A. (2018). Early development of attention to threat-related facial expressions. *PLOS ONE, 13*(5), e0197424.

Lerner, J. S., Gonzalez, R. M., Small, D. A., & Fischhoff, B. (2003). Effects of fear and anger on perceived risks of terrorism: A national field experiment. *Psychological Science, 14*(2), 144–150.

Lerner, J. S., & Keltner, D. (2000). Beyond valence: Toward a model of emotion-specific influences on judgement and choice. *Cognition and Emotion, 14*(4), 473–493.

LeRoy, A. S., Gabert, T., Garcini, L., Murdock, K. W., Heijnen, C., & Fagundes, C. P. (2020). Attachment orientations and loss adjustment among bereaved spouses. *Psychoneuroendocrinology, 112*, 104401.

Levenson, R. W., Carstensen, L. L., Friesen, W. V., & Ekman, P. (1991). Emotion, physiology, and expression in old age. *Psychology and Aging, 6*(1), 28–35.

Levenson, R. W., Ekman, P., Heider, K., & Friesen, W. V. (1992). Emotion and autonomic nervous system activity in the Minangkabau of West Sumatra. *Journal of Personality and Social Psychology, 62*(6), 972–988.

Levine, L. J., Kaplan, R., & Davis, E. (2013). How kids keep their cool. In D. Hermans, B. Rimé, & B. Mesquita (Eds.), *Changing emotions* (pp. 3–9). New York: Psychology Press.

Lewis, M. (1972). State as an infant–environment interaction: An analysis of mother–infant interaction as a function of sex. *Merrill-Palmer Quarterly, 18*(2), 95–121.

Lewis, M. (2014). *The rise of consciousness and the development of emotional life*. New York: Guilford Press.

Lewis, M. (2016a). The emergence of human emotions. In L. F. Barrett, M. Lewis, & J. M. Haviland-Jones (Eds.), *Handbook of emotions* (4th ed., pp. 272–292). New York: Guilford Press.

Lewis, M. (2016b). Self-conscious emotions: Embarrassment, pride, shame, guilt, and hubris. In L. F. Barrett, M. Lewis, & J. M. Haviland-Jones (Eds.), *Handbook of emotions* (4th ed., pp. 792–814). New York: Guilford Press.

Lewis, M. (2019). The self-conscious emotions and the role of shame in psychopathology. In V. LoBue, K. Pérez-Edgar, & K. Buss (Eds.), *Handbook of emotional development* (pp. 311–350). Cham, Switzerland: Springer.

Lewis, M., Alessandri, S. M., & Sullivan, M. W. (1990). Violation of expectancy, loss of control, and anger expressions in young infants. *Developmental Psychology, 26*(5), 745–751.

Lewis, M., & Ramsay, D. (2002). Cortisol response to embarrassment and shame. *Child Development, 73*(4), 1034–1045.

Lewis, M., & Ramsay, D. (2004). Development of self-recognition, personal pronoun use, and pretend play during the 2nd year. *Child Development, 75*(6), 1821–1831.

Lewis, M., Ramsay, D. S., & Sullivan, M. W. (2006). The relation of ANS and HPA activation to infant anger and sadness response to goal blockage. *Developmental Psychology, 48*(5), 397–405.

Lewis, M., Sullivan, M. W., Ramsay, D. S., & Alessandri, S. M. (1992). Individual differences in anger and sad expressions during extinction: Antecedents and consequences. *Infant Behavior and Development, 15*(4), 443–452.

Lewis, M., Sullivan, M. W., Stanger, C., & Weiss, M. (1989). Self development and self-conscious emotions. *Child Development, 60*(1), 146–156.

Lewis, M. D. (2005). Bridging emotion theory and neurobiology through dynamic systems modeling. *Behavioral and Brain Sciences, 28*(2), 169–245.

Lewis, M. D., & Granic, I. (2000). *Emotion, development, and self-organization: Dynamic systems approaches to emotional development.* New York: Cambridge University Press.

Lewis-Morrarty, E., Degnan, K. A., Chronis-Tuscano, A., Rubin, K. H., Cheah, C. S. L., Pine, D. S., . . . Fox, N. A. (2012). Maternal over-control moderates the association between early childhood behavioral inhibition and adolescent social anxiety symptoms. *Journal of Abnormal Child Psychology, 40*(8), 1363–1373.

Li, J.-B., Willems, Y. E., Stok, F. M., Deković, M., Bartels, M., & Finkenauer, C. (2019). Parenting and self-control across early to late adolescence: A three-level meta-analysis. *Perspectives on Psychological Science, 14*(6), 967–1005.

Li, T. M. H., & Wong, P. W. C. (2015). Editorial perspective: Pathological social withdrawal during adolescence: A culture-specific or a global phenomenon? *Journal of Child Psychology and Psychiatry, 56*(10), 1039–1041.

Li, Z., Sturge-Apple, M. L., Martin, M. J., & Davies, P. T. (2019). Interactive effects of family instability and adolescent stress reactivity on socioemotional functioning. *Developmental Psychology, 55*(10), 2193–2202.

Liew, J., Eisenberg, N., & Reiser, M. (2004). Preschoolers' effortful control and negative emotionality, immediate reactions to disappointment, and quality of social functioning. *Journal of Experimental Child Psychology, 89*(4), 298–313.

Lindquist, K. A., Wager, T. D., Kober, H., Bliss-Moreau, E., & Barrett, L. F. (2012). The brain basis of emotion: A meta-analytic review. *Behavioral and Brain Sciences, 35*(3), 121–143.

Lindsey, E. W. (2017). Mutual positive emotion with peers, emotion knowledge, and preschoolers' peer acceptance. *Social Development, 26*(2), 349–366.

Lindsey, E. W. (2020). Relationship context and emotion regulation across the life span. *Emotion, 20*(1), 59–62.

Lionetti, F., Aron, E. N., Aron, A., Klein, D. N., & Pluess, M. (2019). Observer-rated environmental sensitivity moderates children's response to parenting quality in early childhood. *Developmental Psychology, 55*(11), 2389-2402.

Liu, D. Y., & Thompson, R. J. (2017). Selection and implementation of emotion regulation strategies in major depressive disorder: An integrative review. *Clinical Psychology Review, 57,* 183-194.

Liu, Q., He, H., Yang, J., Feng, X., Zhao, F., & Lyu, J. (2020). Changes in the global burden of depression from 1990 to 2017: Findings from the Global Burden of Disease study. *Journal of Psychiatric Research, 126,* 134-140.

Livingstone, K. M., & Isaacowitz, D. M. (2015). Situation selection and modification for emotion regulation in younger and older adults. *Social Psychological and Personality Science, 6*(8), 904-910.

Livingstone, K. M., & Isaacowitz, D. M. (2021). Age and emotion regulation in daily life: Frequency, strategies, tactics, and effectiveness. *Emotion, 31*(1), 39-51.

LoBue, V. (2013). What are we so afraid of? How early attention shapes our most common fears. *Child Development Perspectives, 7*(1), 38-42.

LoBue, V., & Adolph, K. E. (2019). Fear in infancy: Lessons from snakes, spiders, heights, and strangers. *Developmental Psychology, 55*(9), 1889-1907.

LoBue, V., & DeLoache, J. S. (2008). Detecting the snake in the grass: Attention to fear-relevant stimuli by adults and young children. *Psychological Science, 19*(3), 284-289.

LoBue, V., Kim, E., & Delgado, M. (2019). Fear. In V. LoBue, K. Pérez-Edgar, & K. Buss (Eds.), *Handbook of emotional development* (pp. 257-282). Cham, Switzerland: Springer.

LoBue, V., & Rakison, D. H. (2013). What we fear most: A developmental advantage for threat-relevant stimuli. *Developmental Review, 33*(4), 285-303.

LoBue, V., Rakison, D. H., & DeLoache, J. S. (2010). Threat perception across the life span: Evidence for multiple converging pathways. *Current Directions in Psychological Science, 19*(6), 375-379.

Longman, T., Hawes, D. J., & Kohlhoff, J. (2016). Callous–unemotional traits as markers for conduct problem severity in early childhood: A meta-analysis. *Child Psychiatry and Human Development, 47*(2), 326-334.

Lopes, P. N., Mestre, J. M., Guil, R., Kremenitzer, J. P., & Salovey, P. (2012). The role of knowledge and skills for managing emotions in adaptation to school: Social behavior and misconduct in the classroom. *American Educational Research Journal, 49*(4), 710-742.

Lopes, P. N., Salovey, P., & Straus, R. (2003). Emotional intelligence, personality, and the perceived quality of social relationships. *Personality and Individual Differences, 35*(3), 641-658.

Lopez-Duran, N. L., Kovacs, M., & George, C. J. (2009). Hypothalamic–pituitary–adrenal axis dysregulation in depressed children and adolescents: A meta-analysis. *Psychoneuroendocrinology, 34*(9), 1272-1283.

López-Pérez, B., & Pacella, D. (2021). Interpersonal emotion regulation in children: Age, gender, and cross-cultural differences using a serious game. *Emotion, 21*(1), 17-27.

Lorié, Á., Reinero, D. A., Phillips, M., Zhang, L., & Riess, H. (2017). Culture and nonverbal expressions of empathy in clinical settings: A systematic review. *Patient Education and Counseling, 100*(3), 411-424.

Lougheed, J. P., Craig, W. M., Pepler, D., Connolly, J., O'Hara, A., Granic, I., & Hollenstein, T. (2016). Maternal and peer regulation of adolescent emotion: Associations with depressive symptoms. *Journal of Abnormal Child Psychology, 44*(5), 963-974.

Lougheed, J. P., & Hollenstein, T. (2012). A limited repertoire of emotion regulation strategies is associated with internalizing problems in adolescence. *Social Development, 21*(4), 704–721.

Lougheed, J. P., & Hollenstein, T. (2016). Socioemotional flexibility in mother–daughter dyads: Riding the emotional roller coaster across positive and negative contexts. *Emotion, 16*(5), 620–633.

Louie, J. Y., Wang, S.-W., Fung, J., & Lau, A. (2015). Children's emotional expressivity and teacher perceptions of social competence: A cross-cultural comparison. *International Journal of Behavioral Development, 39*(6), 497–507.

Lozada, F. T., Halberstadt, A. G., Craig, A. B., Dennis, P. A., & Dunsmore, J. C. (2016). Parents' beliefs about children's emotions and parents' emotion-related conversations with their children. *Journal of Child and Family Studies, 25*(5), 1525–1538.

Lu, T., Posada, G. E., Trumbell, J. M., & Anaya, L. (2018). Maternal sensitivity and co-construction skills: Concurrent and longitudinal associations with preschoolers' secure base behavior. *Monographs of the Society for Research in Child Development, 83*(4), 74–90.

Luchetti, M., Terracciano, A., Stephan, Y., & Sutin, A. R. (2016). Personality and cognitive decline in older adults: Data from a longitudinal sample and meta-analysis. *Journals of Gerontology: Series B. Psychological Sciences and Social Sciences, 71*(4), 591–601.

Luebbe, A. M., Kiel, E. J., & Buss, K. A. (2011). Toddlers' context-varying emotions, maternal responses to emotions, and internalizing behaviors. *Emotion, 11*(3), 697–703.

Luhmann, M., Hofmann, W., Eid, M., & Lucas, R. E. (2012). Subjective well-being and adaptation to life events: A meta-analysis. *Journal of Personality and Social Psychology, 102*(3), 592–615.

Lwi, S. J., Haase, C. M., Shiota, M. N., Newton, S. L., & Levenson, R. W. (2019). Responding to the emotions of others: Age differences in facial expressions and age-specific associations with relational connectedness. *Emotion, 19*(8), 1437–1449.

MacCann, C., Jiang, Y., Brown, L. E. R., Double, K. S., Bucich, M., & Minbashian, A. (2020). Emotional intelligence predicts academic performance: A meta-analysis. *Psychological Bulletin, 146*(2), 150–186.

MacCormack, J. K., Stein, A., Kang, J., Giovanello, K., Satpute, A., & Lindquist, K. A. (2020). Affect in the aging brain: A neuroimaging meta-analysis of older vs. younger adult affective experience and perception. *Affective Science, 1*, 128–154.

Maciejewski, D. F., van Lier, P. A. C., Branje, S. J. T., Meeus, W. H. J., & Koot, H. M. (2015). A 5-year longitudinal study on mood variability across adolescence using daily diaries. *Child Development, 86*(6), 1908–1921.

Madarasz, T. J., Diaz-Mataix, L., Akhand, O., Ycu, E. A., LeDoux, J. E., & Johansen, J. P. (2016). Evaluation of ambiguous associations in the amygdala by learning the structure of the environment. *Nature Neuroscience, 19*(7), 965–972.

Madhyastha, T. M., Hamaker, E. L., & Gottman, J. M. (2011). Investigating spousal influence using moment-to-moment affect data from marital conflict. *Journal of Family Psychology, 25*(2), 292–300.

Madigan, S., Atkinson, L., Laurin, K., & Benoit, D. (2013). Attachment and internalizing behavior in early childhood: A meta-analysis. *Developmental Psychology, 49*(4), 672–689.

Madigan, S., Brumariu, L. E., Villani, V., Atkinson, L., & Lyons-Ruth, K. (2016). Representational and questionnaire measures of attachment: A meta-analysis of relations to child internalizing and externalizing problems. *Psychological Bulletin, 142*(4), 367–399.

Magai, C., Consedine, N. S., Gillespie, M., O'Neal, C., & Vilker, R. (2004). The differential roles of early emotion socialization and adult attachment in adult emotional
experience: Testing a mediator hypothesis. *Attachment and Human Development, 6*(4),
389-417.

Magai, C., Frias, M. T., & Shaver, P. (2016). Attachment in middle and later life. In J. Cassidy & P. R. Shaver (Eds.), *Handbook of attachment* (3rd ed., pp. 534-552). New York:
Guilford Press.

Mahali, S. C., Beshai, S., Feeney, J. R., & Mishra, S. (2020). Associations of negative
cognitions, emotional regulation, and depression symptoms across four continents: International support for the cognitive model of depression. *BMC Psychiatry,
20*, 18.

Main, A., Paxton, A., & Dale, R. (2016). An exploratory analysis of emotion dynamics
between mothers and adolescents during conflict discussions. *Emotion, 16*(6), 913-
928.

Main, M., Kaplan, N., & Cassidy, J. (1985). Security in infancy, childhood, and adulthood:
A move to the level of representation. *Monographs of the Society for Research in Child
Development, 50*(1-2), 66-104.

Main, M., & Solomon, J. (1986). Discovery of an insecure-disorganized/disoriented
attachment pattern. In T. B. Brazelton & M. W. Yogman (Eds.), *Affective development
in infancy* (pp. 95-124). Westport, CT: Ablex.

Malagón-Amor, Á., Martín-López, L. M., Córcoles, D., González, A., Bellsolà, M., Teo,
A. R., . . . Bergé, D. (2018). A 12-month study of the hikikomori syndrome of social
withdrawal: Clinical characterization and different subtypes proposal. *Psychiatry
Research, 270*, 1039-1046.

Malatesta, C. Z., Culver, C., Tesman, J. R., & Shepard, B. (1989). The development of emotion expression during the first two years of life. *Monographs of the Society for Research
in Child Development, 54*(1-2), 1-104.

Malatesta, C. Z., & Haviland, J. M. (1982). Learning display rules: The socialization of
emotion expression in infancy. *Child Development, 53*(4), 991-1003.

Marino, C., Gini, G., Angelini, F., Vieno, A., & Spada, M. M. (2020). Social norms and
emotions in problematic social media use among adolescents. *Addictive Behaviors
Reports, 11*, 100250.

Marks, A. K., Ejesi, K., & Coll, C. G. (2014). Understanding the U.S. immigrant paradox
in childhood and adolescence. *Child Development Perspectives, 8*(2), 59-64.

Marshall, P. J., & Fox, N. A. (2008). Electrophysiological measures in research on social
and emotional development. In L. A. Schmidt & S. J. Segalowitz (Eds.), *Developmental psychophysiology: Theory, systems, and methods* (pp. 127-149). New York: Cambridge
University Press.

Martin, N. G., Maza, L., McGrath, S. J., & Phelps, A. E. (2014). An examination of referential and affect specificity with five emotions in infancy. *Infant Behavior and Development, 37*(3), 286-297.

Martinez, A. M. (2019). The promises and perils of automated facial action coding in
studying children's emotions. *Developmental Psychology, 55*(9), 1965-1981.

Martinotti, G., Vannini, C., Di Natale, C., Sociali, A., Stigliano, G., Santacroce, R., & di
Giannantonio, M. (2020). Hikikomori: Psychopathology and differential diagnosis
of a condition with epidemic diffusion. *International Journal of Psychiatry in Clinical
Practice, 25*(2), 187-194.

Martins, B., & Mather, M. (2016). Default mode network and later-life emotion regulation:

Linking functional connectivity patterns and emotional outcomes. In A. D. Ong & C. E. Löckenhoff (Eds.), *Emotion, aging, and health* (pp. 9-29). Washington, DC: American Psychological Association.

Martins, B., Ponzio, A., Velasco, R., Kaplan, J., & Mather, M. (2015). Dedifferentiation of emotion regulation strategies in the aging brain. *Social Cognitive and Affective Neuroscience, 10*(6), 840-847.

Masson, M., Bussières, E.-L., East-Richard, C., R-Mercier, A., & Cellard, C. (2015). Neuropsychological profile of children, adolescents and adults experiencing maltreatment: A meta-analysis. *Clinical Neuropsychologist, 29*(5), 573-594.

Masten, C. L., Guyer, A. E., Hodgdon, H. B., McClure, E. B., Charney, D. S., Ernst, M., . . . Monk, C. S. (2008). Recognition of facial emotions among maltreated children with high rates of post-traumatic stress disorder. *Child Abuse and Neglect, 32*(1), 139-153.

Mastropieri, D., & Turkewitz, G. (1999). Prenatal experience and neonatal responsiveness to vocal expressions of emotion. *Developmental Psychobiology, 35*(3), 204-214.

Mather, M. (2016). The affective neuroscience of aging. *Annual Review of Psychology, 67,* 213-238.

Mather, M., & Carstensen, L. L. (2005). Aging and motivated cognition: The positivity effect in attention and memory. *Trends in Cognitive Sciences, 9*(10), 496-502.

Mather, M., Clewett, D., Sakaki, M., & Harley, C. (2016). Norepinephrine ignites local hot spots of neuronal excitation: How arousal amplifies selectivity in perception and memory. *Behavioral and Brain Sciences, 39,* e200.

Mather, M., & Ponzio, A. (2016). Emotion and aging. In L. F. Barrett, M. Lewis, & J. M. Haviland-Jones (Eds.), *Handbook of emotions* (4th ed., pp. 319-335). New York: Guilford Press.

Mathews, B. L., Koehn, A. J., Abtahi, M. M., & Kerns, K. A. (2016). Emotional competence and anxiety in childhood and adolescence: A meta-analytic review. *Clinical Child and Family Psychology Review, 19*(2), 162-184.

Matsumoto, D., & Hwang, H. S. (2012). Culture and emotion: The integration of biological and cultural contributions. *Journal of Cross-Cultural Psychology, 43*(1), 91-118.

Matsumoto, D., Yoo, S. H., Fontaine, J., Anguas-Wong, A. M., Arriola, M., Ataca, B., . . . Grossi, E. (2008). Mapping expressive differences around the world: The relationship between emotional display rules and individualism versus collectivism. *Journal of Cross-Cultural Psychology, 39*(1), 55-74.

Matsumoto, D., Yoo, S. H., Nakagawa, S., & the Multinational Study of Cultural Display Rules. (2008). Culture, emotion regulation, and adjustment. *Journal of Personality and Social Psychology, 94*(6), 925-937.

Mayer, J. D., Caruso, D. R., & Salovey, P. (2016). The ability model of emotional intelligence: Principles and updates. *Emotion Review, 8*(4), 290-300.

Mayer, J. D., Salovey, P., Caruso, D. R., & Sitarenios, G. (2003). Measuring emotional intelligence with the MSCEIT V2.0. *Emotion, 3*(1), 97-105.

Mayes, L. C., & Zigler, E. (1992). An observational study of the affective concomitants of mastery in infants. *Child Psychology and Psychiatry and Allied Disciplines, 33*(4), 659-667.

McClure, E. B. (2000). A meta-analytic review of sex differences in facial expression processing and their development in infants, children, and adolescents. *Psychological Bulletin, 126*(3), 424-453.

McCord, B. L., & Raval, V. V. (2016). Asian Indian immigrant and White American maternal emotion socialization and child socio-emotional functioning. *Journal of Child and Family Studies, 25*(2), 464–474.

McCrae, R. R., & Costa, P. T., Jr. (2003). *Personality in adulthood: A five-factor theory perspective* (2nd ed.). New York: Guilford Press.

McCrae, R. R., & John, O. P. (1992). An introduction to the five-factor model and its applications. *Journal of Personality, 60*(2), 175–215.

McGinley, J. J., & Friedman, B. H. (2017). Autonomic specificity in emotion: The induction method matters. *International Journal of Psychophysiology, 118*, 48–57.

McGuire, A., & Jackson, Y. (2018). A multilevel meta-analysis on academic achievement among maltreated youth. *Clinical Child and Family Psychology Review, 21*(4), 450–465.

McLaughlin, K. A., Peverill, M., Gold, A. L., Alves, S., & Sheridan, M. A. (2015). Child maltreatment and neural systems underlying emotion regulation. *Journal of the American Academy of Child and Adolescent Psychiatry, 54*(9), 753–762.

McLaughlin, K. A., Sheridan, M. A., Alves, S., & Mendes, W. B. (2014). Child maltreatment and autonomic nervous system reactivity: Identifying dysregulated stress reactivity patterns by using the biopsychosocial model of challenge and threat. *Psychosomatic Medicine, 76*(7), 538–546.

McRae, K., & Gross, J. J. (2020). Emotion regulation. *Emotion, 20*(1), 1–9.

Mead, M. (1975). The appalling state of the human sciences: Review of *Darwin and Facial Expression*. *Journal of Communication, 25*(1), 209–213.

Melton, M. A., Hersen, M., Van Sickle, T. D., & Van Hasselt, V. B. (1995). Parameters of marriage in older adults: A review of the literature. *Clinical Psychology Review, 15*(8), 891–904.

Meltzoff, A. N., & Marshall, P. J. (2018). Human infant imitation as a social survival circuit. *Current Opinion in Behavioral Sciences, 24*, 130–136.

Meltzoff, A. N., Murray, L., Simpson, E., Heimann, M., Nagy, E., Nadel, J., . . . Ferrari, P. F. (2018). Re-examination of Oostenbroek et al. (2016): Evidence for neonatal imitation of tongue protrusion. *Developmental Science, 21*(4), 1–8.

Mence, M., Hawes, D. J., Wedgwood, L., Morgan, S., Barnett, B., Kohlhoff, J., & Hunt, C. (2014). Emotional flooding and hostile discipline in the families of toddlers with disruptive behavior problems. *Journal of Family Psychology, 28*(1), 12–21.

Mendes, W. B. (2010). Weakened links between mind and body in older age: The case for maturational dualism in the experience of emotion. *Emotion Review, 2*(3), 240–244.

Mérida-López, S., Extremera, N., Quintana-Orts, C., & Rey, L. (2019). In pursuit of job satisfaction and happiness: Testing the interactive contribution of emotion-regulation ability and workplace social support. *Scandinavian Journal of Psychology, 60*, 59–66.

Mesman, J., & Emmen, R. A. G. (2013). Mary Ainsworth's legacy: A systematic review of observational instruments measuring parental sensitivity. *Attachment and Human Development, 15*(5–6), 485–506.

Mesman, J., Minter, T., Angnged, A., Cissé, I. A. H., Salali, G. D., & Migliano, A. B. (2018). Universality without uniformity: A culturally inclusive approach to sensitive responsiveness in infant caregiving. *Child Development, 89*(3), 837–850.

Mesman, J., van IJzendoorn, M. H., & Bakermans-Kranenburg, M. J. (2009). The many faces of the Still-Face Paradigm: A review and meta-analysis. *Developmental Review, 29*(2), 120–162.

Mesman, J., van IJzendoorn, M. H., & Sagi-Schwartz, A. (2016). Cross-cultural patterns of attachment. In J. Cassidy & P. R. Shaver (Eds.), *Handbook of attachment* (3rd ed., pp. 852–877). New York: Guilford Press.

Mesquita, B., De Leersnyder, J., & Boiger, M. (2016). The cultural psychology of emotions. In L. F. Barrett, M. Lewis, & J. M. Haviland-Jones (Eds.), *Handbook of emotions* (4th ed., pp. 393–411). New York: Guilford Press.

Messinger, D. S., Fogel, A., & Dickson, K. L. (2001). All smiles are positive, but some smiles are more positive than others. *Developmental Psychology, 37*(5), 642–653.

Messinger, D. S., Mattson, W. I., Mahoor, M. H., & Cohn, J. F. (2012). The eyes have it: Making positive expressions more positive and negative expressions more negative. *Emotion, 12*(3), 430–436.

Mian, N. D., Wainwright, L., Briggs-Gowan, M. J., & Carter, A. S. (2011). An ecological risk model for early childhood anxiety: The importance of early child symptoms and temperament. *Journal of Abnormal Child Psychology, 39*(4), 501–512.

Miao, C., Humphrey, R. H., & Qian, S. (2017a). Are the emotionally intelligent good citizens or counterproductive? A meta-analysis of emotional intelligence and its relationships with organizational citizenship behavior and counterproductive work behavior. *Personality and Individual Differences, 116*, 144–156.

Miao, C., Humphrey, R. H., & Qian, S. (2017b). A meta-analysis of emotional intelligence and work attitudes. *Journal of Occupational and Organizational Psychology, 90*(2), 177–202.

Miao, C., Humphrey, R. H., Qian, S., & Pollack, J. M. (2019). The relationship between emotional intelligence and the dark triad personality traits: A meta-analytic review. *Journal of Research in Personality, 78*, 189–197.

Mikels, J. A., Löckenhoff, C. E., Maglio, S. J., Carstensen, L. L., Goldstein, M. K., & Garber, A. (2010). Following your heart or your head: Focusing on emotions versus information differentially influences the decisions of younger and older adults. *Journal of Experimental Psychology: Applied, 16*(1), 87–95.

Mikels, J. A., Shuster, M. M., & Thai, S. T. (2015). Aging, emotion, and decision making. In T. M. Hess, J. Strough, & C. E. Löckenhoff (Eds.), *Aging and decision making: Empirical and applied perspectives* (pp. 169–188). San Diego, CA: Elsevier Academic Press.

Mikulincer, M., & Shaver, P. (2016). Adult attachment and emotion regulation. In J. Cassidy & P. R. Shaver (Eds.), *Handbook of attachment: Theory, research, and applications* (3rd ed., pp. 507–533). New York: Guilford Press.

Milevsky, A., Schlechter, M., Netter, S., & Keehn, D. (2007). Maternal and paternal parenting styles in adolescents: Associations with self-esteem, depression and life-satisfaction. *Journal of Child and Family Studies, 16*(1), 39–47.

Miller, J. G., Chocol, C., Nuselovici, J. N., Utendale, W. T., Simard, M., & Hastings, P. D. (2013). Children's dynamic RSA change during anger and its relations with parenting, temperament, and control of aggression. *Biological Psychology, 92*(2), 417–425.

Miller, J. G., Nuselovici, J. N., & Hastings, P. D. (2016). Nonrandom acts of kindness: Parasympathetic and subjective empathic responses to sadness predict children's prosociality. *Child Development, 87*(6), 1679–1690.

Miller, P., & Sperry, L. L. (1987). The socialization of anger and aggression. *Merrill-Palmer Quarterly, 33*(1), 1–31.

Miller, P. J., Fung, H., Lin, S., Chen, E. C.-H., & Boldt, B. R. (2012). How socialization happens on the ground: Narrative practices as alternate socializing pathways in Taiwanese and European-American families. *Monographs of the Society for Research in Child Development, 77*(1), 1–125.

Milojevich, H. M., Levine, L. J., Cathcart, E. J., & Quas, J. A. (2018). The role of maltreatment in the development of coping strategies. *Journal of Applied Developmental Psychology, 54*, 23–32.

Mingebach, T., Kamp-Becker, I., Christiansen, H., & Weber, L. (2018). Meta-meta-analysis on the effectiveness of parent-based interventions for the treatment of child externalizing behavior problems. *PLOS ONE, 13*(9), e0202855.

Mirabile, S. P., Oertwig, D., & Halberstadt, A. G. (2018). Parent emotion socialization and children's socioemotional adjustment: When is supportiveness no longer supportive? *Social Development, 27*(3), 466–481.

Mischel, W., Shoda, Y., & Peake, P. K. (1988). The nature of adolescent competencies predicted by preschool delay of gratification. *Journal of Personality and Social Psychology, 54*(4), 687–696.

Mischel, W., Shoda, Y., & Rodriguez, M. L. (1989). Delay of gratification in children. *Science, 244*(4907), 933–938.

Mitsven, S., Messinger, D. S., Moffitt, J., & Ahn, Y. (2020). Infant emotional development. In J. Lockman & C. Tamis-Lemonda (Eds.), *Handbook of infant development* (pp. 748–782). Cambridge, UK: Cambridge University Press.

Moed, A., Gershoff, E. T., Eisenberg, N., Hofer, C., Losoya, S., Spinrad, T. L., & Liew, J. (2015). Parent–adolescent conflict as sequences of reciprocal negative emotion: Links with conflict resolution and adolescents' behavior problems. *Journal of Youth and Adolescence, 44*(8), 1607–1622.

Möller, E. L., Nikolić, M., Majdandžić, M., & Bögels, S. M. (2016). Associations between maternal and paternal parenting behaviors, anxiety and its precursors in early childhood: A meta-analysis. *Clinical Psychology Review, 45*, 17–33.

Montirosso, R., Provenzi, L., Fumagalli, M., Sirgiovanni, I., Giorda, R., Pozzoli, U., . . . Borgatti, R. (2016). Serotonin transporter gene (SLC6A4) methylation associates with neonatal intensive care unit stay and 3-month-old temperament in preterm infants. *Child Development, 87*(1), 38–48.

Moors, A. (2014). Flavors of appraisal theories of emotion. *Emotion Review, 6*(4), 303–307.

Morales, S., Brown, K. M., Taber-Thomas, B. C., LoBue, V., Buss, K. A., & Pérez-Edgar, K. E. (2017). Maternal anxiety predicts attentional bias towards threat in infancy. *Emotion, 17*(5), 874–883.

Morales, S., & Fox, N. A. (2019). A neuroscience perspective on emotional development. In V. LoBue, K. Pérez-Edgar, & K. Buss (Eds.), *Handbook of emotional development* (pp. 57–81). Cham, Switzerland: Springer.

Moran, L. R., Lengua, L. J., & Zalewski, M. (2013). The interaction between negative emotionality and effortful control in early social-emotional development. *Social Development, 22*(2), 340–362.

Moreira, J., & Silvers, J. A. (2018). In due time: Neurodevelopmental considerations in the study of emotion regulation. In P. M. Cole & T. Hollenstein (Eds.), *Emotion regulation: A matter of time* (pp. 93–116). New York: Routledge.

Morelen, D., Zeman, J., Perry-Parrish, C., & Anderson, E. (2012). Children's emotion regulation across and within nations: A comparison of Ghanaian, Kenyan, and American youth. *British Journal of Developmental Psychology, 30*(3), 415–431.

Mroczek, D. K., & Almeida, D. M. (2004). The effect of daily stress, personality, and age on daily negative affect. *Journal of Personality, 72*(2), 355–378.

Mroczek, D. K., & Kolarz, C. M. (1998). The effect of age on positive and negative affect: A developmental perspective on happiness. *Journal of Personality and Social Psychology, 75*(5), 1333–1349.

Mueller, S., Wagner, J., Smith, J., Voelkle, M. C., & Gerstorf, D. (2018). The interplay of personality and functional health in old and very old age: Dynamic within-person interrelations across up to 13 years. *Journal of Personality and Social Psychology, 115*(6), 1127–1147.

Mumme, D. L., & Fernald, A. (2003). The infant as onlooker: Learning from emotional reactions observed in a television scenario. *Child Development, 74*(1), 221–237.

Muris, P., & Field, A. (2011). The "normal" development of fear and anxiety. In W. Silverman & A. Field (Eds.), *Anxiety disorders in children and adolescents: Research, assessment and intervention* (2nd ed., pp. 76–89). New York: Cambridge University Press.

Muris, P., Mayer, B., Borth, M., & Vos, M. (2013). Nonverbal and verbal transmission of disgust from mothers to offspring: Effects on children's evaluation of a novel animal. *Behavior Therapy, 44*(2), 293–301.

Murray-Close, D. (2013). Psychophysiology of adolescent peer relations: I. Theory and research findings. *Journal of Research on Adolescence, 23*(2), 236–259.

Nachmias, M., Gunnar, M., Mangelsdorf, S., Parritz, R. H., & Buss, K. (1996). Behavioral inhibition and stress reactivity: The moderating role of attachment security. *Child Development, 67*(2), 508–522.

Nakagawa, A., & Sukigara, M. (2012). Difficulty in disengaging from threat and temperamental negative affectivity in early life: A longitudinal study of infants aged 12–36 months. *Behavioral and Brain Functions, 8*, 40.

Nelson, D. W. (2009). Feeling good and open-minded: The impact of positive affect on cross cultural empathic responding. *Journal of Positive Psychology, 4*(1), 53–63.

Nelson, J. A., & Boyer, B. P. (2018). Maternal responses to negative emotions and child externalizing behavior: Different relations for 5-, 6-, and 7-year-olds. *Social Development, 27*(3), 482–494.

Nelson, J. A., Leerkes, E. M., Perry, N. B., O'Brien, M., Calkins, S. D., & Marcovitch, S. (2013). European-American and African-American mothers' emotion socialization practices relate differently to their children's academic and social-emotional competence. *Social Development, 22*(3), 485–498.

Nelson, N. L., Nowicki, E., Diemer, M. C., Sangster, K., Cheng, C., & Russell, J. A. (2018). Children can create a new emotion category through a process of elimination. *Cognitive Development, 47*, 117–123.

Nelson, N. L., & Russell, J. A. (2011). Preschoolers' use of dynamic facial, bodily, and vocal cues to emotion. *Journal of Experimental Child Psychology, 110*(1), 52–61.

Nelson, N. L., & Russell, J. A. (2013). Universality revisited. *Emotion Review, 5*(1), 8–15.

Neppl, T. K., Conger, R. D., Scaramella, L. V., & Ontai, L. L. (2009). Intergenerational continuity in parenting behavior: Mediating pathways and child effects. *Developmental Psychology, 45*(5), 1241–1256.

Nigg, J. T. (2006). Temperament and developmental psychopathology. *Journal of Child Psychology and Psychiatry, 47*(3–4), 395–422.

Nofech-Mozes, J., Pereira, J., Gonzalez, A., & Atkinson, L. (2019). Cortisol secretion moderates the association between mother–infant attachment at 17 months and child behavior at age 5 years. *Developmental Psychobiology, 61*(2), 239–253.

Noh, S. R., & Isaacowitz, D. M. (2013). Emotional faces in context: Age differences in recognition accuracy and scanning patterns. *Emotion, 13*(2), 238–249.

Noordermeer, S. D. S., Luman, M., & Oosterlaan, J. (2016). A systematic review and meta-analysis of neuroimaging in oppositional defiant disorder (ODD) and conduct disorder (CD) taking attention-deficit hyperactivity disorder (ADHD) into account. *Neuropsychology Review, 26*(1), 44–72.

Norasakkunkit, V., & Uchida, Y. (2014). To conform or to maintain self-consistency? Hikikomori risk in Japan and the deviation from seeking harmony. *Journal of Social and Clinical Psychology, 33*(10), 918–935.

Nozadi, S. S., Spinrad, T. L., Eisenberg, N., & Eggum-Wilkens, N. D. (2015). Associations of anger and fear to later self-regulation and problem behavior symptoms. *Journal of Applied Developmental Psychology, 38*, 60–69.

Öhman, A., & Mineka, S. (2001). Fears, phobias, and preparedness: Toward an evolved module of fear and fear learning. *Psychological Review, 108*(3), 483–522.

O'Kearney, R., Salmon, K., Liwag, M., Fortune, C.-A., & Dawel, A. (2017). Emotional abilities in children with oppositional defiant disorder (ODD): Impairments in perspective-taking and understanding mixed emotions are associated with high callous–unemotional traits. *Child Psychiatry and Human Development, 48*(2), 346–357.

Oldehinkel, A. J., Hartman, C. A., Ferdinand, R. F., Verhulst, F. C., & Ormel, J. (2007). Effortful control as modifier of the association between negative emotionality and adolescents' mental health problems. *Development and Psychopathology, 19*(2), 523–539.

Oostenbroek, J., Suddendorf, T., Nielsen, M., Redshaw, J., Kennedy-Costantini, S., Davis, J., . . . Slaughter, V. (2016). Comprehensive longitudinal study challenges the existence of neonatal imitation in humans. *Current Biology, 26*, 1334–1338.

Opitz, P. C., Rauch, L. C., Terry, D. P., & Urry, H. L. (2012). Prefrontal mediation of age differences in cognitive reappraisal. *Neurobiology of Aging, 33*(4), 645–655.

Oster, H. (2005). The repertoire of infant facial expressions: An ontogenetic perspective. In J. Nadel & D. Muir (Eds.), *Emotional development: Recent research advances* (pp. 261–292). New York: Oxford University Press.

Otto, H., & Keller, H. (2014). *Different faces of attachment: Cultural variations on a universal human need.* New York: Cambridge University Press.

Otto, H., & Keller, H. (2015). A good child is a calm child: Mothers' social status, maternal conceptions of proper demeanor, and stranger anxiety in one-year old Cameroonian Nso children. *Psychological Topics, 24*(1), 1–25.

Otto, L. R., Sin, N. L., Almeida, D. M., & Sloan, R. P. (2018). Trait emotion regulation strategies and diurnal cortisol profiles in healthy adults. *Health Psychology, 37*(3), 301–305.

Palmer, A., Lakhan-Pal, S., & Cicchetti, D. (2019). Emotional development and depression. In V. LoBue, K. Pérez-Edgar, & K. A. Buss (Eds.), *Handbook of emotional development* (pp. 695–748). New York: Springer.

Park, C., Rosenblat, J. D., Lee, Y., Pan, Z., Cao, B., Iacobucci, M., & McIntyre, R. S. (2019). The neural systems of emotion regulation and abnormalities in major depressive disorder. *Behavioural Brain Research, 367*, 181–188.

Park, D. C., & Reuter-Lorenz, P. (2009). The adaptive brain: Aging and neurocognitive scaffolding. *Annual Review of Psychology, 60*, 173–196.

Park, J., Kitayama, S., Miyamoto, Y., & Coe, C. L. (2020). Feeling bad is not always unhealthy: Culture moderates the link between negative affect and diurnal cortisol profiles. *Emotion, 20*(5), 721–733.

Parker, A. E., Halberstadt, A. G., Dunsmore, J. C., Townley, G., Bryant, A., Thompson, J. A., & Beale, K. (2012). "Emotions are a window into one's heart": A qualitative analysis of parental beliefs about children's emotions across three ethnic groups. *Monographs of the Society for Research in Child Development, 77*(3), 81–106.

Parrigon, K., Kerns, K. A., Abtahi, M., & Koehn, A. (2015). Attachment and emotion in middle childhood and adolescence. *Psychological Topics, 24*(1), 27–50.

Patterson, G. R. (1982). *Coercive family process.* Eugene, OR: Castalia.

Peltola, M. J., Hietanen, J. K., Forssman, L., & Leppänen, J. M. (2013). The emergence and stability of the attentional bias to fearful faces in infancy. *Infancy, 18*(6), 905–926.

Peltola, M. J., Leppänen, J. M., Mäki, S., & Hietanen, J. K. (2009). Emergence of enhanced attention to fearful faces between 5 and 7 months of age. *Social Cognitive and Affective Neuroscience, 4*(2), 134–142.

Peng, M., Johnson, C., Pollock, J., Glasspool, R., & Harris, P. (1992). Training young children to acknowledge mixed emotions. *Cognition and Emotion, 6*(5), 387–401.

Pereg, D., & Mikulincer, M. (2004). Attachment style and the regulation of negative affect: Exploring individual differences in mood congruency effects on memory and judgment. *Personality and Social Psychology Bulletin, 30*(1), 67–80.

Pérez-Edgar, K. (2019). Through the looking glass: Temperament and emotion as separate and interwoven constructs. In V. LoBue, K. Pérez-Edgar, & K. Buss (Eds.), *Handbook of emotional development* (pp. 139–168). Cham, Switzerland: Springer.

Pérez-Edgar, K., Morales, S., LoBue, V., Taber-Thomas, B. C., Allen, E. K., Brown, K. M., & Buss, K. A. (2017). The impact of negative affect on attention patterns to threat across the first 2 years of life. *Developmental Psychology, 53*(12), 2219–2232.

Perlman, S. B., Kalish, C. W., & Pollak, S. D. (2008). The role of maltreatment experience in children's understanding of the antecedents of emotion. *Cognition and Emotion, 22*(4), 651–670.

Perlman, S. B., Luna, B., Hein, T. C., & Huppert, T. J. (2014). fNIRS evidence of prefrontal regulation of frustration in early childhood. *NeuroImage, 85*(Part 1), 326–334.

Perry-Parrish, C., & Zeman, J. (2011). Relations among sadness regulation, peer acceptance, and social functioning in early adolescence: The role of gender. *Social Development, 20*(1), 135–153.

Pesowski, M. L., & Friedman, O. (2015). Preschoolers and toddlers use ownership to predict basic emotions. *Emotion, 15*(1), 104–108.

Pessoa, L. (2019). Embracing integration and complexity: Placing emotion within a science of brain and behaviour. *Cognition and Emotion, 33*(1), 55–60.

Pethtel, O., & Chen, Y. (2010). Cross-cultural aging in cognitive and affective components of subjective well-being. *Psychology and Aging, 25*(3), 725–729.

Piaget, J. (1952). *The origins of intelligence in children* (M. Cook, Trans.). New York: Norton.

Piazza, J. R., Charles, S. T., Stawski, R. S., & Almeida, D. M. (2013). Age and the association between negative affective states and diurnal cortisol. *Psychology and Aging, 28*(1), 47–56.

Pine, D. S. (2007). Research review: A neuroscience framework for pediatric anxiety disorders. *Journal of Child Psychology and Psychiatry, 48*(7), 631–648.

Pinquart, M. (2017). Associations of parenting dimensions and styles with internalizing symptoms in children and adolescents: A meta-analysis. *Marriage and Family Review, 53*(7), 613–640.

Planalp, E. M., & Goldsmith, H. H. (2020). Observed profiles of infant temperament: Stability, heritability, and associations with parenting. *Child Development, 91*(3), e563–e580.

Pluess, M. (2015). Individual differences in environmental sensitivity. *Child Development Perspectives, 9*(3), 138–143.

Pluess, M., & Belsky, J. (2013). Vantage sensitivity: Individual differences in response to positive experiences. *Psychological Bulletin, 139*(4), 901–916.

Polk, D. E., Cohen, S., Doyle, W. J., Skoner, D. P., & Kirschbaum, C. (2005). State and trait affect as predictors of salivary cortisol in healthy adults. *Psychoneuroendocrinology, 30*(3), 261–272.

Pollak, S. D., Camras, L. A., & Cole, P. M. (2019). Progress in understanding the emergence of human emotion. *Developmental Psychology, 55*(9), 1801–1811.

Pollak, S. D., Cicchetti, D., Hornung, K., & Reed, A. (2000). Recognizing emotion in faces: Developmental effects of child abuse and neglect. *Developmental Psychology, 36*(5), 679–688.

Pollak, S. D., Messner, M., Kistler, D. J., & Cohn, J. F. (2009). Development of perceptual expertise in emotion recognition. *Cognition, 110*(2), 242–247.

Pollak, S. D., & Sinha, P. (2002). Effects of early experience on children's recognition of facial displays of emotion. *Developmental Psychology, 38*(5), 784–791.

Pons, F., & Harris, P. (2000). *Test of Emotion Comprehension.* Lausanne, Switzerland: Francfort Communication & Partnaires.

Pons, F., & Harris, P. (2019). Children's understanding of emotions or Pascal's "error": Review and prospects. In V. LoBue, K. Pérez-Edgar, & K. Buss (Eds.), *Handbook of emotional development* (pp. 431–449). Cham, Switzerland: Springer.

Pons, F., Harris, P. L., & de Rosnay, M. (2004). Emotion comprehension between 3 and 11 years: Developmental periods and hierarchical organization. *European Journal of Developmental Psychology, 1*(2), 127–152.

Porges, S. W. (2007). The polyvagal perspective. *Biological Psychology, 74*(2), 116–143.

Porges, S. W., & Furman, S. A. (2011). The early development of the autonomic nervous system provides a neural platform for social behaviour: A polyvagal perspective. *Infant and Child Development, 20*(1), 106–118.

Portwood, S. G., Lawler, M. J., & Roberts, M. C. (2021). Science, practice, and policy related to adverse childhood experiences: Framing the conversation. *American Psychologist, 76*(2), 181–187.

Posada, G. E., & Waters, H. S. (2018). Secure base behavior, co-construction, and attachment scripts. *Monographs of the Society for Research in Child Development, 83*(4), 22–34.

Posner, M. I., & Rothbart, M. K. (2007). Research on attention networks as a model for the integration of psychological science. *Annual Review of Psychology, 58*, 1–23.

Potegal, M. (2019). On being mad, sad, and very young. In A. K. Roy, M. A. Brotman, & E. Leibenluft (Eds.), *Irritability in pediatric psychopathology* (pp. 105–145). New York: Oxford University Press.

Potegal, M., & Davidson, R. J. (2003). Temper tantrums in young children: 1. Behavioral composition. *Journal of Developmental and Behavioral Pediatrics, 24*(3), 140–147.

Potter, S., Drewelies, J., Wagner, J., Duezel, S., Brose, A., Demuth, I., . . . Gerstorf, D. (2020). Trajectories of multiple subjective well-being facets across old age: The role of health and personality. *Psychology and Aging, 35*(6), 894–909.

Potthoff, S., Garnefski, N., Miklósi, M., Ubbiali, A., Domínguez-Sánchez, F. J., Martins, E. C., . . . Kraaij, V. (2016). Cognitive emotion regulation and psychopathology across cultures: A comparison between six European countries. *Personality and Individual Differences, 98*, 218–224.

Pressman, S. D., Jenkins, B. N., & Moskowitz, J. T. (2019). Positive affect and health: What do we know and where next should we go? *Annual Review of Psychology, 70*, 627–650.

Provenzi, L., Giusti, L., & Montirosso, R. (2016). Do infants exhibit significant cortisol reactivity to the Face-to-Face Still-Face paradigm? A narrative review and meta-analysis. *Developmental Review, 42*, 34–55.

Pruessner, L., Barnow, S., Holt, D. V., Joormann, J., & Schulze, K. (2020). A cognitive control framework for understanding emotion regulation flexibility. *Emotion, 20*(1), 21-29.

Puente-Martínez, A., Prizmic-Larsen, Z., Larsen, R. J., Ubillos-Landa, S., & Páez-Rovira, D. (2021). Age differences in emotion regulation during ongoing affective life: A naturalistic experience sampling study. *Developmental Psychology, 57*(1), 126-138.

Pushkar, D., Chaikelson, J., Conway, M., Etezadi, J., Giannopoulus, C., Li, K., & Wrosch, C. (2010). Testing continuity and activity variables as predictors of positive and negative affect in retirement. *Journals of Gerontology: Series B. Psychological Sciences and Social Sciences, 65B*(1), 42-49.

Putnam, S. P., Ellis, L. K., & Rothbart, M. K. (2001). The structure of temperament from infancy through adolescence. In A. Eliasz & A. Angleitner (Eds.), *Advances in research on temperament* (pp. 165-182). Lengerich, Germany: Pabst Science.

Putnam, S. P., Gartstein, M. A., & Rothbart, M. K. (2006). Measurement of fine-grained aspects of toddler temperament: The Early Childhood Behavior Questionnaire. *Infant Behavior and Development, 29*(3), 386-401.

Putnam, S. P., & Rothbart, M. K. (2006). Development of Short and Very Short Forms of the Children's Behavior Questionnaire. *Journal of Personality Assessment, 87*(1), 102-112.

Qualter, P., Gardner, K. J., Pope, D. J., Hutchinson, J. M., & Whiteley, H. E. (2012). Ability emotional intelligence, trait emotional intelligence, and academic success in British secondary schools: A 5-year longitudinal study. *Learning and Individual Differences, 22*(1), 83-91.

Quinn, P. C., Anzures, G., Izard, C. E., Lee, K., Pascalis, O., Slater, A. M., & Tanaka, J. W. (2011). Looking across domains to understand infant representation of emotion. *Emotion Review, 3*(2), 197-206.

Quiñones-Camacho, L. E., & Davis, E. L. (2018). Discrete emotion regulation strategy repertoires and parasympathetic physiology characterize psychopathology symptoms in childhood. *Developmental Psychology, 54*(4), 718-730.

Quiñones-Camacho, L. E., & Davis, E. (2020). Children's awareness of the context-appropriate nature of emotion regulation strategies across emotions. *Cognition and Emotion, 34*(5), 977-985.

Rabinowitz, J. A., & Drabick, D. A. G. (2017). Do children fare for better and for worse? Associations among child features and parenting with child competence and symptoms. *Developmental Review, 45*, 1-30.

Ramsden, S. R., & Hubbard, J. A. (2002). Family expressiveness and parental emotion coaching: Their role in children's emotion regulation and aggression. *Journal of Abnormal Child Psychology, 30*(6), 657-667.

Ramsey, E., Patterson, G. R., & Walker, H. M. (1990). Generalization of the antisocial trait from home to school settings. *Journal of Applied Developmental Psychology, 11*(2), 209-223.

Raval, V. V., & Walker, B. L. (2019). Unpacking "culture": Caregiver socialization of emotion and child functioning in diverse families. *Developmental Review, 51*, 146-174.

Ready, R. E., Åkerstedt, A. M., & Mroczek, D. K. (2012). Emotional complexity and emotional well-being in older adults: Risks of high neuroticism. *Aging and Mental Health, 16*(1), 17-26.

Reck, C., Tietz, A., Müller, M., Seibold, K., & Tronick, E. (2018). The impact of maternal anxiety disorder on mother–infant interaction in the postpartum period. *PLOS ONE, 13*(5), e0194763.

Reed, A. E., Chan, L., & Mikels, J. A. (2014). Meta-analysis of the age-related positivity effect: Age differences in preferences for positive over negative information. *Psychology and Aging, 29*(1), 1-15.

Reed, A. E., Mikels, J. A., & Simon, K. I. (2014). Older adults prefer less choice than young adults. *Translational Issues in Psychological Science, 1*(S), 5-10.

Reef, J., van Meurs, I., Verhulst, F. C., & van der Ende, J. (2010). Children's problems predict adults' DSM-IV disorders across 24 years. *Journal of the American Academy of Child and Adolescent Psychiatry, 49*(11), 1117-1124.

Reisenzein, R., Studtmann, M., & Horstmann, G. (2013). Coherence between emotion and facial expression: Evidence from laboratory experiments. *Emotion Review, 5*(1), 16-23.

Reitman, D., Rhode, P. C., Hupp, S. D. A., & Altobello, C. (2002). Development and validation of the Parental Authority Questionnaire—Revised. *Journal of Psychopathology and Behavioral Assessment, 24*(2), 119-127.

Reschke, P. J., Walle, E. A., Flom, R., & Guenther, D. (2017). Twelve-month-old infants' sensitivity to others' emotions following positive and negative events. *Infancy, 22*(6), 874-881.

Resurrección, D. M., Salguero, J. M., & Ruiz-Aranda, D. (2014). Emotional intelligence and psychological maladjustment in adolescence: A systematic review. *Journal of Adolescence, 37*(4), 461-472.

Rhee, S. H., Lahey, B. B., & Waldman, I. D. (2015). Comorbidity among dimensions of childhood psychopathology: Converging evidence from behavior genetics. *Child Development Perspectives, 9*(1), 26-31.

Ridgeway, D., Waters, E., & Kuczaj, S. A. (1985). Acquisition of emotion-descriptive language: Receptive and productive vocabulary norms for ages 18 months to 6 years. *Developmental Psychology, 21*(5), 901-908.

Rigato, S., Menon, E., Johnson, M. H., & Farroni, T. (2011). The interaction between gaze direction and facial expressions in newborns. *European Journal of Developmental Psychology, 8*(5), 624-636.

Rivers, S. E., Brackett, M. A., Reyes, M. R., Elbertson, N. A., & Salovey, P. (2013). Improving the social and emotional climate of classrooms: A clustered randomized controlled trial testing the RULER approach. *Prevention Science, 14*(1), 77-87.

Rivers, S. E., Brackett, M. A., Reyes, M. R., Mayer, J. D., Caruso, D. R., & Salovey, P. (2012). Measuring emotional intelligence in early adolescence with the MSCEIT-YV. *Journal of Psychoeducational Assessment, 30*(4), 344-366.

Roben, C. K. P., Cole, P. M., & Armstrong, L. M. (2013). Longitudinal relations among language skills, anger expression, and regulatory strategies in early childhood. *Child Development, 84*(3), 891-905.

Roberts, B. W., & Nickel, L. B. (2017). A critical evaluation of the neo-socioanalytic model of personality. In J. Specht (Ed.), *Personality development across the lifespan* (pp. 157-177). San Diego, CA: Elsevier Academic Press.

Rodrigues, M., Sokolovic, N., Madigan, S., Luo, Y., Silva, V., Misra, S., & Jenkins, J. (2021). Paternal sensitivity and children's cognitive and socioemotional outcomes: A meta-analytic review. *Child Development, 92*(2), 554-577.

Rogers, A. A., Padilla-Walker, L. M., McLean, R. D., & Hurst, J. L. (2020). Trajectories of perceived parental psychological control across adolescence and implications for the development of depressive and anxiety symptoms. *Journal of Youth and Adolescence, 49*(1), 136-149.

Rogers, A. A., Updegraff, K. A., Iida, M., Dishion, T. J., Doane, L. D., Corbin, W. C., . . .

Ha, T. (2018). Trajectories of positive and negative affect across the transition to college: The role of daily interactions with parents and friends. *Developmental Psychology, 54*(11), 2181-2192.

Romens, S. E., McDonald, J., Svaren, J., & Pollak, S. D. (2015). Associations between early life stress and gene methylation in children. *Child Development, 86*(1), 303-309.

Roos, L. G., Levens, S. M., & Bennett, J. M. (2018). Stressful life events, relationship stressors, and cortisol reactivity: The moderating role of suppression. *Psychoneuroendocrinology, 89,* 69-77.

Roseman, I. J. (2013). Appraisal in the emotion system: Coherence in strategies for coping. *Emotion Review, 5*(2), 141-149.

Rosenthal, N. L., & Kobak, R. (2010). Assessing adolescents' attachment hierarchies: Differences across developmental periods and associations with individual adaptation. *Journal of Research on Adolescence, 20*(3), 678-706.

Rothbart, M. K. (1981). Measurement of temperament in infancy. *Child Development, 52*(2), 569-578.

Rothbart, M. K. (2011). *Becoming who we are: Temperament and personality in development.* New York: Guilford Press.

Rothbart, M. K., Ahadi, S. A., & Evans, D. E. (2000). Temperament and personality: Origins and outcomes. *Journal of Personality and Social Psychology, 78*(1), 122-135.

Rothbart, M. K., Ahadi, S. A., Hershey, K. L., & Fisher, P. (2001). Investigations of temperament at three to seven years: The Children's Behavior Questionnaire. *Child Development, 72*(5), 1394-1408.

Rothbart, M. K., & Bates, J. E. (2006). Temperament. In N. Eisenberg, W. Damon, & R. M. Lerner (Eds.), *Handbook of child psychology: Vol. 3. Social, emotional, and personality development* (6th ed., pp. 99-166). Hoboken, NJ: Wiley.

Rothbart, M. K., Sheese, B. E., Rueda, M. R., & Posner, M. I. (2011). Developing mechanisms of self-regulation in early life. *Emotion Review, 3*(2), 207-213.

Rothbaum, F., Weisz, J., Pott, M., Miyake, K., & Morelli, G. (2000). Attachment and culture: Security in the United States and Japan. *American Psychologist, 55*(10), 1093-1104.

Rothenberg, W. A., Hussong, A. M., Langley, H. A., Egerton, G. A., Halberstadt, A. G., Coffman, J. L., . . . Costanzo, P. R. (2017). Grateful parents raising grateful children: Niche selection and the socialization of child gratitude. *Applied Developmental Science, 21*(2), 106-120.

Rottman, J., DeJesus, J., & Greenebaum, H. (2019). Developing disgust: Theory, measurement, and application. In V. LoBue, K. Pérez-Edgar, & K. Buss (Eds.), *Handbook of emotional development* (pp. 283-309). Cham, Switzerland: Springer.

Rottman, J., Young, L., & Kelemen, D. (2017). The impact of testimony on children's moralization of novel actions. *Emotion, 17*(5), 811-827.

Rozin, P., Guillot, L., Fincher, K., Rozin, A., & Tsukayama, E. (2013). Glad to be sad, and other examples of benign masochism. *Judgment and Decision Making, 8*(4), 439-447.

Rozin, P., Haidt, J., & McCauley, C. R. (2016). Disgust. In L. F. Barrett, M. Lewis, & J. M. Haviland-Jones (Eds.), *Handbook of emotions* (4th ed., pp. 815-834). New York: Guilford Press.

Rozin, P., Lowery, L., Imada, S., & Haidt, J. (1999). The CAD triad hypothesis: A mapping between three moral emotions (contempt, anger, disgust) and three moral codes (community, autonomy, divinity). *Journal of Personality and Social Psychology, 76*(4), 574-586.

Ruba, A. L., Johnson, K. M., Harris, L. T., & Wilbourn, M. P. (2017). Developmental changes in infants' categorization of anger and disgust facial expressions. *Developmental Psychology, 53*(10), 1826–1832.

Ruba, A. L., Meltzoff, A. N., & Repacholi, B. M. (2019). How do you feel? Preverbal infants match negative emotions to events. *Developmental Psychology, 55*(6), 1138–1149.

Ruba, A. L., Meltzoff, A. N., & Repacholi, B. M. (2020). The development of negative event–emotion matching in infancy: Implications for theories in affective science. *Affective Science, 1*, 4–19.

Ruba, A. L., & Pollak, S. D. (2020). The development of emotion reasoning in infancy and early childhood. *Annual Review of Developmental Psychology, 2*, 503–531.

Ruba, A. L., & Repacholi, B. M. (2020). Do preverbal infants understand discrete facial expressions of emotion? *Emotion Review, 12*(4), 235–250.

Rubin, K. H., Burgess, K. B., & Hastings, P. D. (2002). Stability and social-behavioral consequences of toddlers' inhibited temperament and parenting behaviors. *Child Development, 73*(2), 483–495.

Ruby, M. B., Falk, C. F., Heine, S. J., Villa, C., & Silberstein, O. (2012). Not all collectivisms are equal: Opposing preferences for ideal affect between East Asians and Mexicans. *Emotion, 12*(6), 1206–1209.

Rudolph, K. D., Davis, M. M., & Monti, J. D. (2017). Cognition–emotion interaction as a predictor of adolescent depressive symptoms. *Developmental Psychology, 53*(12), 2377–2383.

Ruffman, T., Murray, J., Halberstadt, J., & Taumoepeau, M. (2010). Verbosity and emotion recognition in older adults. *Psychology and Aging, 25*(2), 492–497.

Ruiz-Belda, M.-A., Fernández-Dols, J.-M., Carrera, P., & Barchard, K. (2003). Spontaneous facial expressions of happy bowlers and soccer fans. *Cognition and Emotion, 17*(2), 315–326.

Russell, J., & Barrett, L. F. (1999). Core affect, prototypical emotional episodes and other things called emotion: Dissecting the elephant. *Journal of Personality and Social Psychology, 76*(5), 805–819.

Russell, J. A. (1994). Is there universal recognition of emotion from facial expression? A review of the cross-cultural studies. *Psychological Bulletin, 115*(1), 102–141.

Russell, J. A. (2003). Core affect and the psychological construction of emotion. *Psychological Review, 110*(1), 145–172.

Russell, J. A., & Widen, S. C. (2002). Words versus faces in evoking preschool children's knowledge of the causes of emotions. *International Journal of Behavioral Development, 26*(2), 97–103.

Rutter, M., Graham, P., Chadwick, O. F., & Yule, W. (1976). Adolescent turmoil: Fact or fiction? *Child Psychology and Psychiatry and Allied Disciplines, 17*(1), 35–56.

Ryan, L. H., Newton, N. J., Chauhan, P. K., & Chopik, W. J. (2017). Effects of pre-retirement personality, health and job lock on post-retirement subjective well-being. *Translational Issues in Psychological Science, 3*(4), 378–387.

Saarimäki, H., Gotsopoulos, A., Jääskeläinen, I. P., Lampinen, J., Vuilleumier, P., Hari, R., . . . Nummenmaa, L. (2016). Discrete neural signatures of basic emotions. *Cerebral Cortex, 26*(6), 2563–2573.

Saarni, C. (1979). Children's understanding of display rules for expressive behavior. *Developmental Psychology, 15*(4), 424–429.

Saarni, C. (1984). An observational study of children's attempts to monitor their expressive behavior. *Child Development, 55*, 1504–1513.

Saarni, C. (1999). *The development of emotional competence.* New York: Guilford Press.

Sacks, D. (2003). Age limits and adolescents. *Paediatrics and Child Health, 8*(9), 577. Retrieved from *www.ncbi.nlm.nih.gov/pmc/articles/PMC2794325/#__sec1title.*

Sagi, A., & Hoffman, M. L. (1976). Empathic distress in the newborn. *Developmental Psychology, 12*(2), 175–176.

Sai, L., Luo, S., Ward, A., & Sang, B. (2016). Development of the tendency to use emotion regulation strategies and their relation to depressive symptoms in Chinese adolescents. *Frontiers in Psychology, 7,* 1222.

Sallquist, J., DiDonato, M. D., Hanish, L. D., Martin, C. L., & Fabes, R. A. (2012). The importance of mutual positive expressivity in social adjustment: Understanding the role of peers and gender. *Emotion, 12*(2), 304–313.

Salovey, P., & Mayer, J. D. (1990). Emotional intelligence. *Imagination, Cognition, and Personality, 9,* 185–211.

Samuel, L. J., Roth, D. L., Schwartz, B. S., Thorpe, R. J., & Glass, T. A. (2018). Socioeconomic status, race/ethnicity, and diurnal cortisol trajectories in middle-aged and older adults. *Journals of Gerontology: Series B. Psychological Sciences and Social Sciences, 73*(3), 468–476.

Sánchez-Álvarez, N., Extremera, N., & Fernández-Berrocal, P. (2016). The relation between emotional intelligence and subjective well-being: A meta-analytic investigation. *Journal of Positive Psychology, 11*(3), 276–285.

Sánchez-Pérez, N., Putnam, S. P., Gartstein, M. A., & González-Salinas, C. (2020). ADHD and ODD symptoms in toddlers: Common and specific associations with temperament dimensions. *Child Psychiatry and Human Development, 51*(2), 310–320.

Sands, M., Ngo, N., & Isaacowitz, D. M. (2016). The interplay of motivation and emotion: View from adulthood and old age. In L. F. Barrett, M. Lewis, & J. M. Haviland-Jones (Eds.), *Handbook of emotions* (4th ed., pp. 336–349). New York: Guilford Press.

Sawyer, A. M., Borduin, C. M., & Dopp, A. R. (2015). Long-term effects of prevention and treatment on youth antisocial behavior: A meta-analysis. *Clinical Psychology Review, 42,* 130–144.

Schachter, S., & Singer, J. (1962). Cognitive, social, and physiological determinants of emotional state. *Psychological Review, 69*(5), 379–399.

Schäfer, J. Ö., Naumann, E., Holmes, E. A., Tuschen-Caffier, B., & Samson, A. C. (2017). Emotion regulation strategies in depressive and anxiety symptoms in youth: A meta-analytic review. *Journal of Youth and Adolescence, 46*(2), 261–276.

Scheibe, S., Sheppes, G., & Staudinger, U. M. (2015). Distract or reappraise? Age-related differences in emotion-regulation choice. *Emotion, 15*(6), 677–681.

Scherer, K. R. (1984). Emotion as a multicomponent process: A model and some cross-cultural data. *Review of Personality and Social Psychology, 5,* 37–63.

Scherer, K. R. (2001). Appraisal considered as a process of multilevel sequential checking. In K. R. Scherer, A. Schorr, & T. Johnstone (Eds.), *Appraisal processes in emotion: Theory, methods, research* (pp. 92–120). New York: Oxford University Press.

Scherer, K. R., & Fontaine, J. R. J. (2019). The semantic structure of emotion words across languages is consistent with componential appraisal models of emotion. *Cognition and Emotion, 33*(4), 673–682.

Scherer, K. R., & Moors, A. (2019). The emotion process: Event appraisal and component differentiation. *Annual Review of Psychology, 70,* 719–745.

Scherer, M., & Herrmann-Lingen, C. (2009). Single item on positive affect is associated with 1-year survival in consecutive medical inpatients. *General Hospital Psychiatry, 31*(1), 8–13.

Scherr, S., Mares, M.-L., Bartsch, A., & Götz, M. (2018). On the relevance of parents and TV as socializers of 6-19-year-olds' expressions of emotion: Representative data from Germany. *Journal of Children and Media, 12*(1), 33-50.

Schneirla, T. C. (1959). An evolutionary and developmental theory of biphasic processes underlying approach and withdrawal. In M. R. Jones (Ed.), *Nebraska Symposium on Motivation* (pp. 1-42). Lincoln: University of Nebraska Press.

Schwartz, G., Izard, C. E., & Ansul, S. (1985). The 5-month-old's ability to discriminate facial expressions of emotion. *Infant Behavior and Development, 8*, 65-77.

Schweizer, S., Gotlib, I. H., & Blakemore, S.-J. (2020). The role of affective control in emotion regulation during adolescence. *Emotion, 20*(1), 80-86.

Scott, B. G., Lemery-Chalfant, K., Clifford, S., Tein, J. Y., Stoll, R., & Goldsmith, H. H. (2016). A twin factor mixture modeling approach to childhood temperament: Differential heritability. *Child Development, 87*(6), 1940-1955.

Seddon, J. A., Rodriguez, V. J., Provencher, Y., Raftery-Helmer, J., Hersh, J., Labelle, P. R., & Thomassin, K. (2020). Meta-analysis of the effectiveness of the Trier Social Stress Test in eliciting physiological stress responses in children and adolescents. *Psychoneuroendocrinology, 116*, 104582.

Seider, B. H., Shiota, M. N., Whalen, P., & Levenson, R. W. (2011). Greater sadness reactivity in late life. *Social Cognitive and Affective Neuroscience, 6*(2), 186-194.

Seligman, M. E. (1971). Phobias and preparedness. *Behavior Therapy, 2*(3), 307-320.

Seligman, M. E. P. (2019). Positive psychology: A personal history. *Annual Review of Clinical Psychology, 15*, 1-23.

Sendzik, L., Schäfer, J. Ö., Samson, A. C., Naumann, E., & Tuschen-Caffier, B. (2017). Emotional awareness in depressive and anxiety symptoms in youth: A meta-analytic review. *Journal of Youth and Adolescence, 46*(4), 687-700.

Serrano, J., Iglesias, J., & Loeches, A. (1992). Visual discrimination and recognition of facial expressions of anger, fear, and surprise in 4- to 6-month-old infants. *Developmental Psychobiology, 25*(6), 411-425.

Serrano, J. M., Iglesias, J., & Loeches, A. (1995). Infants' responses to adult static facial expressions. *Infant Behavior and Development, 18*(4), 477-482.

Shackman, A. J., & Fox, A. S. (2016). Contributions of the central extended amygdala to fear and anxiety. *Journal of Neuroscience, 36*(31), 8050-8063.

Shackman, J. E., & Pollak, S. D. (2014). Impact of physical maltreatment on the regulation of negative affect and aggression. *Development and Psychopathology, 26*(4), 1021-1033.

Shaffer, A., Burt, K. B., Obradović, J., Herbers, J. E., & Masten, A. S. (2009). Intergenerational continuity in parenting quality: The mediating role of social competence. *Developmental Psychology, 45*(5), 1227-1240.

Shafir, R., Schwartz, N., Blechert, J., & Sheppes, G. (2015). Emotional intensity influences pre-implementation and implementation of distraction and reappraisal. *Social Cognitive and Affective Neuroscience, 10*(10), 1329-1337.

Shamaskin, A. M., Mikels, J. A., & Reed, A. E. (2010). Getting the message across: Age differences in the positive and negative framing of health care messages. *Psychology and Aging, 25*(3), 746-751.

Shannon, K. E., Beauchaine, T. P., Brenner, S. L., Neuhaus, E., & Gatzke-Kopp, L. (2007). Familial and temperamental predictors of resilience in children at risk for conduct disorder and depression. *Development and Psychopathology, 19*(3), 701-727.

Sheese, B. E., Voelker, P. M., Rothbart, M. K., & Posner, M. I. (2007). Parenting quality interacts with genetic variation in dopamine receptor D4 to influence temperament in early childhood. *Development and Psychopathology, 19*(4), 1039-1046.

Shek, D. T. L. (2007). A longitudinal study of perceived differences in parental control and parent–child relational qualities in Chinese adolescents in Hong Kong. *Journal of Adolescent Research, 22*(2), 156–188.

Sheppes, G., Scheibe, S., Suri, G., & Gross, J. J. (2011). Emotion-regulation choice. *Psychological Science, 22*(11), 1391–1396.

Sheppes, G., Scheibe, S., Suri, G., Radu, P., Blechert, J., & Gross, J. J. (2014). Emotion regulation choice: A conceptual framework and supporting evidence. *Journal of Experimental Psychology: General, 143*(1), 163–181.

Sherman, L. J., Rice, K., & Cassidy, J. (2015). Infant capacities related to building internal working models of attachment figures: A theoretical and empirical review. *Developmental Review, 37*, 109–141.

Shields, S., & Cicchetti, D. (1995, April). *The development of an emotion regulation assessment battery: Reliability and validity among at-risk grade-school children.* Paper presented at the Society for Research in Child Development, Indianapolis, IN.

Shields, S. A., MacArthur, H. J., & McCormick, K. T. (2018). The gendering of emotion and the psychology of women. In C. B. Travis, J. W. White, A. Rutherford, W. S. Williams, S. L. Cook, & K. F. Wyche (Eds.), *APA handbook of the psychology of women: Vol. 1. History, theory, and battlegrounds* (pp. 189–206). Washington, DC: American Psychological Association.

Shiner, R. L., Buss, K. A., McClowry, S. G., Putnam, S. P., Saudino, K. J., & Zentner, M. (2012). What is temperament now? Assessing progress in temperament research on the twenty-fifth anniversary of Goldsmith et al (1987). *Child Development Perspectives, 6*(4), 436–444.

Shiota, M. N., & Levenson, R. W. (2009). Effects of aging on experimentally instructed detached reappraisal, positive reappraisal, and emotional behavior suppression. *Psychology and Aging, 24*(4), 890–900.

Shiota, M. N., & Neufeld, S. L. (2014). My heart will go on: Aging and autonomic nervous system responding in emotion. In P. Verhaeghen & C. Hertzog (Eds.), *Oxford handbook of emotion, social cognition, and problem solving in adulthood* (pp. 225–237). New York: Oxford University Press.

Shipman, K. L., Zeman, J., Nesin, A. E., & Fitzgerald, M. (2003). Children's strategies for displaying anger and sadness: What works with whom? *Merrill-Palmer Quarterly, 49*(1), 100–122.

Shoda, Y., Mischel, W., & Peake, P. (1990). Predicting adolescent cognitive and self-regulatory competencies from preschool delay of gratification: Identifying diagnostic conditions. *Developmental Psychology, 26*(6), 978–986.

Shulman, E. P., Smith, A. R., Silva, K., Icenogle, G., Duell, N., Chein, J., & Steinberg, L. (2016). The dual systems model: Review, reappraisal, and reaffirmation. *Developmental Cognitive Neuroscience, 17*, 103–117.

Shuster, M. M., Camras, L. A., Grabell, A., & Perlman, S. B. (2020). Faces in the wild: A naturalistic study of children's facial expressions in response to an Internet prank. *Cognition and Emotion, 34*(2), 359–366.

Shuster, M. M., Mikels, J. A., & Camras, L. A. (2017). Adult age differences in the interpretation of surprised facial expressions. *Emotion, 17*(2), 191–195.

Siegel, E. H., Sands, M. K., Van den Noortgate, W., Condon, P., Chang, Y., Dy, J., . . . Barrett, L. F. (2018). Emotion fingerprints or emotion populations? A meta-analytic investigation of autonomic features of emotion categories. *Psychological Bulletin, 144*(4), 343–393.

Silvers, J. A., McRae, K., Gabrieli, J. D., Gross, J. J., Remy, K. A., & Ochsner, K. N. (2012).

Age-related differences in emotional reactivity, regulation, and rejection sensitivity in adolescence. *Emotion, 12*(6), 1235-1247.

Simon, R. W., & Nath, L. E. (2004). Gender and emotion in the United States: Do men and women differ in self-reports of feelings and expressive behavior? *American Journal of Sociology, 109*(5), 1137-1176.

Simonds, J., Kieras, J. E., Rueda, M. R., & Rothbart, M. K. (2007). Effortful control, executive attention, and emotional regulation in 7-10-year-old children. *Cognitive Development, 22*(4), 474-488.

Sims, T., Koopmann-Holm, B., Young, H. R., Jiang, D., Fung, H., & Tsai, J. L. (2018). Asian Americans respond less favorably to excitement (vs calm)-focused physicians compared to European Americans. *Cultural Diversity and Ethnic Minority Psychology, 24*(1), 1-14.

Slagt, M., Dubas, J., Deković, M., & van Aken, M. A. G. (2016). Differences in sensitivity to parenting depending on child temperament: A meta-analysis. *Psychological Bulletin, 142*(10), 1068-1110.

Slagt, M., Dubas, J., & van Aken, M. A. G. (2016). Differential susceptibility to parenting in middle childhood: Do impulsivity, effortful control and negative emotionality indicate susceptibility or vulnerability? *Infant and Child Development, 25*(4), 302-324.

Slagt, M., Dubas, J. S., van Aken, M. A. G., Ellis, B. J., & Deković, M. (2018). Sensory processing sensitivity as a marker of differential susceptibility to parenting. *Developmental Psychology, 54*(3), 543-558.

Sliwinski, M. J., & Scott, S. B. (2014). Boundary conditions for emotional well-being in aging: The importance of daily stress. In P. Verhaeghen & C. Hertzog (Eds.), *Oxford handbook of emotion, social cognition, and problem solving in adulthood* (pp. 128-141). New York: Oxford University Press.

Sloan, E., Hall, K., Moulding, R., Bryce, S., Mildred, H., & Staiger, P. K. (2017). Emotion regulation as a transdiagnostic treatment construct across anxiety, depression, substance, eating and borderline personality disorders: A systematic review. *Clinical Psychology Review, 57*, 141-163.

Smetana, J., Crean, H. F., & Campione-Barr, N. (2005). Adolescents' and parents' changing conceptions of parental authority. In J. Smetana (Ed.), *Changing boundaries of parental authority during adolescence* (pp. 31-46). San Francisco: Jossey-Bass.

Smith, C., & Ellsworth, P. (1985). Patterns of cognitive appraisal in emotion. *Journal of Personality and Social Psychology, 48*(4), 813-838.

Smith, J. D., Dishion, T. J., Shaw, D. S., Wilson, M. N., Winter, C. C., & Patterson, G. R. (2014). Coercive family process and early-onset conduct problems from age 2 to school entry. *Development and Psychopathology, 26*(4), 917-932.

Smith, K. A., & Pollak, S. D. (2021). Rethinking concepts and categories for understanding the neurodevelopmental effects of childhood adversity. *Perspectives on Psychological Science, 16*(1), 67-93.

Smith, R., Thayer, J. F., Khalsa, S. S., & Lane, R. D. (2017). The hierarchical basis of neurovisceral integration. *Neuroscience and Biobehavioral Reviews, 75*, 274-296.

Smyth, J. M., Ockenfels, M. C., Gorin, A. A., Catley, D., Porter, L. S., Kirschbaum, C., . . . Stone, A. A. (1997). Individual differences in the diurnal cycle of cortisol. *Psychoneuroendocrinology, 22*(2), 89-105.

Snyder, H. R., Gulley, L. D., Bijttebier, P., Hartman, C. A., Oldehinkel, A. J., Mezulis, A., . . . Hankin, B. L. (2015). Adolescent emotionality and effortful control: Core latent constructs and links to psychopathology and functioning. *Journal of Personality and Social Psychology, 109*(6), 1132-1149.

Snyder, J., Cramer, A., Afrank, J., & Patterson, G. R. (2005). The contributions of ineffective discipline and parental hostile attributions of child misbehavior to the development of conduct problems at home and school. *Developmental Psychology*, *41*(1), 30–41.

Somerville, L. H. (2016). Emotional development in adolescence. In L. F. Barrett, M. Lewis, & J. M. Haviland-Jones (Eds.), *Handbook of emotions* (4th ed., pp. 350–365). New York: Guilford Press.

Somerville, L. H., Hare, T., & Casey, B. J. (2011). Frontostriatal maturation predicts cognitive control failure to appetitive cues in adolescents. *Journal of Cognitive Neuroscience*, *23*(9), 2123–2134.

Somerville, L. H., Jones, R. M., Ruberry, E. J., Dyke, J. P., Glover, G., & Casey, B. J. (2013). The medial prefrontal cortex and the emergence of self-conscious emotion in adolescence. *Psychological Science*, *24*(8), 1554–1562.

Sorce, J., Emde, R., Campos, J. J., & Klinnert, M. (1985). Maternal emotional signaling: Its effect on the visual cliff behavior of 1-year-olds. *Developmental Psychology*, *21*(1), 195–200.

Soto, C. J., & Tackett, J. L. (2015). Personality traits in childhood and adolescence. *Current Directions in Psychological Science*, *24*(5), 358–362.

Soto, J. A., Perez, C. R., Kim, Y.-H., Lee, E. A., & Minnick, M. R. (2011). Is expressive suppression always associated with poorer psychological functioning? A cross-cultural comparison between European Americans and Hong Kong Chinese. *Emotion*, *11*(6), 1450–1455.

Soussignan, R., Dollion, N., Schaal, B., Durand, K., Reissland, N., & Baudouin, J. Y. (2018). Mimicking emotions: How 3–12-month-old infants use the facial expressions and eyes of a model. *Cognition and Emotion*, *32*(4), 827–842.

Soussignan, R., Schaal, B., Marlier, L., & Jiang, T. (1997). Facial and autonomic responses to biological and artificial olfactory stimuli in human neonates: Re-examining early hedonic discrimination of odors. *Physiology and Behavior*, *62*(4), 745–758.

Speisman, J., Lazarus, R., Mordkoff, A., & Davison, L. (1964). Experimental reduction of stress based on ego-defense theory. *Journal of Abnormal and Social Psychology*, *68*(4), 367–380.

Spinrad, T., & Eisenberg, N. (2019). Prosocial emotions. In V. LoBue, K. Pérez-Edgar, & K. Buss (Eds.), *Handbook of emotional development* (pp. 351–372). New York: Springer.

Spinrad, T. L., Eisenberg, N., Gaertner, B., Popp, T., Smith, C. L., Kupfer, A., . . . Hofer, C. (2007). Relations of maternal socialization and toddlers' effortful control to children's adjustment and social competence. *Developmental Psychology*, *43*(5), 1170–1186.

Spruit, A., Schalkwijk, F., van Vugt, E., & Stams, G. J. (2016). The relation between self-conscious emotions and delinquency: A meta-analysis. *Aggression and Violent Behavior*, *28*, 12–20.

Sroufe, L. A. (1977). Wariness of strangers and the study of infant development. *Child Development*, *48*(3), 731–746.

Sroufe, L. A. (1979). The coherence of individual development: Early care, attachment, and subsequent developmental issues. *American Psychologist*, *34*(10), 834–841.

Sroufe, L. A. (1982). The organization of emotional development. *Psychoanalytic Inquiry*, *1*, 575–599.

Sroufe, L. A. (1996). *Emotional development: The organization of emotional life in the early years*. New York: Cambridge University Press.

Sroufe, L. A., Coffino, B., & Carlson, E. A. (2010). Conceptualizing the role of early experience: Lessons from the Minnesota longitudinal study. *Developmental Review,* 30(1), 36–51.

Sroufe, L. A., Waters, E., & Matas, L. (1974). Contextual determinants of infant affective response. In M. Lewis & L. Rosenblum (Eds.), *The origins of behavior: Vol. 2. Fear* (pp. 49–72). New York: Wiley.

Stawski, R. S., Cichy, K. E., Piazza, J. R., & Almeida, D. M. (2013). Associations among daily stressors and salivary cortisol: Findings from the National Study of Daily Experiences. *Psychoneuroendocrinology, 38*(11), 2654–2665.

Steinberg, L. (2008). A social neuroscience perspective on adolescent risk-taking. *Developmental Review, 28*(1), 78–106.

Steinberg, L. (2020). *Adolescence* (12th ed.). New York: McGraw-Hill.

Steinberg, L., Lamborn, S. D., Darling, N., Mounts, N. S., & Dornbusch, S. M. (1994). Overtime changes in adjustment and competence among adolescents from authoritative, authoritarian, indulgent, and neglectful families. *Child Development, 65*(3), 754–770.

Steinberg, L., & Morris, A. S. (2001). Adolescent development. *Annual Review of Psychology, 52,* 83–110.

Stephanou, K., Davey, C. G., Kerestes, R., Whittle, S., & Harrison, B. J. (2017). Hard to look on the bright side: Neural correlates of impaired emotion regulation in depressed youth. *Social Cognitive and Affective Neuroscience, 12*(7), 1138–1148.

Steptoe, A., Deaton, A., & Stone, A. A. (2015). Subjective wellbeing, health, and ageing. *Lancet, 385*(9968), 640–648.

Stern, J. A., & Cassidy, J. (2018). Empathy from infancy to adolescence: An attachment perspective on the development of individual differences. *Developmental Review, 47,* 1–22.

Stern, M., & Karraker, K. H. (1989). Sex stereotyping of infants: A review of gender labeling studies. *Sex Roles: A Journal of Research, 20*(9–10), 501–522.

Stevenson, R. J., Oaten, M. J., Case, T. I., Repacholi, B. M., & Wagland, P. (2010). Children's response to adult disgust elicitors: Development and acquisition. *Developmental Psychology, 46*(1), 165–177.

Stewart, A. J., & Vandewater, E. A. (1993). The Radcliffe class of 1964: Career and family social clock projects in a transitional cohort. In K. D. Hulbert & D. T. Schuster (Eds.), *Women's lives through time: Educated American women of the twentieth century* (pp. 235–258). San Francisco, CA: Jossey-Bass

Stokes, J. E. (2019). Social integration, perceived discrimination, and self-esteem in mid- and later life: Intersections with age and neuroticism. *Aging and Mental Health, 23*(6), 727–735.

Stone, A. A., Schwartz, J. E., Broderick, J. E., & Deaton, A. (2010). A snapshot of the age distribution of psychological well-being in the United States. *Proceedings of the National Academy of Sciences of the USA, 107*(22), 9985–9990.

Subra, B., Muller, D., Fourgassie, L., Chauvin, A., & Alexopoulos, T. (2018). Of guns and snakes: Testing a modern threat superiority effect. *Cognition and Emotion, 32*(1), 81–91.

Sullivan, S., Campbell, A., Hutton, S., & Ruffman, T. (2017). What's good for the goose is not good for the gander: Age and gender differences in scanning emotion faces. *Journal of Gerontology: B. Psychological Sciences, 72*(3), 441–447.

Suri, G., Sheppes, G., Young, G., Abraham, D., McRae, K., & Gross, J. J. (2018). Emotion regulation choice: The role of environmental affordances. *Cognition and Emotion, 32*(5), 963–971.

Sutton, J., Smith, P., & Swettenham, J. (1999). Social cognition and bullying: Social inadequacy or skilled manipulation? *British Journal of Developmental Psychology, 17,* 435–450.

Suveg, C., & Zeman, J. (2004). Emotion regulation in children with anxiety disorders. *Journal of Clinical Child and Adolescent Psychology, 33*(4), 750–759.

Sylvestre, A., Bussières, È.-L., & Bouchard, C. (2016). Language problems among abused and neglected children: A meta-analytic review. *Child Maltreatment, 21*(1), 47–58.

Tamir, M., Schwartz, S. H., Cieciuch, J., Riediger, M., Torres, C., Scollon, C., . . . Vishkin, A. (2016). Desired emotions across cultures: A value-based account. *Journal of Personality and Social Psychology, 111*(1), 67–82.

Tangney, J., Wagner, P., Burggraf, S., Gramzow, R., & Fletcher, C. (1990). *The Test of Self-Conscious Affect for Children (TOSCA-C).* Fairfax, VA: George Mason University.

Tangney, J. P., Wagner, P. E., Hill-Barlow, D., Marschall, D. E., & Gramzow, R. (1996). Relation of shame and guilt to constructive versus destructive responses to anger across the lifespan. *Journal of Personality and Social Psychology, 70*(4), 797–809.

Taylor, R. D., Oberle, E., Durlak, J. A., & Weissberg, R. P. (2017). Promoting positive youth development through school-based social and emotional learning interventions: A meta-analysis of follow-up effects. *Child Development, 88*(4), 1156–1171.

Taylor, Z. E., Eisenberg, N., Spinrad, T. L., Eggum, N. D., & Sulik, M. J. (2013). The relations of ego-resiliency and emotion socialization to the development of empathy and prosocial behavior across early childhood. *Emotion, 13*(5), 822–831.

Telzer, E. H., Jorgensen, N. A., Prinstein, M. J., & Lindquist, K. A. (2021). Neurobiological sensitivity to social rewards and punishments moderates link between peer norms and adolescent risk taking. *Child Development, 92*(2), 731–745.

Thelen, E., & Smith, L. B. (2006). Dynamic systems theories. In R. M. Lerner & W. Damon (Eds.), *Handbook of child psychology: Vol. 1. Theoretical models of human development* (6th ed., pp. 258–312). Hoboken, NJ: Wiley.

Thomas, J. C., Letourneau, N., Campbell, T. S., Tomfohr-Madsen, L., Giesbrecht, G. F., & the APrON Study Team. (2017). Developmental origins of infant emotion regulation: Mediation by temperamental negativity and moderation by maternal sensitivity. *Developmental Psychology, 53*(4), 611–628.

Thompson, R. (1994). Emotion regulation: A theme in search of a definition. *Monographs of the Society for Research on Child Development, 59*(2-3), 25–52.

Thompson, R. A. (2014). Socialization of emotion and emotion regulation in the family. In J. J. Gross (Ed.), *Handbook of emotion regulation* (2nd ed., pp. 173–186). New York: Guilford Press.

Thompson, R. A. (2016). Early attachment and later development: Reframing the questions. In J. Cassidy & P. R. Shaver (Eds.), *The handbook of attachment* (3rd ed., pp. 952–877). New York: Guilford Press.

Thompson, S. F., Zalewski, M., Kiff, C. J., Moran, L., Cortes, R., & Lengua, L. J. (2020). An empirical test of the model of socialization of emotion: Maternal and child contributors to preschoolers' emotion knowledge and adjustment. *Developmental Psychology, 56*(3), 418–430.

Tilley, J. L., Huey, S. J., Jr., Farver, J. M., Lai, M. H. C., & Wang, C. X. (2021). The immigrant paradox in the problem behaviors of youth in the United States: A meta-analysis. *Child Development, 92*(2), 502–516.

Tomkins, S. S. (1962). *Affect, imagery, consciousness: Vol 1. The positive affects.* New York: Springer.

Tompkins, V., Benigno, J. P., Lee, B. L., & Wright, B. M. (2018). The relation between parents' mental state talk and children's social understanding: A meta-analysis. *Social Development, 27*(2), 223–246.

Topa, G., Depolo, M., & Alcover, C.-M. (2018). Early retirement: A meta-analysis of its antecedent and subsequent correlates. *Frontiers in Psychology, 8,* 2157.

Tottenham, N., & Gabard-Durnam, L. J. (2017). The developing amygdala: A student of the world and a teacher of the cortex. *Current Opinion in Psychology, 17,* 55–60.

Tracy, J. L., Robins, R. W., & Schriber, R. A. (2009). Development of a FACS-verified set of basic and self-conscious emotion expressions. *Emotion, 9*(4), 554–559.

Trentacosta, C. J., & Fine, S. E. (2010). Emotion knowledge, social competence, and behavior problems in childhood and adolescence: A meta-analytic review. *Social Development, 19*(1), 1–29.

Trickett, P. K., Gordis, E., Peckins, M. K., & Susman, E. J. (2014). Stress reactivity in maltreated and comparison male and female young adolescents. *Child Maltreatment, 19*(1), 27–37.

Trommsdorff, G., Friedlmeier, W., & Mayer, B. (2007). Sympathy, distress, and prosocial behavior of preschool children in four cultures. *International Journal of Behavioral Development, 31*(3), 284–293.

Tronick, E., Adamson, L., Wise, S., & Brazelton, T. B. (1978). The infant's response to entrapment between contradictory messages in face-to-face interaction. *Journal of the American Academy of Child Psychiatry, 17*(1), 1–13.

Tronick, E., & Beeghly, M. (2011). Infants' meaning-making and the development of mental health problems. *American Psychologist, 66*(2), 107–119.

Tsai, J. L. (2007). Ideal affect: Cultural causes and behavioral consequences. *Perspectives on Psychological Science, 2*(3), 242–259.

Tsai, J. L., Knutson, B., & Fung, H. H. (2006). Cultural variation in affect valuation. *Journal of Personality and Social Psychology, 90*(2), 288–307.

Tsai, J. L., & Sims, T. (2016). Emotional aging in different cultures: Implications of affect valuation theory. In A. D. Ong & C. E. Löckenhoff (Eds.), *Emotion, aging, and health.* (pp. 119–143). Washington, DC: American Psychological Association.

Tsai, J. L., Sims, T., Qu, Y., Thomas, E., Jiang, D., & Fung, H. H. (2018). Valuing excitement makes people look forward to old age less and dread it more. *Psychology and Aging, 33*(7), 975–992.

Tsotsi, S., Broekman, B. F. P., Shek, L. P., Tan, K. H., Chong, Y. S., Chen, H., . . . Rifkin-Graboi, A. E. (2019). Maternal parenting stress, child exuberance, and preschoolers' behavior problems. *Child Development, 90*(1), 136–146.

Uchino, B. N., Birmingham, W., & Berg, C. A. (2010). Are older adults less or more physiologically reactive? A meta-analysis of age-related differences in cardiovascular reactivity to laboratory tasks. *Journals of Gerontology: Series B. Psychological Sciences and Social Sciences, 65B*(2), 154–162.

Urry, H. L., & Gross, J. J. (2010). Emotion regulation in older age. *Current Directions in Psychological Science, 19*(6), 352–357.

Ursache, A., Kiely Gouley, K., Dawson-McClure, S., Barajas-Gonzalez, R. G., Calzada, E. J., Goldfeld, K. S., & Brotman, L. M. (2020). Early emotion knowledge and later academic achievement among children of color in historically disinvested neighborhoods. *Child Development, 91*(6), e1249–e1266.

Vaish, A., Carpenter, M., & Tomasello, M. (2016). The early emergence of guilt-motivated prosocial behavior. *Child Development, 87*(6), 1772–1782.

Vaish, A., Grossmann, T., & Woodward, A. (2008). Not all emotions are created equal:

The negativity bias in social-emotional development. *Psychological Bulletin, 134*(3), 383–403.

Valiente, C., Eisenberg, N., Shepard, S. A., Fabes, R. A., Cumberland, A. J., Losoya, S. H., & Spinrad, T. L. (2004). The relations of mothers' negative expressivity to children's experience and expression of negative emotion. *Journal of Applied Developmental Psychology, 25*(2), 215–235.

Van Assche, L., Luyten, P., Bruffaerts, R., Persoons, P., van de Ven, L., & Vandenbulcke, M. (2013). Attachment in old age: Theoretical assumptions, empirical findings and implications for clinical practice. *Clinical Psychology Review, 33*(1), 67–81.

Van Beveren, M.-L., Mezulis, A., Wante, L., & Braet, C. (2019). Joint contributions of negative emotionality, positive emotionality, and effortful control on depressive symptoms in youth. *Journal of Clinical Child and Adolescent Psychology, 48*(1), 131–142.

Van Bockstaele, B., Verschuere, B., Tibboel, H., De Houwer, J., Crombez, G., & Koster, E. H. W. (2014). A review of current evidence for the causal impact of attentional bias on fear and anxiety. *Psychological Bulletin, 140*(3), 682–721.

Van den Akker, A. L., Briley, D. A., Grotzinger, A. D., Tackett, J. L., Tucker-Drob, E. M., & Harden, K. P. (2021). Adolescent Big Five personality and pubertal development: Pubertal hormone concentrations and self-reported pubertal status. *Developmental Psychology, 57*(1), 60–72.

van der Pol, L. D., Groeneveld, M. G., van Berkel, S. R., Endendijk, J. J., Hallers-Haalboom, E. T., Bakermans-Kranenburg, M. J., & Mesman, J. (2015). Fathers' and mothers' emotion talk with their girls and boys from toddlerhood to preschool age. *Emotion, 15*(6), 854–864.

van Goozen, S. H. M., Fairchild, G., Snoek, H., & Harold, G. T. (2007). The evidence for a neurobiological model of childhood antisocial behavior. *Psychological Bulletin, 133*(1), 149–182.

van IJzendoorn, M. H., & Bakermans-Kranenburg, M. J. (2019). Bridges across the intergenerational transmission of attachment gap. *Current Opinion in Psychology, 25*, 31–36.

van IJzendoorn, M. H., & Sagi, A. (2001). Cultural blindness or selective inattention? *American Psychologist, 56*(10), 824–825.

Vasey, M. W., Harbaugh, C. N., Fisher, L. B., Heath, J. H., Hayes, A. F., & Bijttebier, P. (2014). Temperament synergies in risk for and protection against depressive symptoms: A prospective replication of a three-way interaction. *Journal of Research in Personality, 53*, 134–147.

Venezia, M., Messinger, D. S., Thorp, D., & Mundy, P. (2004). The development of anticipatory smiling. *Infancy, 6*(3), 397–406.

Verhage, M. L., Schuengel, C., Madigan, S., Fearon, R. M. P., Oosterman, M., Cassibba, R., . . . van IJzendoorn, M. H. (2016). Narrowing the transmission gap: A synthesis of three decades of research on intergenerational transmission of attachment. *Psychological Bulletin, 142*(4), 337–366.

Verhoef, R. E. J., Alsem, S. C., Verhulp, E. E., & De Castro, B. O. (2019). Hostile intent attribution and aggressive behavior in children revisited: A meta-analysis. *Child Development, 90*(5), e525–e547.

Vermeulen, A., Vandebosch, H., & Heirman, W. (2018a). Shall I call, text, post it online or just tell it face-to-face? How and why Flemish adolescents choose to share their emotions on- or offline. *Journal of Children and Media, 12*(1), 81–97.

Vermeulen, A., Vandebosch, H., & Heirman, W. (2018b). #Smiling, #venting, or both?

Adolescents' social sharing of emotions on social media. *Computers in Human Behavior*, *84*, 211–219.

Viana, A. G., Dixon, L. J., Stevens, E. N., & Ebesutani, C. (2016). Parental emotion socialization strategies and their interaction with child interpretation biases among children with anxiety disorders. *Cognitive Therapy and Research*, *40*(5), 717–731.

Vine, V., & Aldao, A. (2014). Impaired emotional clarity and psychopathology: A transdiagnostic deficit with symptom-specific pathways through emotion regulation. *Journal of Social and Clinical Psychology*, *33*(4), 319–342.

Visted, E., Vøllestad, J., Nielsen, M. B., & Schanche, E. (2018). Emotion regulation in current and remitted depression: A systematic review and meta-analysis. *Frontiers in Psychology*, *9*, 756.

Voltmer, K., & von Salisch, M. (2017). Three meta-analyses of children's emotion knowledge and their school success. *Learning and Individual Differences*, *59*, 107–118.

von Helversen, B., & Mata, R. (2012). Losing a dime with a satisfied mind: Positive affect predicts less search in sequential decision making. *Psychology and Aging*, *27*(4), 825–839.

von Polier, G. G., Greimel, E., Konrad, K., Großheinrich, N., Kohls, G., Vloet, T. D., . . . Schulte-Rüther, M. (2020). Neural correlates of empathy in boys with early onset conduct disorder. *Frontiers in Psychiatry*, *11*, 178.

Vygotsky, L. S., Rieber, R. W., & Carton, A. S. (1987). *The collected works of L. S. Vygotsky: Vol. 1. Problems of general psychology*. New York: Plenum Press. (Original work published in 1934)

Wager, T. D., Kang, J., Johnson, T. D., Nichols, T. E., Satpute, A., & Barrett, L. F. (2015). A Bayesian model of category-specific emotional brain responses. *PLoS Computational Biology*, *11*(4), e1004066.

Wakschlag, L. S., & Keenan, K. (2001). Clinical significance and correlates of disruptive behavior in environmentally at-risk preschoolers. *Journal of Clinical Child Psychology*, *30*(2), 262–275.

Walker-Andrews, A. S., Krogh-Jespersen, S., Mayhew, E. M. Y., & Coffield, C. N. (2011). Young infants' generalization of emotional expressions: Effects of familiarity. *Emotion*, *11*(4), 842–851.

Walle, E. A., & Dahl, A. (2020). Definitions matter for studying emotional development. *Developmental Psychology*, *56*(4), 837–840.

Walle, E. A., Reschke, P. J., Camras, L. A., & Campos, J. J. (2017). Infant differential behavioral responding to discrete emotions. *Emotion*, *17*(7), 1078–1091.

Waller, R., Wagner, N. J., Barstead, M. G., Subar, A., Petersen, J. L., Hyde, J. S., & Hyde, L. W. (2020). A meta-analysis of the associations between callous–unemotional traits and empathy, prosociality, and guilt. *Clinical Psychology Review*, *75*, 101809.

Waters, S. F., & Thompson, R. A. (2014). Children's perceptions of the effectiveness of strategies for regulating anger and sadness. *International Journal of Behavioral Development*, *38*(2), 174–181.

Watson, D., Clark, L. A., & Tellegen, A. (1988). Development and validation of brief measures of positive and negative affect: The PANAS scales. *Journal of Personality and Social Psychology*, *54*(6), 1063–1070.

Watson, J. B., & Rayner, R. (1920). Conditioned emotional reactions. *Journal of Experimental Psychology*, *3*(1), 1–14.

Watts, T. W., Duncan, G. J., & Quan, H. (2018). Revisiting the marshmallow test: A conceptual replication investigating links between early delay of gratification and later outcomes. *Psychological Science*, *29*(7), 1159–1177.

Webb, S. J., Monk, C. S., & Nelson, C. A. (2001). Mechanisms of postnatal neurobiological development: Implications for human development. *Developmental Neuropsychology*, *19*(2), 147–171.

Webb, T. L., Miles, E., & Sheeran, P. (2012). Dealing with feeling: A meta-analysis of the effectiveness of strategies derived from the process model of emotion regulation. *Psychological Bulletin*, *138*(4), 775–808.

Weems, C. F., Silverman, W. K., Rapee, R. M., & Pina, A. A. (2003). The role of control in childhood anxiety disorders. *Cognitive Therapy and Research*, *27*(5), 557–568.

Weinberger, A. H., Gbedemah, M., Martinez, A. M., Nash, D., Galea, S., & Goodwin, R. D. (2018). Trends in depression prevalence in the USA from 2005 to 2015: Widening disparities in vulnerable groups. *Psychological Medicine*, *48*(8), 1308–1315.

Weinstein, E. (2017). Adolescents' differential responses to social media browsing: Exploring causes and consequences for intervention. *Computers in Human Behavior*, *76*, 396–405.

Wenzler, S., Levine, S., van Dick, R., Oertel-Knöchel, V., & Aviezer, H. (2016). Beyond pleasure and pain: Facial expression ambiguity in adults and children during intense situations. *Emotion*, *16*(6), 807–814.

Wettstein, M., Wahl, H.-W., & Siebert, J. S. (2020). 20-year trajectories of health in midlife and old age: Contrasting the impact of personality and attitudes toward own aging. *Psychology and Aging*, *35*(6), 910–924.

Weymouth, B. B., Buehler, C., Zhou, N., & Henson, R. A. (2016). A meta-analysis of parent–adolescent conflict: Disagreement, hostility, and youth maladjustment. *Journal of Family Theory and Review*, *8*(1), 95–112.

Widen, S. C. (2016). The development of children's concepts of emotion. In L. F. Barrett, M. Lewis, & J. M. Haviland-Jones (Eds.), *Handbook of emotions* (4th ed., pp. 307–318). New York: Guilford Press.

Widen, S. C., & Nelson, N. L. (2022). Differentiation and language acquisition in children's understanding of emotion. In D. Dukes, A. C. Samson, & E. A. Walle (Eds.), *Handbook of emotional development* (pp. 174–187). Oxford, UK: Oxford University Press.

Widen, S. C., & Russell, J. (2002). Gender and preschoolers' perception of emotion. *Merrill-Palmer Quarterly*, *48*(3), 248–262.

Widen, S. C., & Russell, J. A. (2004). The relative power of an emotion's facial expression, label, and behavioral consequence to evoke preschoolers' knowledge of its cause. *Cognitive Development*, *19*(1), 111–125.

Wieck, C., & Kunzmann, U. (2017). Age differences in emotion recognition: A question of modality? *Psychology and Aging*, *32*(5), 401–411.

Wilhelm, I., Born, J., Kudielka, B. M., Schlotz, W., & Wüst, S. (2007). Is the cortisol awakening rise a response to awakening? *Psychoneuroendocrinology*, *32*(4), 358–366.

Williams, B. R., Ponesse, J., Schachar, R., Logan, G., & Tannock, R. (1999). Development of inhibitory control across the life span. *Developmental Psychology*, *35*(1), 205–213.

Williams, K., & McGillicuddy-De Lisi, A. (1999). Coping strategies in adolescents. *Journal of Applied Developmental Psychology*, *20*(4), 537–549.

Willoughby, T., Good, M., Adachi, P. J. C., Hamza, C., & Tavernier, R. (2013). Examining the link between adolescent brain development and risk taking from a social-developmental perspective. *Brain and Cognition*, *83*(3), 315–323.

Wilson, R. S., Krueger, K. R., Arnold, S. E., Barnes, L. L., de Leon, C. F. M., Bienias, J. L., & Bennett, D. A. (2006). Childhood adversity and psychosocial adjustment in old age. *American Journal of Geriatric Psychiatry*, *14*(4), 307–315.

Wilson, T. E., Weedon, J., Cohen, M. H., Golub, E. T., Milam, J., Young, M. A., . . . Fredrickson, B. L. (2017). Positive affect and its association with viral control among women with HIV infection. *Health Psychology, 36*(1), 91–100.

Winecoff, A., LaBar, K. S., Madden, D. J., Cabeza, R., & Huettel, S. A. (2011). Cognitive and neural contributors to emotion regulation in aging. *Social Cognitive and Affective Neuroscience, 6*(2), 165–176.

Wolff, P. H. (1963). Observations on the early development of smiling. In B. Foss (Ed.), *Determinants of infant behavior* (Vol. 2, pp. 113–132). London: Methuen.

Wolff, P. H. (1969). The natural history of crying and other vocalizations in early infancy. In B. Foss (Ed.), *Determinants of infant behavior* (Vol. 4, pp. 81–109). London: Methuen.

Wolff, P. H. (1987). *The development of behavioral states and the expression of emotions in early infancy: New proposals for investigation.* Chicago: University of Chicago Press.

Wols, A., Scholte, R. H. J., & Qualter, P. (2015). Prospective associations between loneliness and emotional intelligence. *Journal of Adolescence, 39*, 40–48.

Wong, B., Cronin-Golomb, A., & Neargarder, S. (2005). Patterns of visual scanning as predictors of emotion identification in normal aging. *Neuropsychology, 19*(6), 739–749.

World Health Organization (2020). Adolescent Health. Retrieved from *www.who.int/health-topics/adolescent-health#tab=tab_1.*

Worldometer. (2020). *Life expectancy of the world population.* Retrieved from *www.worldometers.info/demographics/life-expectancy.*

Wörmann, V., Holodynski, M., Kärtner, J., & Keller, H. (2012). A cross-cultural comparison of the development of the social smile: A longitudinal study of maternal and infant imitation in 6- and 12-week-old infants. *Infant Behavior and Development, 35*(3), 335–347.

Wörmann, V., Holodynski, M., Kärtner, J., & Keller, H. (2014). The emergence of social smiling: The interplay of maternal and infant imitation during the first three months in cross-cultural comparison. *Journal of Cross-Cultural Psychology, 45*(3), 339–361.

Wu, A. F. W., Ooi, J., Wong, P. W. C., Catmur, C., & Lau, J. Y. F. (2019). Evidence of pathological social withdrawal in non-Asian countries: A global health problem? *Lancet Psychiatry, 6*(3), 195–196.

Wu, D. Y. H. (1996). Chinese childhood socialization. In M. H. Bond (Ed.), *Handbook of Chinese psychology* (pp. 143–154). New York: Oxford University Press.

Wu, Y., & Schulz, L. E. (2020). Understanding social display rules: Using one person's emotional expressions to infer the desires of another. *Child Development, 91*(5), 1786–1799.

Xu, F., & Kushnir, T. (2013). Infants are rational constructivist learners. *Current Directions in Psychological Science, 22*(1), 28–32.

Yap, M. B. H., Pilkington, P. D., Ryan, S. M., & Jorm, A. F. (2014). Parental factors associated with depression and anxiety in young people: A systematic review and meta-analysis. *Journal of Affective Disorders, 156*, 8–23.

Yeager, D. S., Dahl, R. E., & Dweck, C. S. (2018). Why interventions to influence adolescent behavior often fail but could succeed. *Perspectives on Psychological Science, 13*(1), 101–122.

Yeh, K. H., Bedford, O., Wu, C. W., Wang, S. Y., & Yen, N. S. (2017). Suppression benefits boys in Taiwan: The relation between gender, emotional regulation strategy, and mental health. *Frontiers in Psychology, 8*, 135.

Young, N. A., & Mikels, J. A. (2020). Paths to positivity: The relationship of age differences in appraisals of control to emotional experience. *Cognition and Emotion, 34*(5), 1010–1019.

Young, N. A., Minton, A., & Mikels, J. A. (2021). The appraisal approach to aging and emotion: An integrative theoretical framework. *Developmental Review, 59,* 100947.

Youssef, G. J., Whittle, S., Allen, N. B., Lubman, D. I., Simmons, J. G., & Yücel, M. (2016). Cognitive control as a moderator of temperamental motivations toward adolescent risk-taking behavior. *Child Development, 87*(2), 395–404.

Zaman, W., & Fivush, R. (2013). Gender differences in elaborative parent–child emotion and play narratives. *Sex Roles, 68*(9–10), 591–604.

Zastrow, B. L., Martel, M. M., & Widiger, T. A. (2018). Preschool oppositional defiant disorder: A disorder of negative affect, surgency, and disagreeableness. *Journal of Clinical Child and Adolescent Psychology, 47*(6), 967–977.

Zeifman, D., & Hazan, C. (2016). Pair bonds as attachments: Mounting evidence in support of Bowlby's hypothesis. In J. Cassidy & P. R. Shaver (Eds.), *Handbook of attachment* (3rd ed., pp. 416–434). New York: Guilford Press.

Zelazo, P. R., & Komer, M. J. (1971). Infant smiling to nonsocial stimuli and the recognition hypothesis. *Child Development, 42*(5), 1327–1339.

Zhang, F., & Labouvie-Vief, G. (2004). Stability and fluctuation in adult attachment style over a 6-year period. *Attachment and Human Development, 6*(4), 419–437.

Zhang, W., Fagan, S. E., & Gao, Y. (2017). Respiratory sinus arrhythmia activity predicts internalizing and externalizing behaviors in non-referred boys. *Frontiers in Psychology, 8,* 1496.

Zhang, Z., Zhang, J., Zhao, N., & Yang, Y. (2019). Social network size and subjective well-being: The mediating role of future time perspective among community-dwelling retirees. *Frontiers in Psychology, 10,* 2590.

Zhou, Q., Eisenberg, N., Losoya, S. H., Fabes, R. A., Reiser, M., Guthrie, I. K., . . . Shepard, S. A. (2002). The relations of parental warmth and positive expressiveness to children's empathy-related responding and social functioning: A longitudinal study. *Child Development, 73*(3), 893–915.

Zimmer-Gembeck, M., & Skinner, E. (2011). The development of coping across childhood and adolescence: An integrative review and critique of research. *International Journal of Behavioral Development, 35*(1), 1–17.

Zimmermann, P. (2004). Attachment representations and characteristics of friendship relations during adolescence. *Journal of Experimental Child Psychology, 88*(1), 83–101.

Zimmermann, P., & Iwanski, A. (2014). Emotion regulation from early adolescence to emerging adulthood and middle adulthood. *International Journal of Behavioral Development, 38*(2), 182–194.

Zimmermann, P., Maier, M. A., Winter, M., & Grossmann, K. E. (2001). Attachment and adolescents' emotion regulation during a joint problem-solving task with a friend. *International Journal of Behavioral Development, 25*(4), 331–343.

Zsido, A. N., Deak, A., & Bernath, L. (2019). Is a snake scarier than a gun? The ontogenetic–phylogenetic dispute from a new perspective: The role of arousal. *Emotion, 19*(4), 726–732.

Zuckerman, M. (1994). *Behavioral expressions and biosocial bases of sensation seeking.* New York: Cambridge University Press.

Index

Note. *f* following a page number indicates a figure.
Page references in **bold** indicate glossary entries.

Ability EI, 133–136, 138, 173–175, 177, **297**. *See also* Emotional intelligence (EI)
Abuse, 220, 251–252, **297**. *See also* Adverse childhood experiences (ACEs); Maltreatment
Academic problems, 43, 68, 113–114, 135
Acceptingness, 43, 122–123, **297**
Accessibility, 43, **297**
Acculturation, 125–126. *See also* Cultural factors
Adjustment, 135–136, 137, 162–163, 280–281, 289
Adolescence
  acculturation and, 125–126
  attachment and, 110–113
  cultural factors and, 125–126
  depression and, 270–271
  emotion regulation and, 118–125
  emotion understanding and, 133–136
  emotional expression and experience, 104–107
  empathy and, 225
  gender and, 126–128
  neurobiological factors, 128–133
  overview, 103–104, 136–138
  social interactions and, 113–118
  temperament and, 108–110
Adult Attachment Interview (AAI), 110, 147–148
Adult Temperament Questionnaire (ATQ), 146
Adulthood. *See also* Later adulthood
  attachment and, 147–149
  cultural factors and, 158–165
  disgust and, 245–246
  emotion regulation and, 152–158
  emotional expression and experience, 139–141
  emotional intelligence (EI) and, 173–175
  emotion-related parenting behaviors and, 149–151
  facial expressions and, 140–145

gender and, 165–167
  neurobiological factors, 167–173
  overview, 139, 175–177
  socialization of emotion-related parenting behaviors and, 149–151
  from temperament to personality, 145–147
Adverse childhood experiences (ACEs), 186–187, 251–252, 287, **297**. *See also* Abuse; Maltreatment; Neglect
Adversity, 251–252
Affect. *See also* Subjective well-being (SWB)
  adolescence and, 104–105, 106–107
  affect sharing, 34, 226
  arousal and, 201–202
  compared to core affect, 9–10
  complexity, 185–186
  definition of, **297**
  infancy and, 64
  mirroring/modeling, 17
  overview, 29–34, 139–140
  parent–adolescent conflicts and, 114–115
Affect balance score, 179, **298**
Affect programs, 6–7, **298**
Affect valuation theory (AVT), 162, 201, **298**
AFFEX (System for Identifying Affect Expressions by Holistic Judgments), 30–33, **298**
Aggression, 220, 242–243, 250, 256, 272–279
Aging. *See* Later adulthood
Agreeableness
  adulthood and, 176
  emotional regulation in adulthood and, 155–156
  later adulthood and, 184–186, 212
  ODD and CD and, 273
  overview, 145–147

Alexithymia, 261, **298**
Allostasis, 10, **298**
Amae, 247–248
Ambivalent attachment. *See* Resistant/
    ambivalent attachment
Amygdala. *See also* Brain functioning
    anxiety and, 266
    depression and, 271
    infancy and, 52–53, 64
    later adulthood and, 203–204, 213
    maltreatment and, 258
    temperament during infancy and, 40
Anger
    adolescence and, 127–128
    appraisals and, 8
    cultural factors and, 160–161
    gender and, 165, 166–167
    infancy and, 61–63
    maltreatment and, 219–220, 256
    overview, 238–244, 250
Anticipatory smile, **298**. *See also* Smiling
Antisocial behavior, 272–279
Antisocial coping strategies, 256
Anxiety, 262–267, 270–271, 288
Anxiety disorders, 261, 262, 267
Anxious/preoccupied attachment, 187–189,
    190–191, **298**. *See also* Attachment
Appeal function, 17, **298**
Appraisal theories. *See also* Theories of emotion
    definition of, **298**
    functionalist/relational perspective and, 25
    overview, 5–6, 7–9, 27
Appraisals. *See also* Reappraisal
    anger and aggression and, 243
    bias and, 192
    cultural factors and, 160–161
    decision making during later adulthood and,
        193
    definition of, **298**
    functionalist/relational perspective and, 25
    later adulthood and, 212
    overview, 6, 7–8, 27
Arousal/regulatory systems, 122–123, 193, 261
Attachment. *See also* Anxious/preoccupied
    attachment; Dismissing/avoidant
    attachment; Fearful attachment; Relational
    factors; Resistant/ambivalent attachment;
    Secure attachment style
    adolescence and, 110–113, 137
    adulthood and, 147–149, 176
    anxiety and, 264
    childhood and, 71–72
    cortisol and, 55
    cultural factors and, 47–48, 64
    depression and, 269–270
    emotion regulation during childhood and,
        84
    empathy and, 224
    environmental sensitivity and, 253–254
    infancy and, 40–43, 47–48, 55, 63–64
    later adulthood and, 187–191, 212

socialization and regulation during infancy
    and, 44–45
transmission gap, 149, **316**
Attentional bias, 233–235
Attentional deployment, 153, 196, **299**. *See also*
    Strategy use
Attention-deficit/hyperactivity disorder
    (ADHD), 39
Authoritarian parenting style, 150–151, 270, **299**.
    See also Parenting
Authoritative parenting style, 150–151, **299**. *See
    also* Parenting
Autonomic nervous system (ANS). *See also*
    Neurobiological factors
    adolescence and, 131–132, 138
    adulthood and, 170–171, 177
    anxiety and, 267
    childhood and, 93–94
    definition of, **299**
    depression and, 271–272
    infancy and, 53–54, 64
    later adulthood and, 207–208
    maltreatment and, 258
    overview, 2
Avoidance, 122–123, 246, 256
Avoidant attachment, 42, 84, **299**. *See also*
    Attachment; Dismissing/avoidant
    attachment

Basic (or discrete) emotion theories. *See also*
    Discrete emotion theories; Theories of
    emotion
    childhood and, 67
    definition of, **299**
    functionalist/relational perspective and, 24–26
    infancy and, 64
    overview, 5–7, 27
Basic emotions, 18, 20–21, 26–27, 190–192
Behavioral inhibition (BI)
    anxiety and, 262–263
    definition of, **299**
    environmental sensitivity and, 255
    temperament during adolescence and, 109–110
    temperament during childhood and, 70–71
    temperament during infancy and, 37–38,
        39–40
Behavioral observation, 80–81, 293–294
Beliefs, 77–78, 87–88
Benign masochism, 244–245, **299**
Biases
    anxiety and, 265
    later adulthood and, 193–194, 210–211
    maltreatment and, 259–260
    threats and fear and, 233–235
Big Five/Five-Factor model. *See also*
    Temperament
    adulthood and, 175–176
    definition of, **299**
    gender and, 165
    later adulthood and, 184–186, 212
    overview, 146

Big Six emotions
  adulthood and, 142, 144, 176
  definition of, **299**
  overview, 6, 215–216
Blame, 220
Borderline personality disorder, 261
Brain functioning. *See also* Neurobiological
    factors
  adolescence and, 128–133, 138
  adulthood and, 167–169
  childhood and, 90–93, 102
  infancy and, 51–53, 64
  later adulthood and, 203–207
  maltreatment and, 257–259
Broaden-and-build theory (BBT), 229–231, 249,
    300
Broad-to-differentiated hypothesis, 97–98, **300**

Callous unemotionality (CU)
  ability EI and, 135
  adolescence and, 135
  definition of, **300**
  ODD and CD and, 274–275
  overview, 273, 288–289
Caregiving behaviors. *See also* Parenting
  attachment during infancy and, 42–43
  contingent responding and, 74–75
  cultural factors and, 48
  discussion of emotions and, 75–76
  exposure to emotion-inducing experiences
    and, 76–77
  gender and, 50–51
  HPA system and, 95
  later adulthood and, 182–183
  socialization and regulation during infancy
    and, 44–45
Categorization, 55–63
Child abuse. *See* Abuse; Adverse childhood
    experiences (ACEs); Maltreatment
Child Behavior Checklist (CBCL)
  adolescence and, 104–105
  anger and, 241–242
  definition of, **300**
  ODD and CD and, 277
  psychopathology and, 261–262
  temperament during childhood and, 69
Child Behavior Questionnaire (CBQ), 112–113
Childhood
  anger and, 239–241
  attachment and, 71–72
  cultural factors and, 85–88, 102
  disgust and, 244–246
  emotion regulation and, 78–84, 85, 101–102
  emotion understanding and, 95–100
  emotional expression and experience, 65–68, 101
  empathy and, 223–226
  gender and, 88–90, 102
  neurobiological factors, 90–95, 102
  overview, 65, 100–102
  self-conscious emotions and, 217–219
  socialization and, 72–78, 86–87, 101

temperament and, 69–71, 85–86, 101, 102
  threats and fear and, 237–238
Childhood maltreatment. *See* Maltreatment
Child-oriented school-based programs, 284–286,
    289–290
Children's Behavior Questionnaire (CBQ), 242,
    273
Code-switching, 125–126, **300**
Cognitive change. *See also* Reappraisal; Strategy
    use
  definition of, **300**
  later adulthood and, 196, 197, 198–199
  maltreatment and, 257–258
  overview, 153
Cognitive factors, 3, 26, 83–84, 210, 261, 292
Cognitive reappraisal. *See also* Reappraisal
  adulthood and, 154–155
  definition of, **300**
  depression and, 268–269
  overview, 91, 101, 153
Cognitive-developmental theory, 12, 18
Coherence, 170, **300**
Collectivism, 160, 161–162, **300**. *See also*
    Individualism/collectivism
Common method variance, 151, **301**
Comorbidity, 260, **301**
Conduct disorder (CD)
  cultural factors and, 280
  definition of, **301**
  overview, 241–242, 272–279, 288–289
Conflict, 113–115
Conscientiousness
  adulthood and, 175–176
  emotional regulation in adulthood and, 155
  later adulthood and, 184–186, 212
  ODD and CD and, 273
  overview, 145–147
Constructivist theories, 9, 171. *See also*
    Psychological construction theories; Social
    construction theories
Contempt, 156
Contempt–anger–disgust (CAD) theory, 247, **301**
Contextual factors, 17, 106–107, 109–110,
    136–137. *See also* Environmental factors
Contingent responding, 20–21, 73–75, **301**
Cooperativeness, 43, **301**
Coping strategies, 82, 242, 256, 269
Coping with Children's Negative Emotions Scale
    (CCNES), 74, 86–87, 149–150, 225–226
Coping with Toddlers' Negative Emotions Scale,
    149–150
Core affect, 9, 31–34, 261, **301**
Cortisol
  adolescence and, 132–133
  adulthood and, 171–173
  depression and, 272
  environmental sensitivity and, 253–255
  infancy and, 54–55, 64
  later adulthood and, 208–209, 214
  maltreatment and, 258–259
  ODD and CD and, 278

Cortisol awakening response (CAR), 54–55,
132–133, 208, **301**
Cry face, 31–33, **301**. *See also* Facial expressions
Cultural dimensions theory, 160, **301**
Cultural factors. *See also* WEIRD (Western,
educated, industrialized, rich demographic)
populations
adolescence and, 125–126
adulthood and, 158–165, 176–177
childhood and, 85–88, 102
culture-specific emotions, 247–248, 250, 292
empathy and, 227–229
HPA system and, 172–173
infancy and, 45–48, 64
later adulthood and, 199–202, 213
overview, 26–27, 292
psychopathology and, 279–282, 289
self-conscious emotions and, 221
subjective well-being (SWB) and, 140–141
temperament during infancy and, 40
threats and fear and, 238
Cultural norm hypothesis, 280
Cyberbullying, 115. *See also* Social media

Decision making, 192–195, 212
Dedifferentiation, 206, **302**
Delay of gratification tasks, 80–81, 123–125,
138, **302**
Demonstrative modeling, 72–73, **302**
Depression
alexithymia and, 261
cultural factors and, 163–164, 280, 281
later adulthood and, 182–183
overview, 267–272, 288
parent–adolescent conflicts and, 114–115
socialization and regulation during infancy
and, 45
Detachment, 197, 257–258
Developmental theories. *See also* Theories of
emotion
affective and/or cognitive pre-emotion
precursors, 17–26
basic emotions as foundations of development,
13–17
future research directions and, 291–295
history of, 12
overview, 11, 13, 27
Dexamethasone suppression test (DST), 272, **302**
Diagnosis, 260–261, 279–282
*Diagnostic and Statistical Manual of Mental
Disorders* (DSM-5)
behavioral problems and, 272–273
cultural factors and, 279–280
definition of, **302**
depression and, 267
overview, 260
temper tantrums and, 240
Dialect theory of emotional expression, 159, **302**
Diathesis–stress model, 252–255, **302**
Differential emotions theory (DET)
anger and, 238
definition of, **302**

overview, 13–15, 27–28
theory of emotion and consciousness and,
20–21
Differential susceptibility model, 252–255, **302**
Disappointing present procedure, 82–83, **302**
Discrete emotion theories, 30–34, 35–36, 177. *See
also* Basic (or discrete) emotion theories
Discrete emotional facial expressions, 30–31, 66.
See also Facial expressions
Discrimination, 55–63, 64, **302**
Discussion of emotions, 73, 75–76, 95–98, **303**
Disengagement, 256
Disgust, 61–63, 244–247, 250
Dismissing/avoidant attachment, 187–189,
190–191, **303**. *See also* Attachment; Avoidant
attachment
Disorganized attachment, 42, **303**. *See also*
Attachment
Display rules, 7, **303**
Disruptive behavior, 272–279
Dissociative behavior, 261
Distraction
adolescence and, 122–123
adulthood and, 154–155
later adulthood and, 199, 213
maltreatment and, 256
Distress reactions, 74, **303**
Distress to limitations, 239, **303**
Distress to novelty, 239, **303**
Dot-probe paradigm, 234–235, **303**
Dual systems model, 129, 193, **303**
Duchenne smile, 34, **303**. *See also* Smiling
Dynamical systems (DS) perspective, 23–24, **304**

Early childhood. *See* Childhood
Eating disorders, 261
Ecological validity, 130–131, **304**
Effect size, **304**
Effortful control (EC)
adolescence and, 108–109, 119–120, 137–138
adulthood and, 152, 154, 175–176
childhood and, 69, 83–84
definition of, **304**
depression and, 268
infancy and, 37
self-conscious emotions and, 219
temperament and, 37, 69, 108–109, 146
Egocentric language, 16, **304**
Electroencephalography (EEG)
childhood and, 91–92, 102
definition of, **304**
empathy and, 226
infancy and, 53
overview, 52
Elicitor-response processes, 26–27
Embarrassment, 216–217, 218–219
Emotion competence, 263–264, **304**
Emotion contagion, 221–223, 226–227
Emotion disconnection, 261
Emotion knowledge, 56, **304**
stage theory of, 98–100
Emotion processing, 90–92

Emotion recognition, 16–17, 95–100
Emotion regulation. *See also* Regulation; Self-regulation; Strategy use
  adolescence and, 118–125, 137–138
  adulthood and, 152–158, 175–176
  anger and, 242
  anxiety and, 263
  childhood and, 78–84, 101–102
  cortisol levels and, 172
  cultural factors and, 162–163, 281–282
  definition of, **304**
  depression and, 268–269
  disgust and, 245
  gender and, 202–203
  later adulthood and, 196–199, 202–203, 212–213
  maltreatment and, 256
  ODD and CD and, 273–274
  overview, 78–79
  psychopathology and, 261
Emotion Regulation Checklist (ERC), 81
Emotion Regulation Questionnaire (ERQ), 162–163, 197
Emotion schema, 14, **305**
Emotion socialization. *See also* Socialization
  anger and, 242
  childhood and, 72–78, 86–87
  empathy and, 224–226
  future research directions and, 292–293
Emotion understanding. *See also* Categorization; Discrimination; Recognition
  adolescence and, 133–136
  childhood and, 95–100, 102
  definition of, **305**
  gender and, 89–90
  infancy and, 64
  later adulthood and, 209–211
  maltreatment and, 259–260
  ODD and CD and, 279
  overview, 56
Emotional clarity, 261
Emotional complexity, 185–186
Emotional go/no-go task, 120, 130, **305**
Emotional intelligence (EI). *See also* Ability EI
  adolescence and, 128, 133–136, 138
  adulthood and, 167, 173–175, 177
  definition of, **305**
  gender and, 167
  later adulthood and, 203, 211
  overview, 133
Emotional labor, 157, **305**
Emotional oddball task, 257
Emotional reactivity, 108–109, 256–257. *See also* Reactivity
Emotional roller coaster task, 115, **305**
Emotional self-awareness, 263, **305**
Emotional well-being, 115–118, 154, 178–180, 181–183. *See also* Subjective well-being (SWB)
Emotion-focused reactions, 74, **304**
Emotion-related discussions. *See* Discussion of emotions

Emotion-related information processing, 191–192
Emotion-related socialization behaviors (ERSBs), 72–73, **305**
Empathic concern. *See* Sympathy
Empathy
  callous unemotionality (CU) and, 274, 276–277
  cultural factors and, 227–229
  definition of, **305**
  neurobiological factors, 226–227
  overview, 221–229, 248–249
Employment functioning, 157–158, 173–174
Endogenous smile, 33, **305**. *See also* Smiling
Environmental factors. *See also* Contextual factors
  appraisals and, 8–9
  depression and, 268
  environmental sensitivity and, 252–255
  functionalist/relational perspective and, 25–26
  temperament during adolescence and, 109–110
  theory of emotion and consciousness and, 21
Environmental sensitivity, 252–255, **306**
Event-related potential (ERP), 52, 53, **306**
Evidence-based programs, 283, **306**
Evolutionary factors, 3–4, 230
Executive functioning skills, 226
Exogenous smile, 33, **306**. *See also* Smiling
Experience sampling methodology (ESM), 104–107, 196–197, 294, **306**
Experiences in Close Relationships (ECR) scale, 148
Exposure to emotion-inducing experiences, 73, 76–77, 216–217, **306**
Expression, emotional. *See also* Facial expressions; Negative emotional expressions; Positive emotional expressions
  adolescence, 104–107, 136
  adulthood and, 147
  childhood and, 65–68, 85, 101
  cultural factors and, 158–165
  gender and, 165–166
  infancy and, 29–34, 46–47, 59–60
  later adulthood and, 178–184, 212
Expressive encouragement, 74, **306**
Expressive regulation, 82–83. *See also* Emotion regulation
Expressive responses, 6–7, 12, 48
Expressive suppression. *See also* Suppression
  adolescence and, 120–122, 137
  adulthood and, 154–155
  cultural factors and, 163–164, 281
  definition of, **306**
  gender and, 202–203
  later adulthood and, 202–203
  maltreatment and, 256
  overview, 121
Externalizing problems
  adolescence and, 125–126
  definition of, **306**
  depression and, 269
  empathy and, 225
  environmental sensitivity and, 253–255

Externalizing problems (cont.)
future research directions and, 293
ODD and CD and, 277–278
parent–adolescent conflicts and, 113–114
psychopathology and, 261–262
temperament during childhood and, 69
Extraversion
emotional regulation in adulthood and, 155
later adulthood and, 184–186, 212
ODD and CD and, 273
overview, 145–147
temperament and, 146

Facial Action Coding System (FACS), 92–93,
145, 183
Facial expressions. See also Expression,
emotional; Prototypic emotional facial
expressions; Smiling
adulthood and, 140–145, 176–177
anger and, 238–239
childhood and, 65, 66–67, 92–93
cultural factors and, 46–47, 158–159, 176–177
disgust and, 246
infancy and, 30–33, 46–47, 57–60
later adulthood and, 209–211, 212, 214
maltreatment and, 257, 260
theories of emotion and, 3–5, 4f, 6–7
threats and fear and, 233–236
Facial feedback hypothesis, 170, 306
Families of emotion regulation strategies,
152–153, 307. See also Emotion regulation
Family factors. See also Parent factors
adverse childhood experiences (ACEs) and,
251–252
attachment during adolescence and, 111
emotion understanding during childhood
and, 96
parent–adolescent conflicts, 113–115
respiratory sinus arrhythmia (RSA) and,
131–132
Fear, 69–70, 219, 221–222, 233–238, 249–250
Fear of missing out (FOMO), 117–118, 307. See
also Social media
Fear Survey Schedule for Children (FSSC-II), 237
Fearful attachment, 187–189, 190–191, 307. See
also Attachment
Female advantage
ability EI and, 136
adolescence and, 128, 136
adulthood and, 167
definition of, 307
later adulthood and, 203
overview, 89–90
Five-factor model. See Big Five/Five-Factor model
Forced-choice method, 142, 307
Four Horsemen, 156, 307
Functional magnetic resonance imaging (fMRI)
adolescence and, 130
adulthood and, 168–169
childhood and, 91, 102
definition of, 307
empathy and, 226

infancy and, 52–53
later adulthood and, 204, 205
maltreatment and, 257
overview, 51–52
Functional near-infrared spectroscopy (fNIRS),
92, 102
Functionalist/relational perspective, 24–26, 62,
307
Future directions, 291–295

Gender
adolescence and, 126–128, 138
adulthood and, 165–167, 177
callous unemotionality (CU) and, 276–277
childhood and, 83, 88–90, 102
infancy and, 41, 49–51, 64
later adulthood and, 202–203, 213
threats and fear and, 238
Gender similarity hypothesis, 49, 307
Gender-labeling effect, 50–51, 64
Genetic factors, 254–255
Glutamate amplifies noradernergic effects
(GANE) model, 206–207, 307
Goals, 25–26, 77–78, 87–88
Go/no-go task, emotional, 120, 130, 305
Gratification delay. See Delay of gratification
tasks
Guilt, 166, 218–219, 221, 248

Habit-based behaviors, 261
Happiness, 209–211
Harris and Pons' stage theory, 98–100
Health, 194–195, 231–232
Heterochronic development, 23–24, 308
Hikikomori, 281, 308
Hippocampal volume, 203–204
Hormonal factors, 107
Hostile attribution bias, 243, 308
Household dysfunction, 251–252. See also
Adverse childhood experiences (ACEs)
Hygge, 247–248
Hypothalamic–pituitary–adrenal (HPA) system.
See also Cortisol; Neurobiological factors
adolescence and, 132–133, 138
adulthood and, 171–173
anxiety and, 267
childhood and, 94–95, 102
cultural factors and, 172–173
definition of, 308
depression and, 272
infancy and, 54–55, 64
later adulthood and, 208–209, 214
maltreatment and, 258–259
ODD and CD and, 278
overview, 28

Ideal affect, 201, 308
Imbalance model, 129–130, 308
"Immigrant paradox," 125–126
Incidental affect, 192–193, 212, 308
Independent/interdependent, 88, 160, 161–162,
308. See also Individualism/collectivism

Individual differences. *See also* Temperament
adolescence and, 108
adulthood and, 146–147
childhood and, 69
developmental theories and, 12
environmental sensitivity and, 252–255
future research directions and, 292
infancy and, 36–37, 63
later adulthood and, 184–186
self-conscious emotions and, 219
Individualism/collectivism, 88, 160, 161–162,
308. *See also* Collectivism; Independent/
interdependent
Infancy
anger and, 238–240
attachment and, 40–43, 47–48
culture and emotion and, 45–48
discrimination, categorization, and recognition
of emotional expressions and, 55–63
disgust and, 245
emotion regulation and, 44, 45, 79–80
emotional expression and experience, 29–34,
46–47
environmental sensitivity and, 253–255
future research directions and, 292
gender and, 49–51
neurobiological factors, 51–55
overview, 29, 63–64
self-conscious emotions and, 216–217
social referencing and, 60–61
socialization and regulation, 44–45
temperament and, 35–40
theory of emotion and consciousness and,
19–21
threats and fear and, 233–237
Infant Behavior Questionnaire (IBQ), 37,
238–239
Infant–caregiver social interactions, 63
Information processing, 191–192, 200–201, 212,
244
Ingroup advantage, 229, 308
Inhibitory control, 70, 119–120, 273. *See also*
Behavioral inhibition (BI); Effortful control
(EC)
Insecure attachment, 42. *See also* Attachment;
Avoidant attachment; Disorganized
attachment; Resistant/ambivalent
attachment
Instrumental action, 5, 308
Integral affect, 192–193, 309
Intellect/openness to experience, 145–147,
155–156, 184–186, 212
Interdependent. *See* Independent/
interdependent
Intergenerational transmission, 148–149,
150–151, 309
Internal working model (IWM)
adolescence and, 110, 112
childhood and, 71
definition of, 309
empathy and, 224
infancy and, 43

Internalizing problems
adolescence and, 125–126
definition of, 309
depression and, 269
environmental sensitivity and, 253–255
future research directions and, 293
ODD and CD and, 277–278
parent–adolescent conflicts and, 113–114
psychopathology and, 261–262
temperament during childhood and, 69
International core patterns (ICPs), 159, 309
Intervention programs, 260–261, 282–287,
289–290
Intrusive parenting. *See* Parenting
Inventory of Callous–Unemotional Traits,
274–275

Job satisfaction. *See* Workplace
Joint storytelling task, 71, 309

Labeling emotion, 97–98. *See also* Language;
Linguistic labeling
Laboratory Temperament Assessment Battery
(Lab-TAB), 35–36, 37, 69, 239, 273
Language
development of, 26
differential emotions theory (DET) and, 14
emotion regulation during childhood and, 84
emotion understanding during childhood and,
95–98
sociocultural internalization model and, 16–17
Later adulthood. *See also* Adulthood
attachment and, 187–191
cultural factors and, 199–202
decision making and, 192–195
emotion regulation and, 196–199
emotion understanding during, 209–211
emotional expression and experience, 178–184
emotion-related information processing and,
191–192
gender and, 202–203
neurobiological factors, 203–209
overview, 178, 211–214
personality and, 184–187
Life satisfaction, 140–141, 163–164, 175, 181–183.
See also Subjective well-being (SWB)
Linguistic labeling, 22, 97–98. *See also* Language
Locationist view, 168–169, 309

Magnetic resonance imaging (MRI), 51–52, 309
Maltreatment, 219–220, 255–260, 287, 309. *See
also* Abuse; Adverse childhood experiences
(ACEs); Neglect
Marshmallow task, 124–125, 309
Maternal Emotions Style Questionnaire, 74
Maternal factors, 41–42, 45, 111, 225, 270. *See
also* Parent factors
Maturational dualism theory, 204
MAX (Maximally Discriminative Facial
Movement Coding System), 30–33, 310
Mayer–Salovey–Caruso Emotional Intelligence
Test (MSCEIT), 134–135, 174–175, 177

Medial prefrontal cortex (mPFC), 226, 271
Memory, 203–204
Mental stage, 99
Meta-analysis, 310
Methodology, 293–294
Minimization, 74, 310
Mirror-recognition task, 216, 310
Moderation effect, 77, 78, 310
Moodiness, 105–106
Moral emotions, 219, 246–247
Multivoxel pattern analysis (MVPA), 168–169
Mutual regulation model, 44–45, 310

Natural kinds, 169, 310
Near-infrared spectroscopy (NIRS), 52, 310
Negative emotional expressions. *See also*
    Expression, emotional
  adolescence and, 104–105, 114–115, 136
  childhood and, 67
  infancy and, 61–63
  later adulthood and, 179–180, 191
  maltreatment and, 260
  school environment and, 68
Negative reactivity, 36–37, 262–263, 310. *See also*
    Reactivity
Negative valence systems, 260–261
Negativity bias, 233–235, 310
Neglect, 219, 255, 311. *See also* Adverse childhood
    experiences (ACEs); Maltreatment
NEO Personality Inventory, 146, 165
Neonate, 57–58, 311. *See also* Infancy
Neurobiological factors. *See also* Autonomic
    nervous system (ANS); Brain functioning;
    Hypothalamic–pituitary–adrenal (HPA)
    system
  adolescence and, 128–133, 138
  adulthood and, 167–173, 177
  anxiety and, 266–267
  childhood and, 90–95, 102
  depression and, 270–272
  empathy and, 226–227
  infancy and, 51–55, 64
  later adulthood and, 203–209, 213–214
  maltreatment and, 257–259
  ODD and CD and, 276–278
  overview, 26
  temperament during infancy and, 40
  theories of emotion and, 2
Neuroticism
  adulthood and, 176
  emotional regulation in adulthood and, 155
  later adulthood and, 184–186, 212
  ODD and CD and, 273
  overview, 145–147
Normative changes, 146–147, 184–186, 292

Objective self-awareness, 19, 216, 311
Observational methods, 80–81, 293–294
Occupational functioning, 157–158, 173–174
Older adults. *See* Later adulthood
Older children. *See* Childhood

Open-mouth smiles, 34. *See also* Smiling
Openness to experience, 145–147, 155–156,
    184–186, 212
Oppositional defiant disorder (ODD), 240,
    272–279, 288–289, 311
Organizational perspective, 17–19, 27–28
Orienting/regulation, 36–37, 146, 311
Overlap procedure, 233, 311
Overprotective parenting. *See* Parenting

Parasocial attachment figures, 190, 311
Parasympathetic nervous system (PNS), 54, 93,
    267, 311
Parent factors. *See also* Family factors
  attachment during adolescence and, 111
  depression and, 269–270
  emotion understanding during childhood
    and, 96
  parental warmth, 270
  respiratory sinus arrhythmia (RSA) and,
    131–132
  socialization and, 77–78, 87–88
Parent–adolescent conflicts, 113–115, 137
Parent–child attachments, 111–112, 224. *See also*
    Attachment
Parent–Child Interaction Therapy (PCIT),
    282–283, 289
Parenting. *See also* Attachment; Caregiving
    behaviors; Socialization
  anxiety and, 264–265
  childhood and, 70–71, 85–86, 87–88, 101
  contingent responding and, 74–75
  cultural factors and, 48
  depression and, 269–270
  discussion of emotions and, 75–76
  emotion-related parenting behaviors and,
    149–151, 176
  empathy and, 223–224, 225
  environmental sensitivity and, 254
  exposure to emotion-inducing experiences
    and, 76–77
  gender and, 50–51
  HPA system and, 95
  infancy and, 36, 39–40, 42–43, 44–45
  intervention programs, 282–283
  ODD and CD and, 275–276
  self-conscious emotions and, 219
  temperament and, 36, 39–40, 70–71, 85–86,
    101
Paternal factors, 291–292. *See also* Parent factors
PATHS (Promoting Alternative Thinking
    Strategies), 285, 290, 311
PCIT (Parent–Child Interaction Therapy), 311
Peer relationships
  adolescence and, 107, 115–118, 132, 137
  attachment during adolescence and, 111–112
  overview, 291–292
  social media and texting and, 115–118
Performance orientation, 218
Permissive parenting style, 150–151, 311. *See also*
    Parenting

Personal distress, 223, **312**
Personality
    adulthood and, 145–147, 175–176
    emotion schemas and, 14
    emotional regulation in adulthood and,
        155–156
    gender and, 165–166
    later adulthood and, 184–187, 212
    ODD and CD and, 273–274
    temperament and, 145–147
Physical abuse. *See* Abuse; Adverse childhood
    experiences (ACEs); Maltreatment
Play smiles, 34. *See also* Smiling
Polyvagal theory, 54, **312**
Positive and Negative Affect Scales (PANAS),
    200, 228–229, **312**
Positive emotional expressions. *See also*
    Expression, emotional
    adolescence and, 104–105, 136
    adulthood and, 140–141
    empathy and, 225
    infancy and, 61
    later adulthood and, 179–180, 191, 209–211
    maltreatment and, 260
    parent-adolescent conflicts and, 114–115
    school environment and, 68
Positive emotions, 229–232, 249
Positive psychology, **312**
Positive reappraisal, 197, 198. *See also* Reappraisal
Positive valence systems, 261
Positivity bias, 193–194
Positivity effect
    cultural factors and, 200–201
    decision making during later adulthood and,
        193–194
    definition of, **312**
    later adulthood and, 191, 200–201, 212
    overview, 191
Postpartum mental health, 45
Prefrontal cortex (PFC). *See also* Brain
    functioning
    anxiety and, 266
    childhood and, 90–91
    depression and, 271
    empathy and, 226
    infancy and, 52–53
    later adulthood and, 204, 205–206, 213
    maltreatment and, 258
Preoccupied attachment. *See* Anxious/
    preoccupied attachment
Preschool children. *See* Childhood
Pride, 165–166, 218–219
Proactive aggression, 242–243, **312**. *See also*
    Aggression
Problem solving, 122–123, 155, 269
Problem-focused reactions, 74, **312**
Prosocial behaviors
    anger and aggression and, 243
    definition of, **312**
    empathy and, 223, 225–226, 228
    overview, 76

Prototypic emotional facial expressions, 4–5,
    4*f*, 66–67, 158–159, **312**. *See also* Facial
    expressions
Psychological abuse. *See* Adverse childhood
    experiences (ACEs); Maltreatment
Psychological construction theories, 5–6,
    9–10, **312**. *See also* Constructivist theories;
    Theories of emotion; Theory of constructed
    emotion
Psychological control, 264, 270, 288
Psychopathology, 3, 260–262, 279–282, 288. *See
    also individual disorders and conditions*
Puberty, 103–104, 128–133. *See also* Adolescence
Punitive reactions, 74, **312**

Reactive aggression, 242–243, 250, **313**. *See also*
    Aggression
Reactivity. *See also* Emotional reactivity; Negative
    reactivity
    adolescence and, 107, 108–109, 118–119
    anger and, 238–240
    anxiety and, 262–263, 266
    childhood and, 69, 101
    depression and, 271
    infancy and, 37–38, 39–40
    maltreatment and, 256–257
    temperament and, 37–38, 39–40, 69, 108–109
Reappraisal. *See also* Appraisals; Cognitive
    reappraisal; Strategy use
    adolescence and, 120–123, 137
    adulthood and, 154–155
    anxiety and, 266
    definition of, **313**
    depression and, 268–269, 271
    gender and, 203
    later adulthood and, 196, 197, 198–199, 203,
        213
    maltreatment and, 256
Recognition, 55–63, 64, 142–143, **313**
Referential communication, 60, **313**
Regulation, 44–45, 63, 69. *See also* Emotion
    regulation; Orienting/regulation; Self-
    regulation
Relational factors. *See also* Attachment
    attachment during infancy and, 40–43
    emotional intelligence (EI) and, 174–175
    emotional regulation in adulthood and, 156
    functionalist/relational perspective and, 24–26
    overview, 8, 28
    parent-adolescent conflicts, 113–115
Research directions, 291–295
Research Domain Criteria (RDoC) framework,
    260–261, 288, **313**
Resiliency, 82, 225–226
Resistant/ambivalent attachment, 42, 84, **313**.
    See also Attachment
Respiratory sinus arrhythmia (RSA)
    adolescence and, 131–132, 138
    childhood and, 93–94, 102
    definition of, **313**
    depression and, 271–272

Respiratory sinus arrhythmia (cont.)
    environmental sensitivity and, 255
    infancy and, 64
    ODD and CD and, 277-278
    overview, 54
Response bias, 259-260
Response modulation, 153, 196, **313**. See also
        Strategy use
Retirement, 181-183. See also Later adulthood
Revised Early Adolescent Temperament
        Questionnaire (EATQ-R), 108-109
Reward system, 129, 130, 237, **313**
Risk taking, 128-131, 138
Romantic relationships, 111-112
Rothenberg Test of Social Sensitivity, 96
RULER (Recognizing, Understanding, Labeling,
        Expressing, and Regulating Emotion),
        285-286, 290, **313**
Rumination, 122-123, 268-269

Sadness, 144-145, 219-220, 256
Satisfaction, life. See Life satisfaction; Subjective
        well-being (SWB)
Schachter–Singer theory of emotion, 3, 9, **314**
Schadenfreude, 247-248
Schemas, 14, **305**
School factors, 43, 68. See also Academic
        problems
School-based interventions, 283-287, 289-290
Secure attachment style. See also Attachment
    adulthood and, 148
    attachment during adolescence and, 112
    attachment during infancy and, 42
    definition of, **314**
    empathy and, 224
    later adulthood and, 187-189, 190-191
Secure base behavior, 41, 71, **314**
Selection, optimization, and compensation
        (SOC) theory, 180-181, **314**
Self-blame, 220
Self-conscious emotions, 21, 165-166, 216-221, **314**
Self-consciousness, 21, 106
Self-regulation. See also Emotion regulation;
        Regulation
    anger and, 241
    crying during infancy and, 32
    empathy and, 223-224
    functionalist/relational perspective and, 26
    infancy and, 44-45, 63
Sensitive parenting, 149-150. See also Parenting
Sensitivity, 42-43, 48, **314**
Sexual abuse. See Adverse childhood experiences
        (ACEs)
Shame, 218-220, 221, 248
Shifting, 119-120. See also Effortful control (EC)
Situation modification, 153, 196, **314**. See also
        Strategy use
Situation selection, 152-153, 196, **314**. See also
        Strategy use
Smiling, 33-34, 46-47, 48, 143-145. See also
        Facial expressions

SOC–emotion regulation model (SOC-ER),
        180-181, **314**
Social anxiety disorder, 268-269
Social buffering effect, 55, 95, **315**
Social construction theories, 5-6, 11, **315**. See
        also Constructivist theories; Theories of
        emotion
Social factors, 83-84, 113-118, 261
Social information processing, 244, 250
Social media, 115-118, 137
Social referencing, 17, 60-61, **315**
Social smiles, 33-34, 46, **315**. See also Smiling
Social support, 122-123
Social-emotional adjustment, 48
Socialization. See also Emotion socialization
    adolescence and, 127-128
    anger and, 241-242
    anxiety and, 264-266
    childhood and, 72-78, 86-87, 101
    depression and, 269-270
    disgust and, 246
    emotion-related parenting behaviors and,
        149-151
    empathy and, 224-226
    gender and, 50-51, 89, 166-167, 177
    infancy and, 44-45
    ODD and CD and, 275-276
    self-conscious emotions and, 218-219, 221
    socialization model, 72-77
Sociocultural internalization model, 15-17
Socioeconomic status (SES), 238
Socioemotional adjustment, 70-71
Socioemotional information processing model,
        244
Socioemotional learning (SEL) programs,
        284-287, 290, **315**
Socioemotional selectivity theory (SST)
    cultural factors and, 199-200
    definition of, **315**
    later adulthood and, 180-181, 191, 197-198,
        199-200, 204, 211-212, 213
Spontaneous expressions, 143-145. See also Facial
        expressions; Smiling
Sroufe's organizational model. See Organizational
        perspective
Standards, rules, and goals (SRGs), 21, 216-217,
        315
Stereotyping
    adolescence and, 105-107, 127-128, 138
    gender and, 50-51, 166-167, 177
    later adulthood and, 184
Still-face paradigm, 44, 48, **315**
Stonewalling, 156
Strange Situation procedure, 42, 43, **315**
Strategy use, 26, 122-123, 152-155, 196-199,
        212-213. See also Attentional deployment;
        Cognitive change; Emotion regulation;
        Reappraisal; Response modulation;
        Situation modification; Situation selection
Strength and vulnerability integration (SVI)
        theory, 180-181, **315**

Stress, 107, 109–110
Subjective well-being (SWB). *See also* Affect;
    Emotional well-being
    definition of, **315**
    emotional intelligence (EI) and, 173–175
    later adulthood and, 183
    overview, 139–140
Substance use, 256
Suicide attempts, 256
Suppression, 122–123, 256, 268–269. *See also*
    Expressive suppression
Surgency, 36–37, **316**
Sympathetic nervous system (SNS)
    anxiety and, 267
    childhood and, 93
    definition of, **316**
    depression and, 272
    maltreatment and, 258
    overview, 54
Sympathy, 223–224, 226–229, **316**

Tantrums, temper, 239–240
Task orientation, 218
TCIT-U (Teacher–Child Interaction Training–
    Universal), 284, 289–290, **316**
Teacher-oriented school-based programs,
    283–284, 289
Temper tantrums, 239–240, 250
Temperament. *See also* Big Five/Five-Factor
    model
    adolescence and, 108–110, 126, 137
    adulthood and, 145–147, 175–176
    anger and, 238–239, 241–242
    anxiety and, 262–263
    childhood and, 69–71, 83–84, 85–86, 88, 101,
        102
    definition of, **316**
    depression and, 268
    empathy and, 223–224
    gender and, 49
    infancy and, 35–40, 63
    ODD and CD and, 273–274

overview, 35–38
personality and, 145–147
self-conscious emotions and, 219
stability of, 38–40
Temporo-parietal junction, 226
Test of Emotion Comprehension (TEC), 100, 135
Test of Self-Conscious Affect for Children
    (TOSCA-C), 219, 220
Texting, 115–118, 137
Theories of emotion. *See also* Appraisal theories;
    Basic (or discrete) emotion theories;
    Developmental theories; Psychological
    construction theories; Social construction
    theories
    adult-oriented theories, 5–11
    future research directions and, 291–295
    history of, 2–5, 4*f*
    overview, 1, 5, 26–28
Theory of constructed emotion, 10, 21–23, 169,
    316. *See also* Psychological construction
    theories
Theory of emotion and consciousness, 19–21
Threats and fear, 233–238, 249. *See also* Fear
Treatment, 260–261, 282–287, 289–290
Trier Social Stress Test (TSST), 106

Valence, 9, 64, 260–261, **316**
Values, 40, 77–78, 87–88, 158–165
Vantage sensitivity model, 252–255, **316**
Ventromedial prefrontal cortex (vmPFC),
    203–204, 213, 226, 271
Veridical empathic distress, 22. *See also* Empathy
Violent behavior, 220, 256. *See also* Aggression;
    Behavior
Vocal emotional expression, 58, 59–60, 145

WEIRD (Western, educated, industrialized, rich
    demographic) populations, 45–46, 140, **316**.
    See also Cultural factors
Well-being, 189–190. *See also* Emotional well-
    being; Subjective well-being (SWB)
Workplace, 157–158, 173–174

About the Author

Linda A. Camras, PhD, is Professor Emerita at DePaul University, where she taught both graduate and undergraduate courses on developmental psychology and social and emotional development. In 2021, she was appointed Co-Editor in Chief of the journal *Affective Science*. She has served as Associate Editor for both *Emotion Review* and *Cognition and Emotion*. Dr. Camras's research has focused on the development of emotional expression in infants and children from both Western and Asian cultures. Her work has contributed to the recent revival of interest in constructivist approaches to emotion and emotional development. More recently, she has investigated how American and Chinese children's perceptions of their parents' behaviors affect their emotional well-being.